MEDICAL RADIOLOGY

Diagnostic Imaging

Springer-Verlag Berlin Heidelberg GmbH

A. M. De Schepper · F. Vanhoenacker (Eds.)

Medical Imaging of the Spleen

With Contributions by

H. Aibe · E.C. Benya · J.L. Bloem · H. Bortier · B. Corthouts · A.I. De Backer · M. De Roo
A.M. De Schepper · F. Deckers · H. Degryse · J. Delanote · A. Drevelengas · S.E. Falbo
L. Hendrickx · C.C. Hoeffel · H. Honda · H. Irie · K. Ito · Z.H. Jafri · M. Kunnen · T. Kuroiwa
K. Masuda · P.J. Mergo · D.G. Mitchell · K. Mortelé · B. Op De Beeck · H. Rigauts
P.R. Ros · A. Spilt · W.J. Stevens · L. Steyaert · T. Tajima · E. Totté · R. Van Hee · L. Van Hoe
F. Van Meir · D. Vanbeckevoort · F. Vanhoenacker · P. Vanhoenacker · H. Vereycken
G. Verswijvel · K. Yoshimitsu

Series Editor's Foreword by

A.L. Baert

With 182 Figures in 308 Separate Illustrations, Some in Color

Springer

ARTHUR M. DE SCHEPPER, MD, PhD, Professor
FILIP VANHOENACKER, MD
Department of Radiology
University Hospital Antwerp
Wilrijkstraat 10
B-2650 Edegem
Belgium

MEDICAL RADIOLOGY · Diagnostic Imaging and Radiation Oncology

Continuation of
Handbuch der medizinischen Radiologie
Encyclopedia of Medical Radiology

ISBN 978-3-642-62997-6 ISBN 978-3-642-57045-2 (eBook)
DOI 10.1007/978-3-642-57045-2

Library of Congress Cataloging-in-Publication Data. Medical imaging of the spleen / A. M. De Schepper, F. Vanhoenacker (eds.) ; with contributions by H. Aibe ... [et al.]. p. cm. - (Medical radiology) Includes bibliographical references and index. ISBN 978-3-642-62997-6 1. Spleen–Imaging. 2. Spleen–Diseases–Diagnosis. I. Schepper, A.M.A. de, 1937–. II. Vanhoenacker, F. (Filip), 1962–. III. Series. [DNLM: 1. Spleen–pathology. 2. Diagnostic Imaging. 3. Splenic Diseases–diagnosis. WH 600 M489 2000] RC645.M43 2000 616.4'10754–dc21 DNLM/DLC for Library of Congress 99-40699 CIP

Originally published by Springer-Verlag Berlin Heidelberg New York in 2000
Softcover reprint of the hardcover 1st edition 2000

Typesetting: Best-set Typesetter Ltd., Hong Kong

SPIN: 106 737 24 21/3135 – 5 4 3 2 1 0 – Printed on acid-free paper

Foreword

I would like to express my great appreciation to the editors of this volume, Prof. A. De Schepper and Dr. F. Vanhoenacker, for all their efforts and their enthusiastic commitment to this book. I am very grateful to them for managing to involve so many leading experts, resulting in a much-needed high-quality and absolutely up-to-date textbook on the spleen, an organ which has not always received the attention it deserves from radiologists.

As series editor, I am particularly grateful to the volume editors for adhering strictly to the planed schedule. Their punctuality enabled Springer-Verlag to reduce the production time of this volume to a minimum.

I am very much convinced that this volume on the spleen responds to an important need within the radiological community and that many radiologists will greatly benefit from it. However, surgeons and internal medicine specialists will also be interested in this excellent comprehensive overview of modern radiological imaging of splenic disorders.

Leuven

Albert L. Baert

Preface

Not infrequently, the spleen is regarded as the "silent and forgotten" organ of the abdomen. Though primary splenic diseases are rare, the spleen is a frequent site of secondary manifestations in a wide range of hematological, immunological, oncological, infectious, vascular and systemic disorders. Despite this broad spectrum of splenic diseases, radiological literature on splenic pathology is rather sparse.

Before the advent of cross-sectional imaging methods, the spleen was difficult to display on imaging studies. Plain X-ray films of the upper abdomen (or even tomographs) provide only limited information; they allow detection of intrasplenic calcifications and approximation of the splenic volume. Indirect signs of splenic enlargement can also be found on contrast examinations (barium studies and intravenous urography). In the early 1950s, direct splenoportography was used in the evaluation of splenoportal hypertension. This technique was replaced, in the 1960s, by selective catheter angiography of the splenic artery, which also provided information concerning splenoportal circulation on late (venous phase) images. Catheter angiography was not only used in the diagnosis of vascular lesions; it also proved to be of great value in patients with splenic tumors or after splenic trauma.

The introduction of cross-sectional imaging modalities opened new diagnostic horizons. Ultrasound (US) rapidly became a suitable method for screening abdominal pathology. Despite a low specificity, US provides a high sensitivity for the identification of focal splenic lesions. During the 1980s, due to its superior contrast resolution, computed tomography (CT) became the gold standard for splenic imaging. Nowadays, helical, volumetric CT scanning with bolus injection of contrast material is considered the state-of-the-art imaging modality for evaluation of the spleen. Magnetic resonance (MR) imaging has shown great promise due to its superior tissue-characterization ability in selected cases.

In recent years, there has been a renewed interest in this "forgotten organ", not only from clinicians but also from radiologists. This revival has been sparked by new insights in the physiology and pathophysiology of the spleen, new interest in spleen-sparing surgery and the introduction of new, non-invasive diagnostic modalities. It is in this context that the Scientific Board of the series "Medical Radiology" (edited by A. L. Baert) decided to publish a volume on the spleen, with the purpose of updating our knowledge about radiology of the spleen. When we were offered the opportunity to edit this volume, we accepted the challenge. We have been very fortunate to have been able to find and assemble a group of eminent radiologists who not only share an interest in splenic imaging but who are also excellent scientific authors. We would like to thank all the authors of this volume for submitting well-prepared manuscripts which have made our editing work less time-consuming than initially expected. Without their excellent contributions, this book would never have been written, and the spleen would still be a "silent and forgotten" organ.

In Chaps. 1 and 2, normal anatomy, recent insights in the physiology of the spleen and normal imaging findings are reviewed. Chapters 3 through 11 provide an overview of medical imaging of the spleen in congenital, traumatic, infectious, hematological, vascular-tumoral and systemic diseases. A separate chapter (Chap. 12) is devoted to splenic disorders in infancy and childhood. No book on the spleen would be complete without a chapter dedicated to interventional procedures in managing patients with splenic disorders (Chap. 13). Finally, in the last chapter, we propose a series of diagnostic tables. We hope they will serve as a quick reference for clinicians and radiologists in the interpretation of imaging findings, such as reflectivity (US), attenuation (CT) and signal intensity (MR) of solitary and multiple lesions in normal or enlarged spleens. The role of scintigraphy has been greatly reduced due to the introduction of more sensitive and more specific imaging modalities; for the sake of completeness, scintigraphy is discussed in an appendix.

We gratefully thank all those who have been involved in the preparation of this book, and we hope that this book will help to fill the "splenic hole in the abdominal universe".

Antwerp

ARTHUR M. DE SCHEPPER
FILIP VANHOENACKER

Contents

1 Anatomy, Embryology, Histology and Physiology of the Spleen

W.J. Stevens, H. Bortier, and F. Van Meir

CONTENTS

1.1 Introduction

The spleen is the largest lymphoid organ in the body and is interposed within the circulatory system. The spleen has multiple functions in the human body:

1. It clears the circulation of micro-organisms, particulate antigens and other foreign material.
2. It makes the majority of antibodies and enhances cellular immunity to antigens.
3. It removes normal and abnormal blood cells from the circulation.
4. It plays an important role in extramedullary haematopoiesis.

Part of the splenic circulation is an open circulation, in which the capillaries end in an open system and are not surrounded by endothelium; thus, macrophages can interact freely with the blood cells before the venous system takes up the blood again.

The spleen contains about 25% of the exchangeable T-lymphocyte pool and about 15% of the exchangeable B-lymphocyte pool. T cells stay about 4–6h in the spleen, B cells at least 16h. T cells can stay longer in the periarteriolar lymphatic sheaths (PALS) after antigen contact; in the PALS, they meet the B-lymphocytes easily (Pabst and Westermann 1991).

Splenic phagocytosis involves at least three different processes:

1. Phagocytosis of particulate material or micro-organisms from the blood stream
2. Phagocytosis of circulating immune complexes
3. Elimination of older red and white blood cells

Conversely, antibody production [especially immunoglobulin M (IgM) production] to antigens present in the circulation is the primary function of the spleen. Antibody production starts as early as 16h after introduction of the antigen. The spleen seems to be very important in the primary immune response to antigens transported via the blood stream; hence, antibody production to these antigens is diminished after anatomical or functional splenectomy. However, splenectomy does not significantly alter the immune response to antigens administered via subcutaneous, intradermal, intramuscular and intraperitoneal routes. The spleen is also very important for the immunological memory of T- and B-lymphocytes; production of IgM antibody to antigens is rather normal, but there is a deficient switch from IgM to IgG antibodies after splenectomy. Another important function of the spleen, although not exclusive, is the production of complement components in macrophages of the spleen. A large number of the spleen's functions can probably be taken over by other components of the immune system, such as the thymus, the bone marrow and the lymph nodes (also gut-associated lymphoid tissue and bronchial-associated lymphoid tissue).

1.2 Anatomy and Embryology

The adult spleen is situated in the left hypochondrium at the level of the tenth rib. The spleen has its greatest axis from posterosuperior to anteroinferior. The size of the spleen is about the size of a cupped hand. The length of the spleen is about

W.J. Stevens; University of Antwerp (campus UIA), Universiteitsplein 1, B-2610 Antwerp, Belgium
H. Bortier, F. Van Meir; University of Antwerp (campus RUCA), Groenenborgerlaan 171, B-2020 Antwerp, Belgium

10 cm, the width is about 5 cm and the spleen is about 3–4 cm thick. The diaphragm separates the diaphragmatic surface of the spleen from the pleura, the left lung and the 9th, 10th and 11th ribs. The anterior surface of the spleen lies dorsal to the stomach. The posterior surface lies posterosuperior and is sharper than the anterior surface. The superior surface of the spleen lies anterosuperior and is indented. The inferior surface lies posteroinferior to the splenic flexure. The left kidney lies medial to the spleen. The tail of the pancreas reaches the hilum of the spleen.

The gastric surface of the spleen lies between the hilum and the superior border. The renal surface of the spleen lies between the hilum and the inferior border. The colic surface of the spleen lies between the hilum and the anterior margin. Vessels and nerves enter and leave the spleen at the hilum of the spleen. The splenic artery is one of the three main branches of the celiac trunk. The splenic artery divides into splenic branches, which end in the small brushy arteries. The splenic vein is joined by the superior mesenteric vein to form the portal vein.

The boundaries of the splenic hilum are ligamentous. The phrenicosplenic ligament is a dorsosuperior peritoneal fold between the diaphragm and the concave surface of the spleen. The gastrosplenic (gastrolienal) ligament is an anterosuperior peritoneal fold between the greater curvature of the stomach and the hilum of the spleen. In the gastrosplenic ligament lie the short gastric arteries and the left gastroepiploic artery. The splenorenal (lienorenal) ligament is a peritoneal fold between the spleen and the left kidney (Vellguth et al. 1985).

The spleen develops during the fifth week of embryogenesis. In contrast to the gut organs, the cells of the spleen are mesodermal in origin (Fig. 1.1; Dodds et al. 1990). Multiple aggregations of mesodermal cells are found between the layers of the dorsal mesogastrium. In the second month, the aggregations of mesodermal cells fuse to form the spleen.

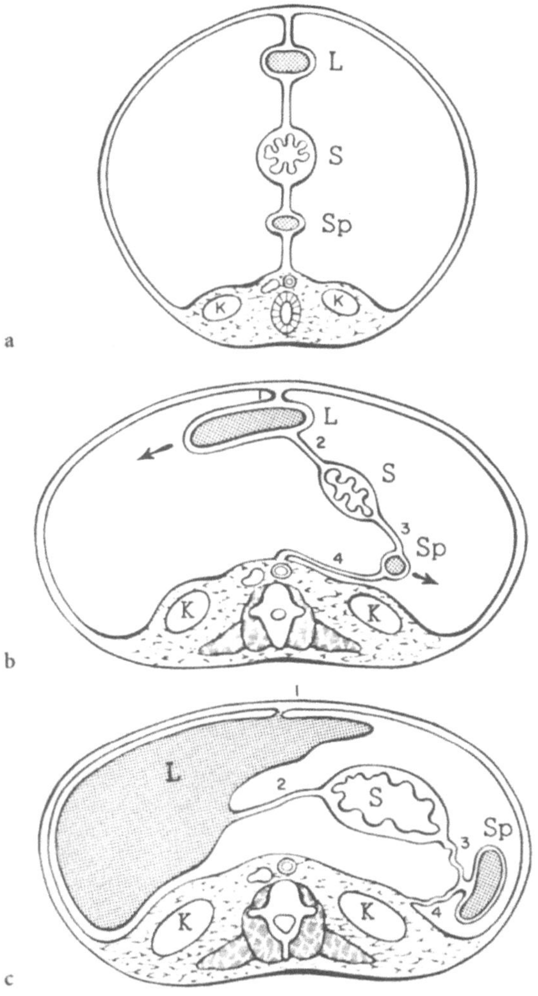

Fig. 1.1. Embryology. Schematic cross-sections of the upper abdomen of the embryo and the foetus. **a** Five-week embryo. The stomach is supported by a dorsal mesentery (or dorsal mesogastrium) and a ventral mesentery (or ventral mesogastrium). The spleen develops within the dorsal mesogastrium, while the liver develops within the ventral mesogastrium. **b** Five-week embryo. As the liver enlarges and turns to the right, the spleen and the stomach turn leftward to form the lesser peritoneal sac. The liver divides the ventral mesogastrium into the falciform (*1*) and gastrohepatic (*2*) ligaments. The spleen divides the dorsal mesogastrium into the gastro-splenic ligament (*3*), and the splenorenal ligament (*4*); part of the gastrosplenic ligament will become the splenorenal ligament. The latter normally lies against and fuses with the posterior peritoneum to form the short splenorenal ligament. Failure of this fusion leads to a long splenic mesentery and a wandering spleen. **c** Mature foetus. Almost all of the posterior part of the dorsal mesogastrium has fused with the posterior peritoneum to leave a short splenorenal ligament (*4*). The gastrosplenic ligament, the spleen and the splenorenal ligament form the lateral margin of the lesser peritoneal sac. *K*, kidney; *L*, liver; *S*, stomach; *Sp*, spleen; *1*, falciform ligament; *2*, gastrohepatic ligament; *3*, gastrosplenic ligament; *4*, splenorenal ligament (Dodds et al. 1990)

The spleen lies close to the stomach, the left kidney, the tail of the pancreas and the left gonadal ridge. The greater curvature of the stomach is initially directed posteriorly. Rotation of this greater curvature and the asymmetrical development of the stomach move the spleen up laterally, in the direction of the greater curvature of the stomach. The movements of the stomach and the spleen form the omental bursa (lesser sac). The anterior surface of the spleen lies dorsal, in contact with the stomach. In a whole embryo, the white mass of the spleen can easily be distinguished from the darker mass of the gastric wall. A small indentation separates the anterior surface of the spleen from the stomach. Enlargement of the omental bursa and several smaller recess ultimately separates the spleen from the stomach. The anterior part of the dorsal mesogastrium, which extends from the greater curvature of the stomach to the spleen, becomes the gastrosplenal (gastrolienal) ligament. The posterior part of the dorsal mesogastrium, which extends from the spleen to the left kidney, becomes the splenorenal ligament. Branches of blood vessels enter the dorsal mesogastrium and reach the spleen, creating the hilum of the spleen. In the seventh and eighth weeks, dark clusters of pigmented cells develop, and the spleen becomes lobular. In the ninth week, small arterial branches grow into these dark areas, and erythropoiesis starts. As the darker areas fuse, the surface of the spleen becomes homogeneously brown, although the indentations at the surface remain visible. In the fifth month, erythropoiesis in the spleen ceases. The remnants of the indentations are clearly visible in new-borns. In adults, these indentations are usually invisible except for the indentations at the superior surface.

During development, the spleen shrinks and grows, then shrinks and grows again. The individual morphology varies. In the third through the eighth weeks, the spleen enlarges 20 times; in the eight through the tenth weeks, the spleen enlarges another four times.

Aplasia or hypoplasia of the spleen are rare, as these situations are usually accompanied by other severe anomalies. Accessory spleens are frequent (4–33%) and are found most commonly near the hilum of the spleen. Multiple accessory spleens can also be found in the neighbourhood of the spleen. These multiple accessory spleens are more or less fused to the spleen and are irrigated by branches of the splenic artery. Deep indentations can give rise to two or three spleens or more. Accessory spleens can also be found in the tail of the pancreas, the splenic mesentery, the omentum, the jejunal and ileal mesenteries and in the neighbourhood of the left ovary or the testicle, as the spleen develops in the vicinity of these organs, close to the gonadal ridge. Accessory spleens distant from the original spleen are usually irrigated by their own vascular structures.

1.3 Microscopic Structure

The spleen is surrounded by a capsule of dense, collagenous tissue (*capsula fibrosa*) that sends out trabeculae dividing the parenchyma, or splenic pulp (*pulpa lienalis*), into incomplete compartments. At the hilum on the medial surface of the spleen, the capsule gives rise to many branching trabeculae carrying nerves and arteries into the splenic pulp. Veins derived from the parenchyma and lymphatic vessels originating in the trabeculae leave through the hilum.

The stroma is composed of a fine mesh of reticular fibres that attach to and blend with the inner surface of the capsule, the trabeculae and the walls of the blood vessels. This fine supporting network contains all of the cellular elements that make up the splenic parenchyma. To understand the functional histology of the spleen, the structure can be explained by (a) discussing the structures encountered when making a fresh cut through the spleen or (b) following the blood supply of the spleen (Van Rooijen et al. 1989).

1.3.1 The Splenic Pulp

1.3.1.1 The White Pulp and Marginal Zone

The white pulp contains arterioles surrounded by a sheath of densely packed small lymphocytes subdivided into the central, intermediate and peripheral marginal zones. The central and intermediate zones are called the PALS (Fig. 1.2). The central zone contains primarily CD4+ T-helper lymphocytes that lie in contact with the interdigitating cells. The intermediate follicular zone is the B-lymphocyte zone, which also contains germinal centres with B-lymphocytes and macrophages. Germinal centres are reaction centres formed in response to antigen exposure; many B-lymphoblasts, B-lymphocytes, macrophages and reticular cells are present (Tarlinton 1998). In humans, the germinal centres may become ex-

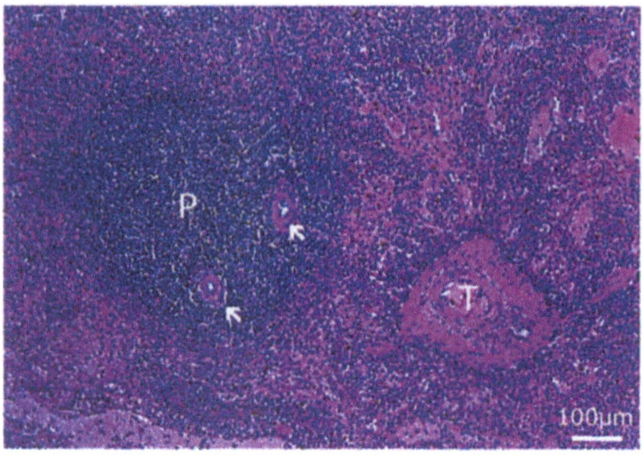

Fig. 1.2. Haematoxylin and eosin-stained section of the human spleen. White pulp: central arterioles (*arrows*) surrounded by the periarteriolar lymphocyte sheath (*P*); *T*, trabecular artery. *Scale bar* 200 µm

tremely large; as the nodules become visible to the naked eye, they are called splenic nodules or Malpighian corpuscles. Between the white pulp and the red pulp lies a peripheral marginal zone consisting of a sparse reticular scaffold and anastomosing fine-vascular channels, the marginal sinuses of which are surrounded by interdigitating dendritic antigen-presenting cells. The peripheral marginal zone also consists of B-lymphocytes with membrane (IgM but lacking membrane IgD), which allows them to react with thymus-independent antigens and macrophages. The B-lymphocytes contact the follicular dendritic cells. Most antigens are recognised by the marginal B-lymphocytes, which degrade the antigens and present them to their surfaces. B-lymphocytes migrate to the border of the PALS, where all the cells necessary for a good immunological response are present (Camacho et al. 1998). Finally, B-lymphocytes differentiate into plasma cells, which remain for longer periods in the vicinity of the red pulp. The marginal zone lies in contact with the red pulp. In the spleen, particulate and soluble antigens follow a different road – soluble antigens are skimmed off with plasma and supplied to the germinal centres in the white pulp. Particulate antigens are transported (with the red blood cells) to the macrophages and subsequently presented to the germinal centres. Although the liver is the major phagocytosing organ, phagocytosis of foreign material is an important function of the spleen, especially with the help of opsonins (antibodies, complement fractions).

1.3.1.2
The Red Pulp

Due to its large number of red blood cells, the red pulp has a red appearance in the fresh state as well as in haematoxylin and eosin-stained histological sections (Fig. 1.3). Essentially, the red pulp consists of large, thin-walled splenic sinuses that are filled with blood and separated by thin plates or cords of lymphoid tissue, the cords of Billroth. These splenic cords consist of a loose network of reticular cells and reticular fibres that contain a large number of macrophages, lymphocytes, plasma cells, granulocytes, red blood cells and platelets.

Macrophages are an important site of red blood cell and platelet destruction in the spleen (Fig. 1.4). At the termination of both platelet and red blood cell life spans, surface changes occur that are recognised as "foreign"; the cell surfaces are coated with antibodies. Phagocytosis is initiated by subsequent binding of the macrophage receptors to the Fc portion of the antibodies coating the blood cells. The iron from destroyed red blood cells is re-utilised when new red blood cells are formed; the splenic macrophages begin the process of haemoglobin breakdown and iron retrieval.

The removal of aged and diseased red blood cells by phagocytosis is just one event taking place in the cords of Billroth. Mature red blood cells can be treated by a process known as "pitting"; inclusions, such as malaria-causing organisms and Heinz bodies (aggregates of denatured haemoglobin), are removed during transit between endothelial sinusoidal cells. Reticulocytes (immature red blood cells released from the bone marrow) are retained in the red pulp for one or two days in a process of normal maturation.

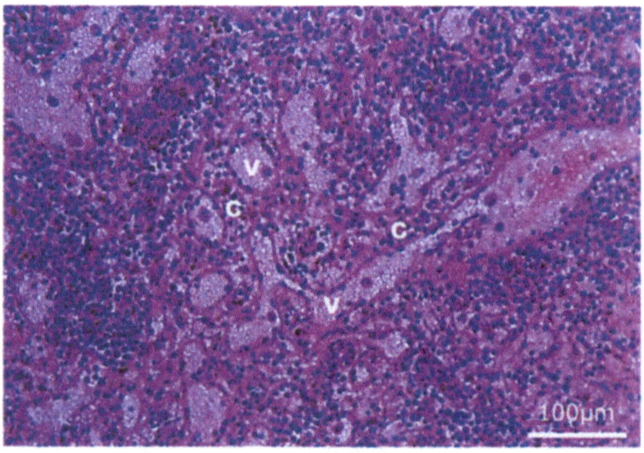

Fig. 1.3. Haematoxylin and eosin-stained section of the human spleen. Red pulp with venous sinuses (*V*) and splenic cords of Billroth (*C*). *Scale bar* 200 µm

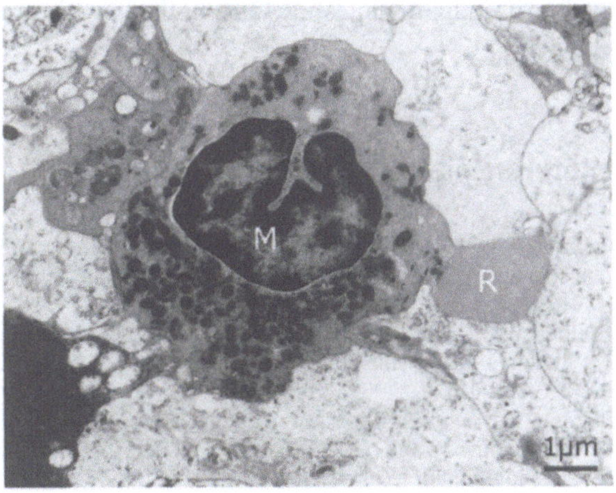

Fig. 1.4. Electron micrograph of a macrophage (*M*) tasting a red blood cell (*R*) in the splenic pulp. *Scale bar* 1 µm

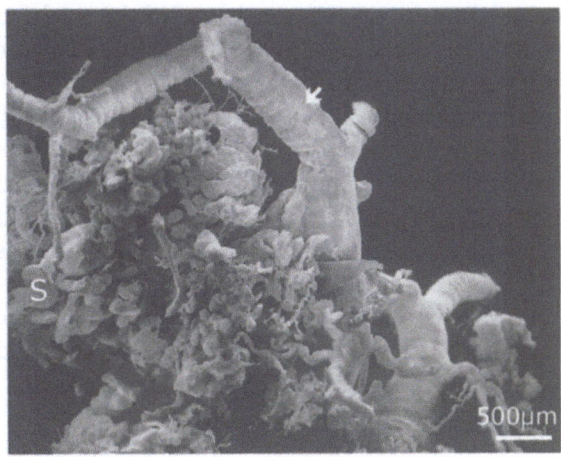

Fig. 1.5. Scanning electron microscopy of splenic human blood vessels. *Arrow*, central artery; *S*, sinus

Blood cells within the red pulp cords represent a pool that is in dynamic equilibrium with cells in the general circulation. Only 3% of red blood cells (but as many as 30% of platelets) are pooled in the spleen. Enlarged spleens can hold up to 72% of the total platelet mass, thus depleting the general circulation.

1.3.2 Splenic Circulation

The structure of the spleen is built around its blood supply. However, disagreement has existed for decades over the pathway taken by the blood as it passes from the arterial system to the venous system. The manner in which this is accomplished has led to two proposed (and later confirmed) models of circulation: the open and the closed circulation models (Kashimura and Fujita 1987).

The central arteries lead to strands of arterioles and capillaries supplying the white pulp, and arterioles and capillaries that run directly into a system of marginal-zone sinuses. These marginal-zone sinuses are arranged concentrically around the white pulp in the perilymphoid marginal zone. Perfusion studies on the human spleen have defined three concentric systems: the marginal-zone network, the marginal sinuses and the perimarginal cavernous sinus (Fig. 1.5). In this area, blood comes into contact with dendritic antigen-presenting cells, and foreign antigens can be trapped and presented to appropriate lymphoid cells. Most of the marginal-zone sinuses drain into the venous sinuses, forming a closed circulatory system.

The central arteries also continue into the red pulp, where they branch into several relatively straight arterioles called penicilli (Fig. 1.6.). When this vessel is thickened by a reticular sheath, it is described as an ellipsoid sheathed capillary. Its sheath is infiltrated by macrophages and lymphocytes; its endothelium is continuous, but the basal lamina is discontinuous. Most of the sheathed capillaries drain into the splenic parenchyma proper, which consists of the stellate reticular network of the splenic cords. This pathway is the open circulatory system. A small proportion of the sheathed capillaries also drain directly into the perimarginal cavernous sinuses.

Washout kinetic studies and quantitative intravital microscopy suggested that 90% of the red blood cells entering the spleen pass through a small, fast

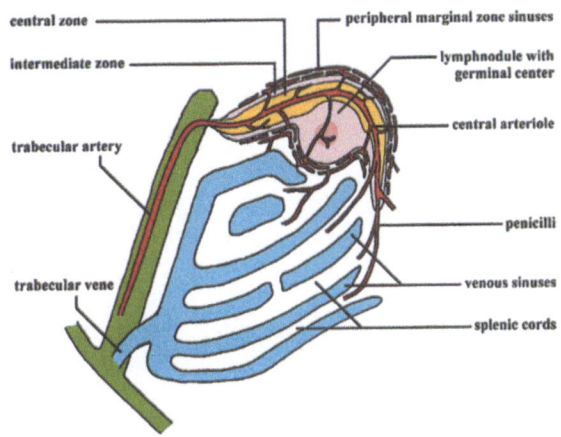

Fig.1.6. Diagram showing the splenic circulation in relation to white and red pulp

compartment containing only 9% of the total red blood cells in the organ; 10% passes through a large or intermediate slow compartment containing 91% of the red blood cells (Groom et al. 1991). The small, fast compartment represents blood flow through the central arteries, which drain (via mainly marginal sinuses or penicilli and bypassing the perilymphoid parenchyma) directly into the venous sinuses; this is the closed circulatory system. The large and intermediate slow compartments represent the splenic cords, where blood enters from mainly penicilli and drains into the venous sinuses; this is the open circulatory system.

The venous return consists of venous sinuses that anastomose freely throughout the red pulp, dividing it into the pulp cords. These blood sinuses have irregular lumina that are easily distended and have a discontinuous endothelial lining. Reticular fibres of the incomplete basal lamina encircle the sinuses like hoops of a wooden barrel. These features facilitate easy, rapid movement of cells between the red pulp and the sinuses. The various sinuses confluence to form pulp veins, which enter the trabeculae to become the trabecular veins. At the hilus, these veins unite to form the splenic vein, which joins with the veins draining the intestine to form the hepatic portal vein.

References

Camacho SA, Kosco-Vilbois MH, Berek C (1998) The dynamic structure of the germinal center. Immonol Today 19:511–514

Dodds WJ, Taylor AJ, Erickson SJ, et al. (1990) Radiologic imaging of splenic anomalies. AJR Am J Roentgenol 155:805–810

Groom AC, Schmidt EE, Macdonald IC (1991) Microcirculatory pathways and blood flow in spleen: new insights from washout kinetics, corrosion casts, and quantitative intravital videomicroscopy. Scanning Microsc 5:159–174

Kashimura M, Fujita T. (1987) A scanning electron microscopy study of human spleen: relationship between the microcirculation and functions. Scanning Microsc 1:841–851

Pabst R, Westermann J (1991) The role of the spleen in lymphocyte migration. Scanning Microsc 5:1075–1089

Tarlinton D (1998) Germinal centers: form and function. Curr Opin Immunol 10:245–251

Van Rooijen N, Claassen E, Kraal G, et al. (1989) Cytological basis of immune functions of the spleen. Prog Histochem Cytochem 19:1–71

Vellguth S, Van Gaudedecker B, Muller-Hermelinck HK (1985) The development of the human spleen. Cell Tissue Res 242:579–592

2 The Normal Spleen on Different Imaging Modalities

S.E. Falbo and Z.H. Jafri

CONTENTS

This chapter discusses the appearance of the normal spleen on various imaging modalities, including plain films, ultrasound, computed tomography, magnetic resonance imaging and angiography. A brief review of the normal appearance of the fetal and pediatric spleens is also included.

2.1 Introduction

Before the development of more advanced imaging modalities, such as computed tomography (CT) and magnetic resonance (MR) imaging, the spleen was an "invisible" organ to the radiologist, often poorly visualized on routine plain films. Pathologic conditions of the spleen were difficult to detect. However, current cross-sectional imaging techniques allow for detailed evaluation of splenic anatomy and pathology. This chapter discusses the appearance of the normal spleen on various imaging modalities including routine plain radiographs, ultrasound, CT, MR imaging and angiography.

S.E. Falbo, Z.H. Jafri; Department of Diagnostic Radiology, William Beaumont Hospital, 3601 W. Thirteen Mile Rd., Royal Oak, Michigan 48073, USA

2.2 Plain Films

Because of variations in size and shape, the spleen often must be markedly enlarged to be seen on plain radiographs. The superior pole of the spleen lies beneath the posterior margin of the left hemidiaphragm. The inferior pole extends anteriorly to the left costal margin, lateral to the body of the stomach. Normally, the spleen does not extend below the left costal margin, and the long axis of the organ usually parallels the posterior ribs (Dachman and Friedman 1993). In one series, the splenic tip was seen in only 44% of plain films (Brogdon and Cros 1959). Fat of the greater omentum and transverse colon often outlines the spleen on plain radiographs (Fig. 2.1). An air-filled stomach or splenic flexure may outline a portion of the spleen (Fig. 2.2). Splenic granulomas, calcified cysts, hematomas, and splenic artery calcifications (Fig. 2.3) are often detected on plain films.

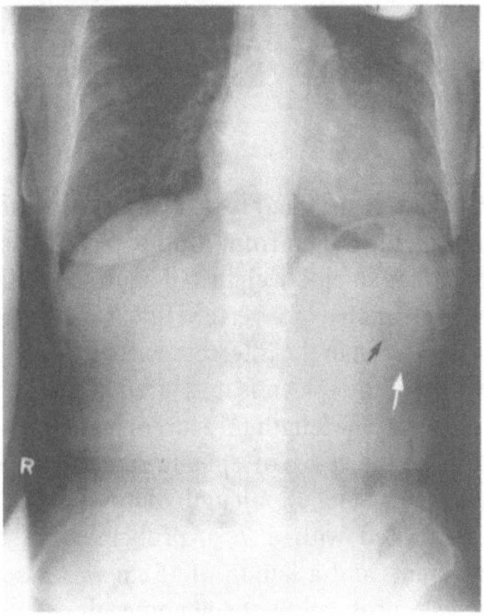

Fig. 2.1. The inferior half of the spleen (*arrows*) is visualized on a plain upright film of the abdomen

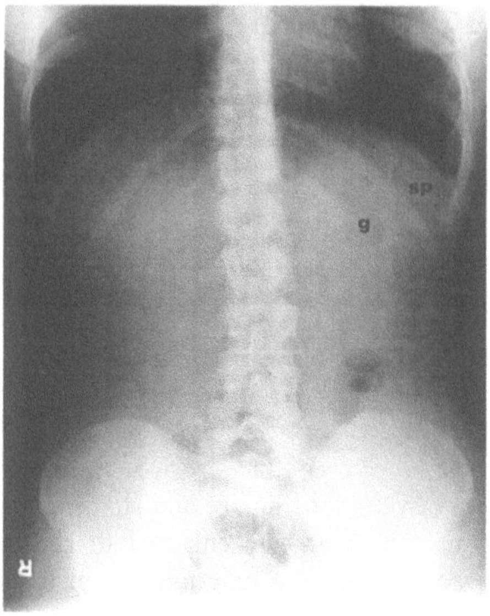

Fig. 2.2. The gastric air bubble (*g*) is visualized just medial to the spleen (*sp*) in the left upper quadrant

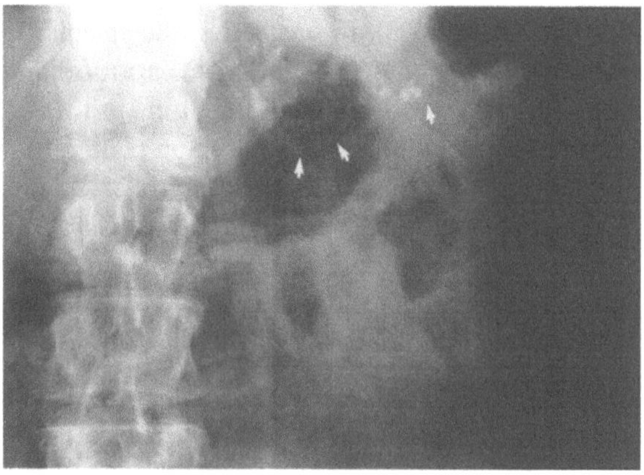

Fig. 2.3. Calcifications (*arrows*) of the splenic artery are commonly visualized

Whitley et al. (1966) described a method for predicting splenic weight from routine plain films using the formula: splenic weight = length × width. The length is estimated by a vertical line from the inferior tip of the spleen to the intercept with the diaphragm. The width of the spleen is measured at the midpoint of the length. The length measurement alone was the single best indicator of splenic size, according to Whitley et al. (1966). A length of more than 11.3 cm was associated with a 70% probability of spleen enlargement, and a length of 15 cm was associated with a 98% probability of splenomegaly.

2.3 Ultrasound

Ultrasound can be particularly useful in the evaluation of the spleen. A normal-sized spleen is best examined with the patient rolled onto the right side at a 45–90° angle, in a left-side-up decubitus position. The sonographic window to the spleen can be maximized with various degrees of inspiration, using an intercostal or subcostal approach. Rib shadowing can be minimized using an oblique plane of scanning along the intercostal space. Anterior scanning with the patient supine is often limited by artifacts from gastric or colonic gas, although filling the stomach with fluid may improve visualization. In patients with hepatomegaly, the left lobe of the liver may provide a window for visualization of the spleen. The spleen may be better visualized from an anterolateral approach if there is ascites or a left pleural effusion.

The spleen should be examined in both the coronal (longitudinal) and axial planes. The coronal plane (Fig. 2.4) is highly accurate for assessment of splenic lesions and documentation of approximate splenic size (Mathieson and Cooperberg 1998). The plane of section should be swept posterior to anterior to view the entire organ. The superior margin of the spleen is marked by the smooth echogenic line of the diaphragm. The inferior–medial margin is identified using the left kidney. Occasionally, the inferior portion of the spleen may extend posterior to the upper pole of the left kidney, yielding a "retrorenal spleen", which is a normal variant. This anomaly must be considered when performing percutaneous procedures, such as placement of a nephrostomy tube in the left kidney. Using a lateral, intercostal approach, axial scanning may help localize lesions in the anterior or posterior aspect of the

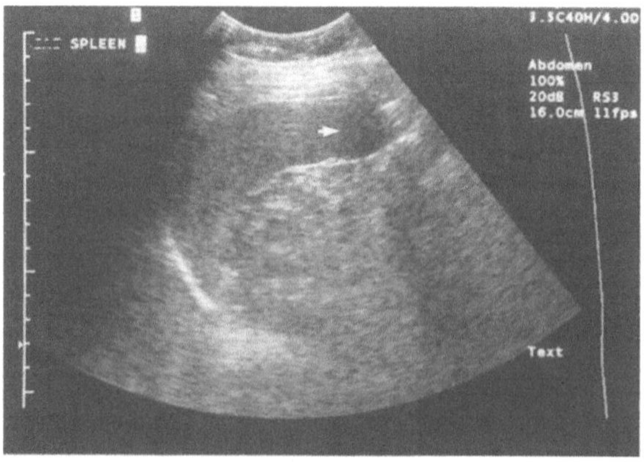

Fig. 2.4. Coronal scan of a normal spleen. The lower pole is partially obscured by a rib shadow (*arrow*)

spleen (MATHIESON and COOPERBERG 1998). The splenic parenchyma should produce homogeneous mid- to low-level echotexture. Occasional bright echoes represent blood vessels (Fig. 2.5). The splenic echogenicity is normally higher than that in the liver. Splenic echogenicity increases with splenomegaly.

The shape of the spleen is highly variable. MATHIESON and COOPERBERG (1998) describe the typical fat "inverted-comma" shape on transverse scanning at the superior aspect of the organ (Fig. 2.6). The complex shape of the organ makes it difficult to establish normal dimensions. FRANK et al. (1986) studied nearly 800 normal patients and found that the length of the spleen was less than 12 cm in 95% of patients. ISHIBASHI et al. (1991) developed a grading system based on a spleen index, which is calculated by multiplying the transverse diameter by the vertical diameter (using measurements taken from images showing the maximum sonographic cross-sectional area). KOGA and MORIKAWA (1975) reported the accuracy of measuring the area of the spleen along the longitudinal axis. RODRIGUES et al. (1995) examined 32 normal spleens from adult corpses and estimated an ultrasound volume using the formula volume = 0.52 × ultrasound height × breadth × width. The spleen has been shown to decrease in size with age and to increase in size with body weight (MESSINEZY et al. 1997), and these factors must be taken into account when assessing spleen size.

The splenic vascular pedicle and intrasplenic vessels can be seen with color-Doppler (Fig. 2.7) and power-Doppler imaging (Figs. 2.8, 2.9). The splenic vein is a useful landmark for identifying the splenic hilum. The pancreatic tail lies adjacent to the splenic artery and vein and may simulate a mass at the splenic hilum. Localization of the splenic artery and vein may be helpful in confirming this pseudo-mass as the normal tail of the pancreas (MATHIESON and COOPERBERG 1998).

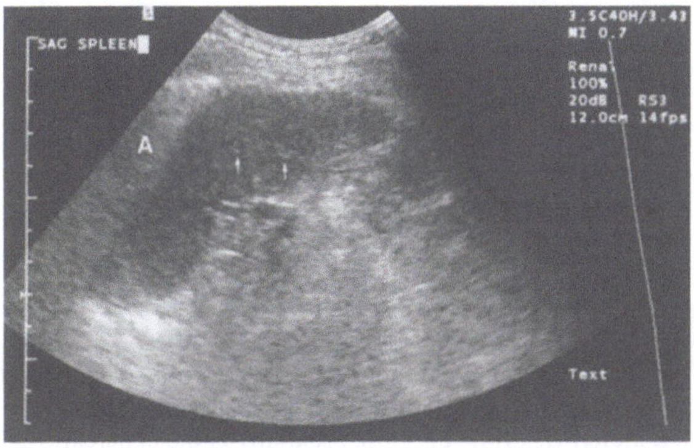

Fig. 2.5. Occasional bright echoes (*arrows*) in the homogeneous splenic parenchyma represent blood vessels. Air in the lung (*A*) obscures the superior margin

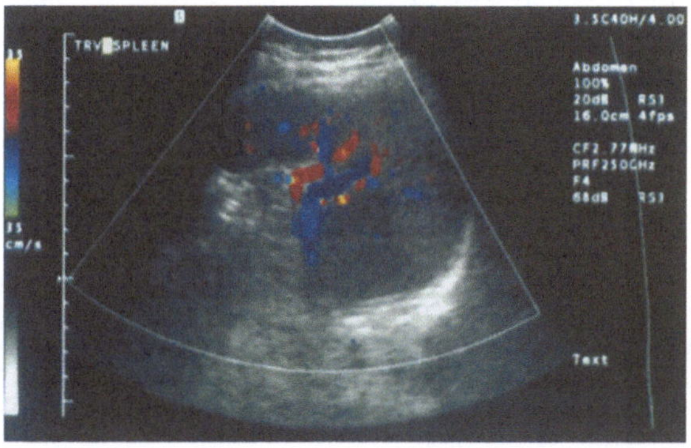

Fig. 2.7. A color Doppler scan demonstrates the vessels of the splenic hilum

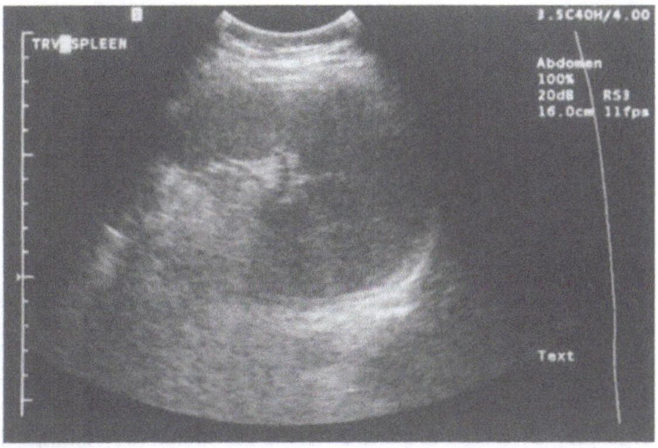

Fig. 2.6. Transverse scan of a normal "inverted comma" - shaped spleen

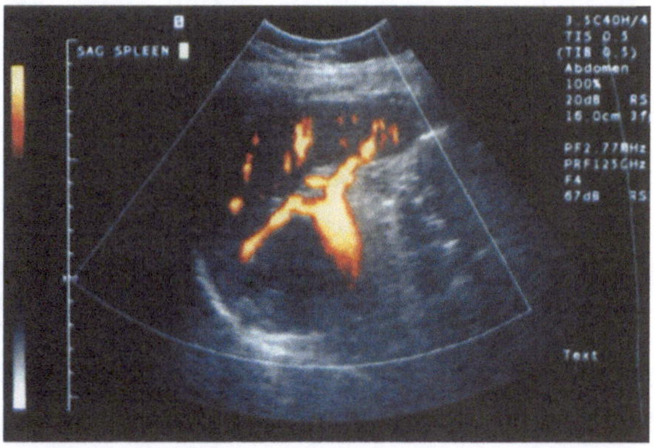

Fig. 2.8. Power Doppler imaging of normal vessels at splenic hilum

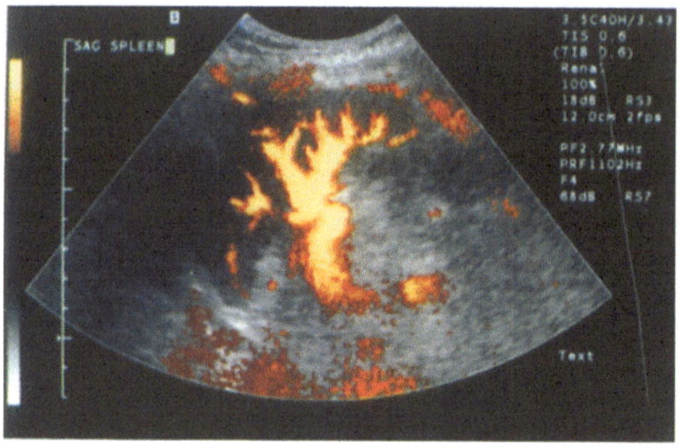

Fig. 2.9. A power Doppler image shows the splenic vascular pedicle and intrasplenic vessels. Note the motion noise surrounding the splenic margin

2.4 Computed Tomography

CT demonstrates the size, configuration, and location of the normal spleen and the relationship of the spleen to adjacent organs. With the advent of helical CT using the single breath-hold technique, motion artifacts and data misregistration are minimized (HEIKEN et al. 1993). Typically, 120 ml of contrast material is injected with a power injector at a rate of 2–3 ml/s. Scanning begins 40–60 s after the beginning of the injection. Images are obtained with 5–7 mm collimation.

The spleen is located posterolaterally in the left upper quadrant, under the leaf of the left hemidiaphragm (Fig. 2.10). The diaphragmatic surface is convex and faces posterolaterally. The spleen sits lateral to the stomach, and the gastric surface of the spleen is concave and faces anteromedially. The renal surface of the spleen is often concave, facing posteromedially (Fig. 2.11). The hilum is most commonly at the gastric surface but can, rarely, be seen at the renal surface. Often, two or more hila are seen (Fig. 2.12). Varying amounts of peritoneal and perirenal fat surround the spleen. At progressively lower axial sections, the amount of perirenal fat increases. In 15–20% of individuals, a retrorenal spleen is seen, with the posterior border of the spleen behind the left kidney (Fig. 2.13; DODDS et al. 1990). Occasionally, the gastrosplenic, splenorenal, or splenocolic ligaments are seen on CT (Figs. 2.14, 2.15). The shape of the spleen on CT varies from a

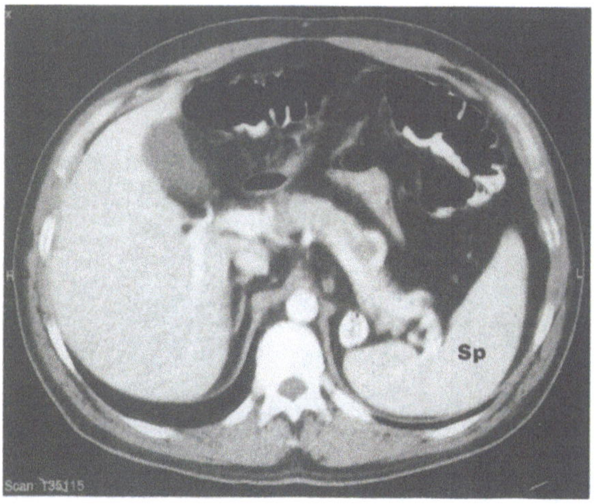

Fig. 2.10. Enhanced helical computed tomography scan through the spleen (*sp*) shows the convex diaphragmatic surface of the spleen, separated from the diaphragm by a small rim of fat

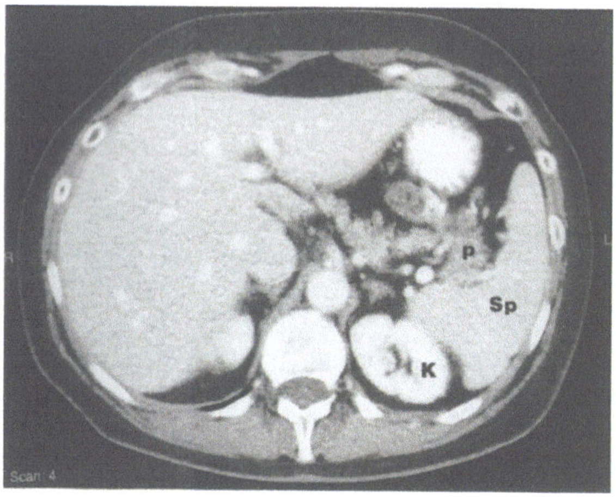

Fig. 2.11. Computed tomography at the mid-splenic level shows the concave renal surface of the spleen (*Sp*) abutting the left kidney (*K*). Note the close proximity of the pancreatic tail (*p*) to the splenic hilum

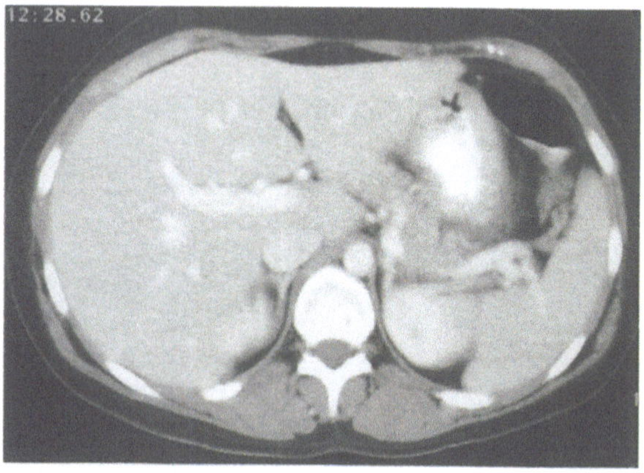

Fig. 2.12. Two hilar arteries entering the spleen are visualized on this contrast-enhanced computed-tomography image

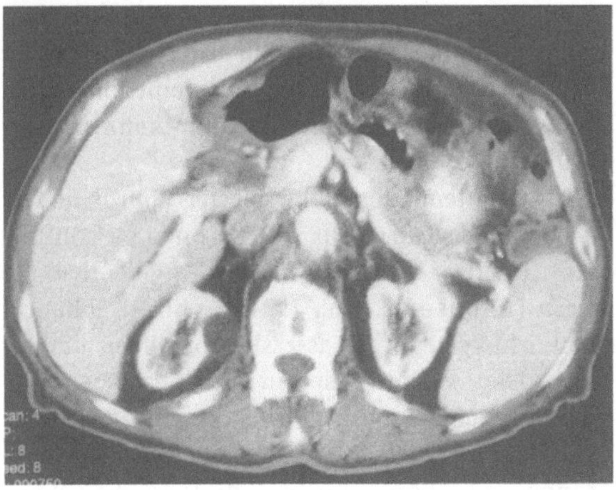

Fig. 2.13. A "retrorenal spleen", with the spleen located behind the left kidney

slender "banana" shape (Fig. 2.15) to a rather plump, round structure. Bizarre shapes occur with lobulated or sharp borders (Fig. 2.16). A prominent medial "tubercle" may be seen at the upper medial pole (Fig. 2.17), simulating a mass (MITTELSTAEDT 1987). Often, congenital clefts extend from fetal lobulations and should not be mistaken for splenic fractures due to trauma (Figs. 2.18, 2.19). Most clefts occur on the diaphragmatic surface. Occasionally, accessory spleens may be seen. Ten percent of the population has one or more accessory spleens, most often located in the vicinity of the splenic hilum (Fig. 2.23).

A splenic index has been described in defining splenic size on CT (STRIJK et al. 1985). The index is

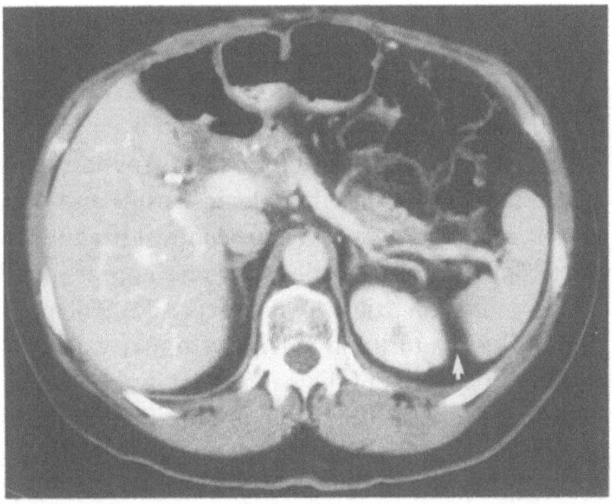

Fig. 2.14. The splenorenal ligament (*arrow*) is occasionally visualized on computed tomography

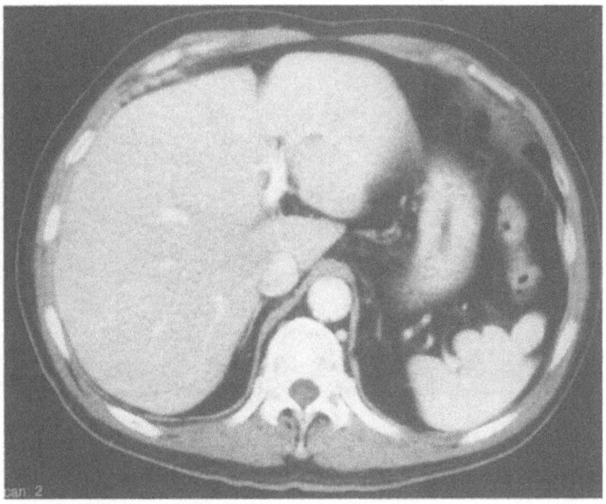

Fig. 2.16. An unusually shaped normal spleen with multiple lobulations

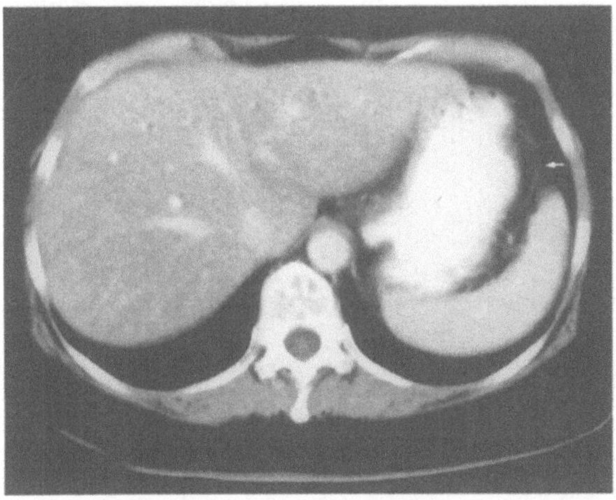

Fig. 2.15. A "banana"-shaped spleen on helical computed tomography. Note the gastrosplenic ligament (*arrow*)

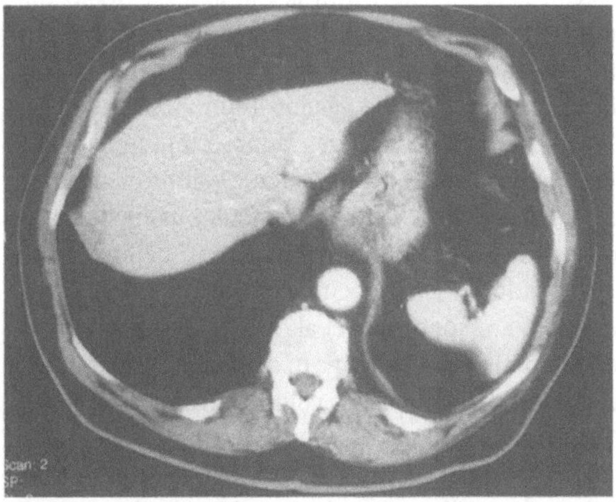

Fig. 2.17. A prominent medial tubercle, which may simulate a mass

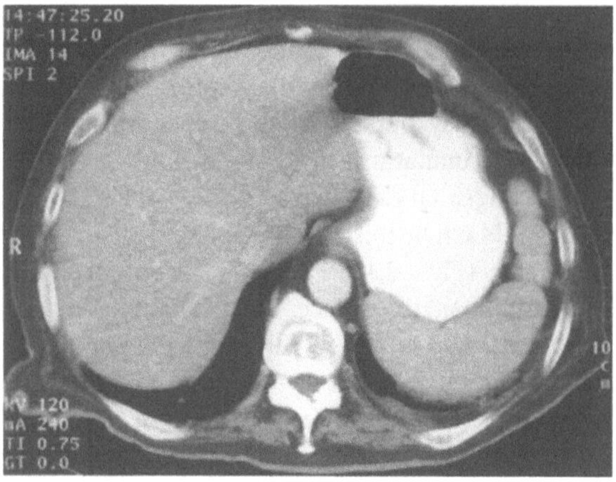

Fig. 2.18. Multiple fetal lobulations of the spleen

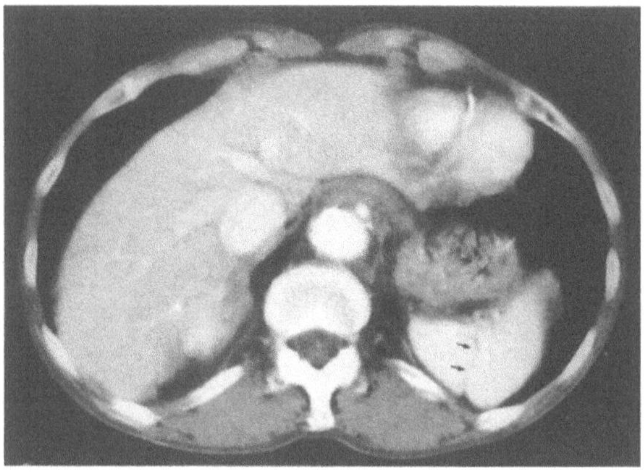

Fig. 2.19. A deep cleft (*arrows*) of the spleen may simulate a splenic laceration

obtained by multiplying spleen thickness, width, and length as visualized on CT. The length is determined by adding all section-thicknesses on which the spleen is seen. The width is the longest organ diameter in the axial scanning plane. The thickness is the distance between the center and peripheral surfaces, measured at the splenic hilum. LACKNER et al. (1980) found splenic index values ranging from 120 to 480 for normal spleens. Splenic volume can also be calculated from CT measurements, using the proposed formula: volume (in cubic centimeters) = 30 + 0.58 (width × length × maximum thickness at the hilum (PRASSOPOULOS et al. 1997). Based on a study of 140 patients, PRASSOPOULOS et al. (1997) found a range of normal splenic volumes from 107.2 cm^3 to 314.5 cm^3.

There can be variation in the position of the spleen depending on patient position in the scanner. BALL et al. (1980) described the ventral and caudal position change of both the liver and spleen when CT scanning was performed in the prone rather than supine position. The spleen can also contract under heavy adrenergic stimulation, a phenomenon seen in trauma patients (GOODMAN and APRAHAMIAN 1990).

The CT attenuation of the spleen is approximately 40–60 Hounsfield units (HU) on non-contrast scans. The liver is normally 5–10 HU higher than the spleen (RABUSHKA et al. 1994). Contrast enhancement is indicated when assessing for splenic pathology. The normal spleen can show quite inhomogeneous contrast enhancement after bolus injection (Fig. 2.20). Fast injection rates yield more pronounced inhomogeneity. With time, the splenic enhancement becomes more uniform (Fig. 2.21). GLAZER et al. (1981) described a homogeneous appearance within 2 min after bolus injection. MILES et al. (1995) confirmed that the heterogeneous pattern observed in the first minute of contrast enhancement is due to differential perfusion rates, which have been attributed to variable rates of blood flow through the cords of the red pulp.

The omental and mesenteric fat surrounding the spleen sharply outlines the splenic capsule and hilar vessels even before intravenous contrast is administered. The tortuous splenic artery may appear round or curvilinear on axial sections (Fig. 2.22). The position of the less tortuous splenic vein may vary relative to the position of the pancreas (Fig. 2.23).

A "bare" area of the spleen has been described as a consistent finding on CT in patients with ascites (VIBHAKAR and BELLON 1984). This so-called bare

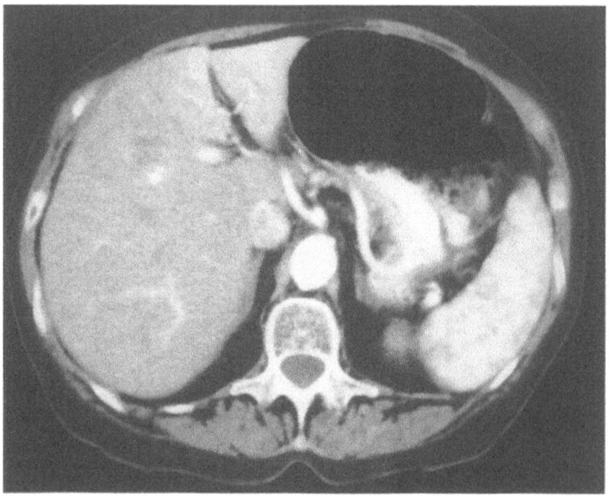

Fig. 2.20. Dynamic contrast-enhanced computed tomography (after bolus contrast injection) shows normal heterogeneous enhancement of the spleen

a 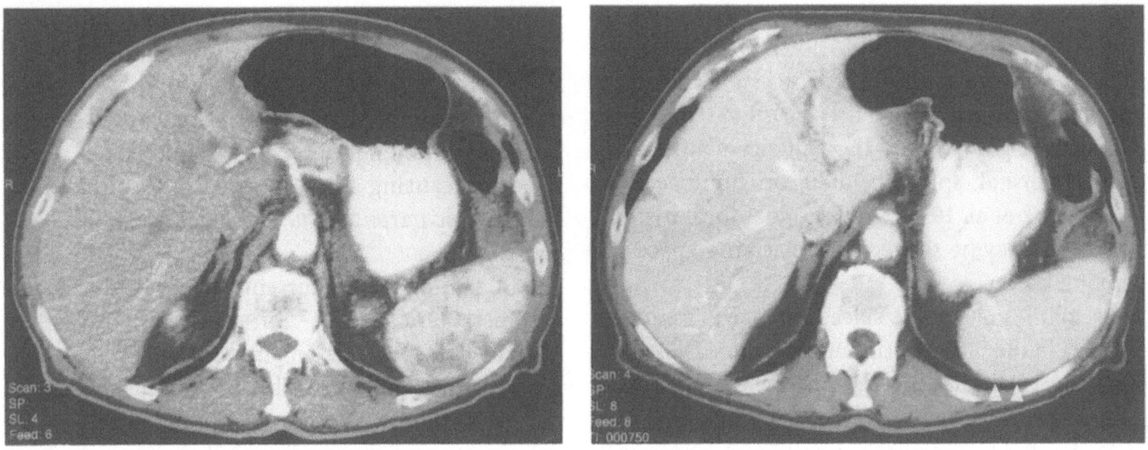 b

Fig. 2.21. **a** Marked inhomogeneity of splenic enhancement with early scanning after bolus injection. **b** Delayed scanning of the patient in **a** shows a homogeneous splenic appearance. Note the “bare” area of the spleen abutting the pleural space (*arrowheads*)

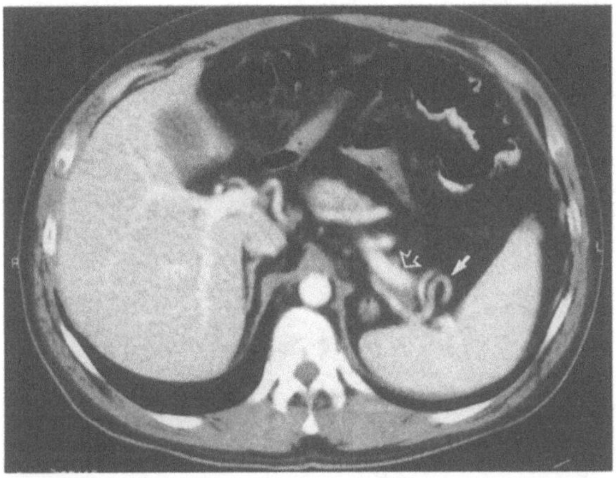

Fig. 2.22. The tortuous splenic artery (*closed arrow*) is visualized adjacent to the splenic vein (*open arrow*), which runs a more linear course

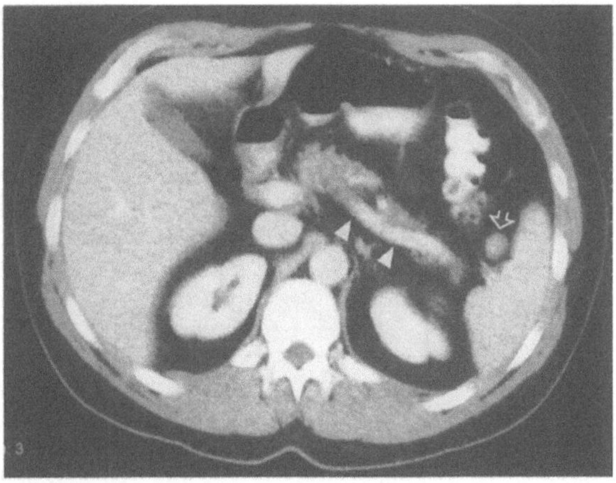

Fig. 2.23. The splenic vein (*arrowheads*) courses along the posterior aspect of the upper pancreatic body. Note the small accessory spleen (*open arrow*)

area is not surrounded by the ascites, as is the remainder of the spleen. This “bare” area is approximately 2–3 cm long and may be outlined by air in the posterior costophrenic sulcus (Fig. 2.21b). The bare area may be helpful in differentiating pleural effusion from ascites, since ascites cannot reach the bare area.

2.5 MR Imaging

The spleen is often evaluated with both T1- and T2-weighted sequences. On T1-weighted sequences, the signal intensity of the spleen is normally less than that of the liver and slightly higher than that of muscle (Fig. 2.24). The spleen is of higher signal intensity than the liver on T2-weighted images (Fig. 2.25). The splenic signal intensity is closely related to paravertebral muscle on T1-weighted images and subcutaneous fat or kidney on T2-weighted images (Mirowitz et al. 1991). The spleen has a homogeneous signal intensity on conventional spin-echo images. However, after contrast injection with gadolinium, the normal spleen often shows mottled inhomogeneous enhancement (Figs. 2.26, 2.27) similar to the phenomenon seen with contrast-enhanced CT. This pattern may be secondary to variable rates of blood flow through the red pulp cords. Another potential reason for the mottled appearance is slow enhancement of white pulp and rapid enhancement of red pulp (Semelka et al. 1992). Delayed repeat imaging will show a homogeneous signal intensity of splenic parenchyma (Fig. 2.26). By 1 min after injection of gadolinium, the enhancement pattern of the normal spleen should be homogeneous (Mirowitz et al. 1991). Any residual focal hypointense area may be suspected to harbor a space-occupying lesion.

Pseudo-lesions of the spleen can occur from flow artifacts in the phase-encoding direction. These artifacts can be limited by exchanging the phase and frequency-encoding directions, although the artifacts may still be visualized anterior and posterior to the aorta (Ito et al. 1996).

Although gadolinium is the most commonly used contrast agent, superparamagnetic iron-oxide agents may be used to evaluate the spleen. These agents are specifically distributed to the reticuloendothelial cells, decreasing T2 relaxation time and causing a loss of signal intensity of normal splenic parenchyma (Weissleder et al. 1988; Fig. 2.28).

MR angiography is currently being used to evaluate mesenteric vessels. Shirkhoda et al. (1998) described a contrast-enhanced, breath-hold, fat-suppressed, three-dimensional technique that allows the evaluation of mesenteric vessels, including the splenic artery and vein (Figs. 2.29, 2.30).

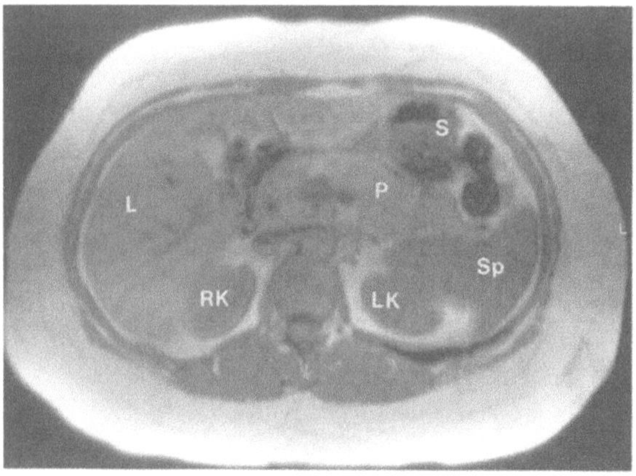

Fig. 2.24. This T1-weighted sequence shows a normal spleen (*Sp*) of lower signal intensity than the liver (*L*). The adjacent pancreas (*P*), stomach (*S*), and kidneys (*RK*, *LK*) are seen

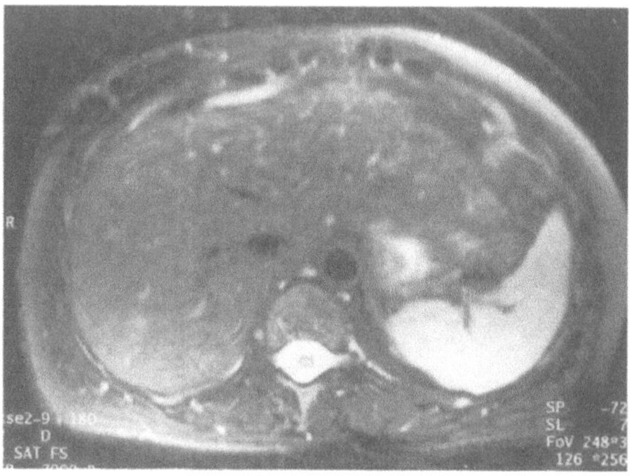

Fig. 2.25. This T2-weighted fast spin-echo sequence with fat saturation shows a hyperintense signal intensity of the normal spleen relative to the liver

a 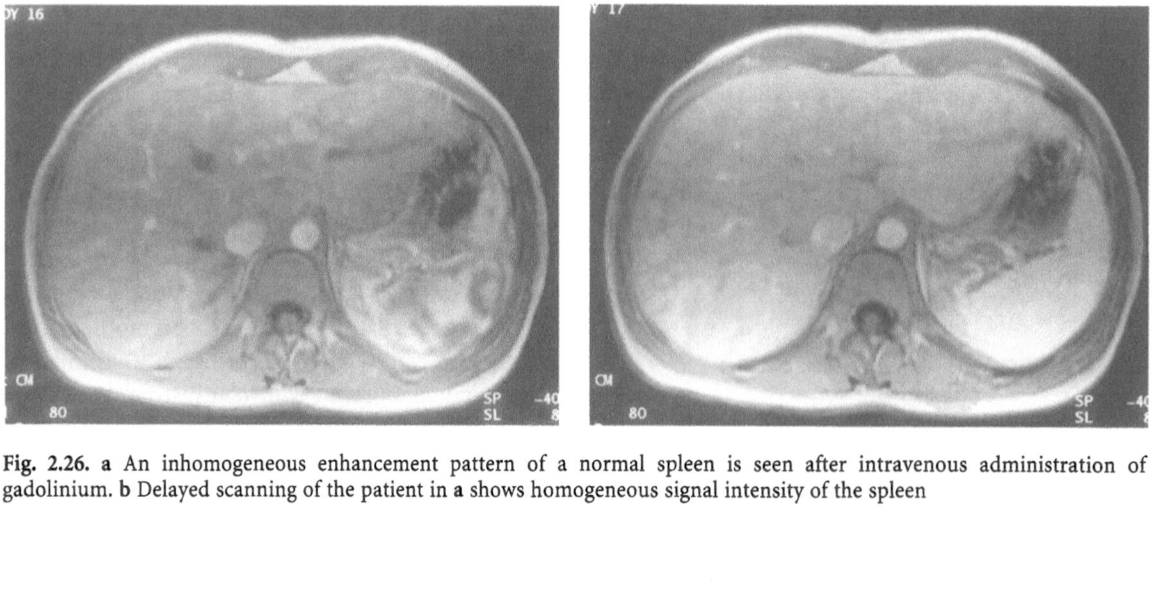 b

Fig. 2.26. a An inhomogeneous enhancement pattern of a normal spleen is seen after intravenous administration of gadolinium. **b** Delayed scanning of the patient in **a** shows homogeneous signal intensity of the spleen

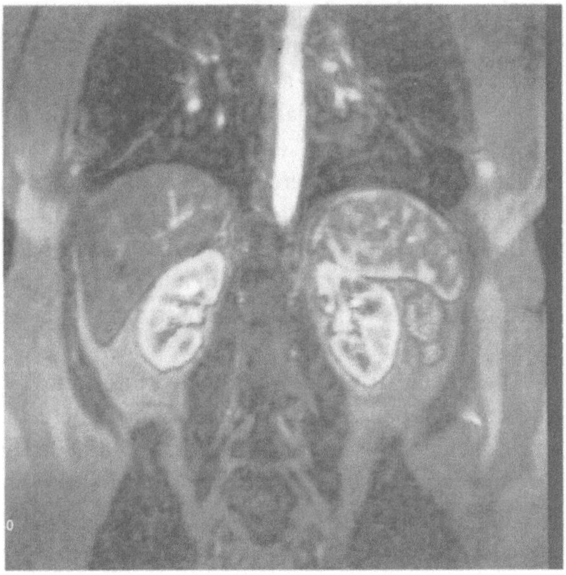

Fig. 2.27. A coronal magnetic resonance image shows heterogeneous enhancement of a normal spleen during the early phase of a dynamic study

a

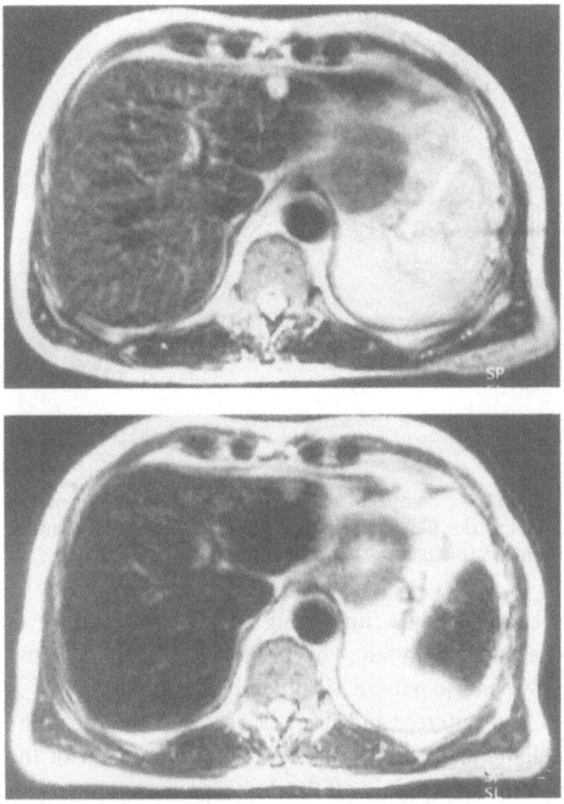

b

Fig. 2.28. **a** Turbo spin echo (TSE) T2-weighted image before administration of superparamagnetic iron oxide [SPIO, a reticuloendothelial system (RES) contrast agent]. The signal intensity (SI) of the normal spleen is higher than that of the liver. **b** TSE T2-weighted image after administration of SPIO. There is a marked decrease of the SI of liver and spleen, due to uptake of SPIO contrast in the RES of the liver and spleen. A hemangioma is seen within the left liver

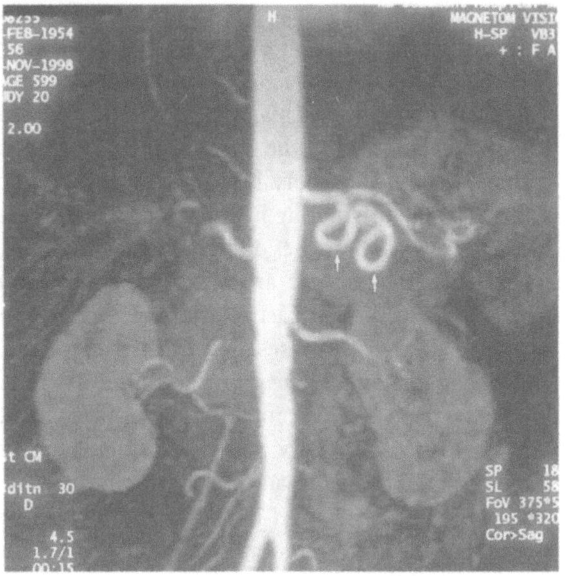

Fig. 2.29. The arterial phase of a contrast-enhanced magnetic resonance angiography study shows a very tortuous splenic artery (*arrows*) entering the spleen

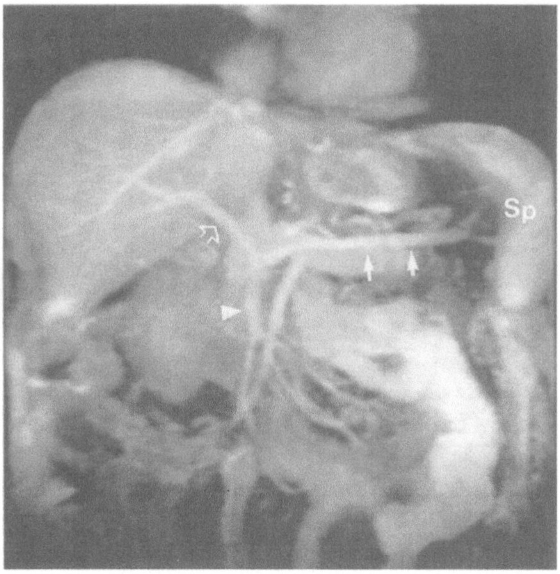

Fig. 2.30. The venous phase image from a contrast-enhanced magnetic resonance angiography study shows the splenic vein (*closed arrows*) arising from the spleen (*Sp*). The splenic vein joins the superior mesenteric vein (*arrowhead*) to form the portal vein (*open arrow*)

2.6 Angiography

The splenic artery is remarkable for its large size relative to the size of the organ and its tortuous course. The splenic artery is a branch of the celiac artery, usually originating just distal to the left gastric artery, which branches off first. Most commonly, the splenic and hepatic arteries form a common trunk distal to the left gastric artery (Fig. 2.31). In approximately 25% of cases, the left gastric, splenic, and hepatic arteries arise from a common trunk, forming a tripod celiac configuration (Abrams and Meyerovitz 1997). Very rarely, the splenic artery may originate from the aorta, superior mesenteric artery, or the right aspect of the celiac axis. These vessels may need injection when a celiac angiogram fails to reveal the splenic artery.

The arterial blood supply to the spleen is quite varied. In 100 human dissections, Michels (1942) found no two patterns alike. Classically, two basic types of splenic arterial patterns have been described. A "distributed" arterial pattern has a short splenic artery with numerous small branches coming off the trunk and entering 75% of the medial surface of the spleen. The "compact" arterial pattern has a relatively long splenic artery with a few, large terminal branches entering 30% of the spleen's medial surface (Fig. 2.32).

The splenic artery can be divided into four segments: suprapancreatic, pancreatic, prepancreatic, and prehilar (Abrams and Meyerovitz 1997). The suprapancreatic segment involves the first 1–3 cm after the origin of the artery. The pancreatic portion is the most tortuous and runs along the pancreas, supplying small pancreatic branches. The prepancreatic segment runs along the anterior surface of the pancreatic tail. The prehilar segment is found between the pancreatic tail and spleen.

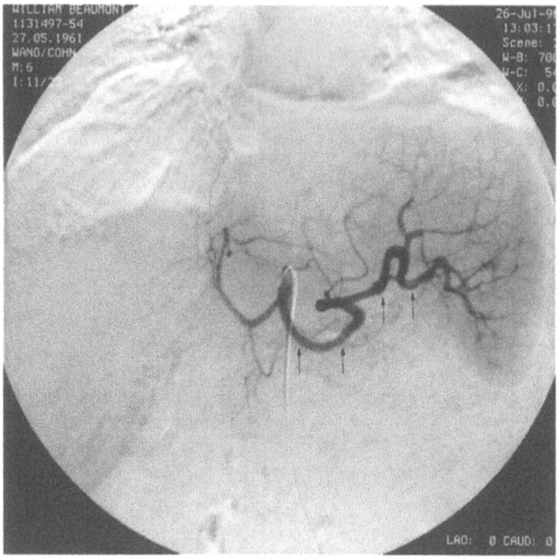

Fig. 2.31. This selective celiac injection shows a normal tortuous splenic artery (*arrows*) arising from the celiac artery

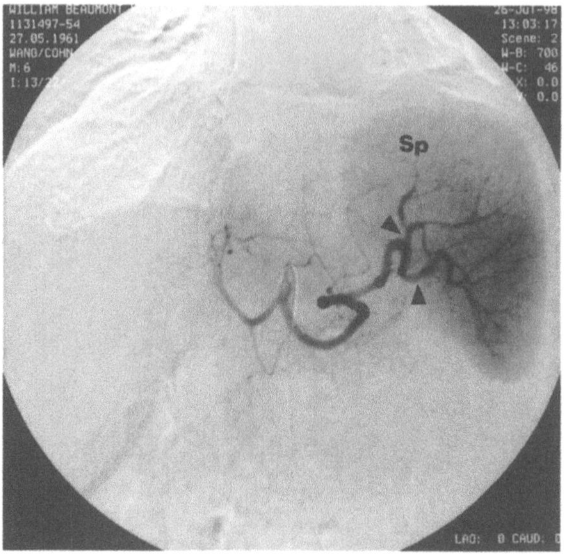

Fig. 2.32. A "compact" arterial pattern of the splenic artery, showing the long splenic artery with a few large terminal branches (*arrowheads*) entering the spleen

The splenic artery travels a serpentine course along the superior border of the pancreatic body. The average length of the artery is 13 cm (range 8–32 cm), and the average width 7.5 mm (range 5–12 mm; Abrams and Meyerovitz 1997). The splenic artery tortuosity is unique among normal arteries. Often, arteries become tortuous due to atherosclerotic disease or as a result of acting as a collateral vessel, but the normal splenic artery can be quite tortuous and may be characterized by loops and spirals. The splenic artery often becomes more tortuous with age (Michels 1942).

The pancreas and stomach receive branches of the splenic artery. The suprapancreatic segment of the splenic artery gives off the dorsal pancreatic artery in 40% of persons (Reuter et al. 1986), and this artery supplies the dorsal surface and branches into the uncinate process. Multiple small pancreatic arteries arise from the splenic artery throughout its course. The largest is the pancreatica magna artery arising in the midportion, which supplies the pancreatic tail.

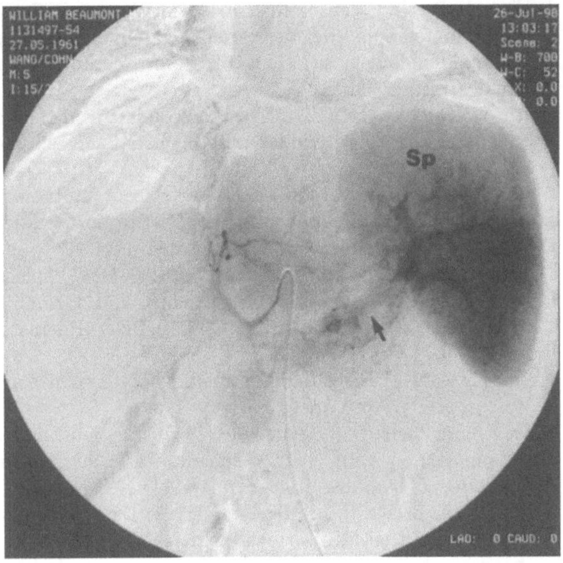

Fig. 2.33. The venous phase of a celiac arteriogram shows early opacification of the splenic vein (*arrow*) and homogeneous enhancement of the splenic parenchyma (*Sp*)

The caudal pancreatic artery arises from the distal splenic artery. The splenic artery also yields short gastric arteries. The left gastroepiploic artery often arises from the inferior splenic artery or its branches.

The splenic vein is formed by variable branches from the spleen, omentum, and gastric fundus that coalesce at the splenic hilum. The splenic vein lies caudal to the artery and joins the superior mesenteric vein to the right of midline to form the portal vein (Fig. 2.33). The splenic vein often receives the inferior mesenteric vein and tiny tributary veins from the pancreatic tail and body.

Abrams and Meyerovitz (1997) noted a wide variation in the transit time of contrast travelling from the splenic artery to the splenic vein, where it is visualized. The range was 3–36 s, with an average circulation time of 8.3 s. The parenchymal phase of the splenic arteriogram may be homogeneous or slightly patchy.

2.7 Imaging the Fetal and Pediatric Spleens

Obstetrical ultrasound examinations can reveal the fetal spleen from 20 weeks. At less than 20 weeks, fetal motion prevents optimal visualization (Aoki et al. 1992). In the transverse plane through the fetal upper abdomen, the fetal spleen is identified as a triangular or crescent-shaped structure posterior to the fluid-filled stomach (Fig. 2.34) and lateral to the left adrenal gland. Aoki et al. (1992) generated normal ranges for splenic length, circumference, and area measurements for estimating the growth of the fetal spleen. Transient contraction of the fetal spleen has been described during vaginal delivery and after cesarean section.

Rosenberg et al. (1991) generated normal values for splenic size from infancy to age 20 years using a one-step measurement of the greatest longitudinal length of the spleen using ultrasound. Loftus and Metreweli (1998) describe a method for detecting splenomegaly in pediatric patients; this method does not require reference to a table of normal values. These authors state that splenomegaly should be suspected in children if the spleen is more than 1.25 times longer than the adjacent kidney, as measured using sonographic lengths of each organ.

Schlesinger et al. (1993) developed standards for the normal volume of the spleen in children, as measured on CT scans. The volume of the spleen correlated better with body weight than with age in their study of 48 children. A recent study of 307 pediatric patients showed a strong correlation between patient height and sonographic splenic length (Konus et al. 1998). These researchers found no statistically significant difference between the longitudinal dimension of the spleen in boys and that in girls.

Marked changes occur in the MR appearance of the normal spleen during childhood. In the neonate, the signal intensity of the spleen is equal to or mildly less than that of the liver on T2-weighted images. The T2-signal intensity of the spleen gradually increases and, by approximately 8 months of age, resembles

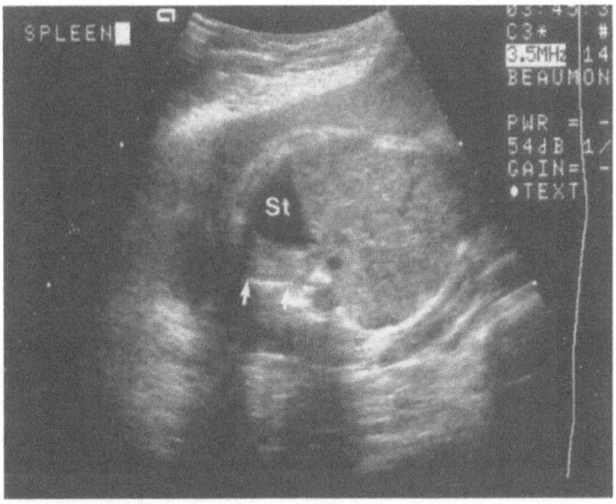

Fig. 2.34. The normal fetal spleen (*arrows*) is seen posterior to the fluid-filled stomach (*St*) (courtesy of C. Comstock)

that of an adult (Donnelly et al. 1996). On T1-weighted images the neonatal-spleen signal intensity is approximately equal to that of the liver and decreases by 1 month of age, becoming lower than the signal intensity of the adult liver (Donnelly et al. 1996). The changes in the neonatal spleen appear to correlate with changes in the white-pulp and red-pulp ratios. At birth, most of the splenic tissue is red pulp and, with increasing age, the lymphoid follicles grow and mature, increasing the amount of white pulp. The large volumes of red pulp in the normal neonatal spleen may be the cause of the low signal intensity on T2-weighted sequences. Nonthrombosed blood (which is present in the red-pulp sinusoids) is dark on T2-weighted sequences (Donnelly et al. 1996).

References

Abrams HL, Meyerovitz MF (1997) Splenic arteriography. In: Baum (ed) Abrams' angiography, 4th edn. Little Brown and Company, Boston, pp 1457–1495

Aoki S, Hata T, Kitao M (1992) Ultrasonographic assessment of fetal and neonatal spleen. Am J Perinatol 9:361–367

Ball WS, Wicks JD, Mettler FA (1980) Prone-supine change in organ position. AJR Am J Roentgenol 135:815–820

Brogdon BG, Cros NE (1959) Observations on the normal spleen. Radiology 72:412–414

Dachman A, Friedman A (1993) Radiology of the spleen. Mosby, St Louis, pp 1–38

Dodds WJ, Taylor AJ, Erickson SJ, et al. (1990) Radiologic imaging of splenic anomalies. AJR Am J Roentgenol 155:805–810

Donnelly LF, Emery KH, Bove KE, et al. (1996) Normal changes in the MR appearance of the spleen during early childhood. AJR Am J Roentgenol 166:635–639

Frank K, Linhart P, Kortsik C, et al. (1986) Sonographic determination of spleen size: normal dimensions in adults with a healthy spleen. Ultraschall Med 7:134–137

Glazer GM, Axel L, Goldberg HI, et al. (1981) Dynamic CT of the normal spleen. AJR Am J Roentgenol 137:343–346

Goodman LR, Aprahamian C (1990) Changes in splenic size after abdominal trauma. Radiology 176:629–632

Heiken JP, Brink JA, Vannier MW (1993) Spiral (helical) CT. Radiology 189:647–656

Ishibashi H, Higuchi N, Shimamura R, et al. (1991) Sonographic assessment and grading of spleen size. J Clin Ultrasound 19:21–25

Ito K, Mitchell DG, Honjo K, et al. (1996) Gadolinium-enhanced MR imaging of the spleen: artifacts and pitfalls. AJR Am J Roentgenol 167:1147–1157

Koga T, Morikawa Y (1975) Ultrasonographic determination of the splenic size and its clinical usefulness in various liver diseases. Radiology 115:157–161

Konus ÖL, Özdemir A, Akkaya A, et al. (1998) Normal liver, spleen, and kidney dimensions in neonates, infants, and children: evaluation with sonography. AJR Am J Roentgenol 171:1693–1698

Lackner K, Brecht G, Janson R, et al. (1980) Wertigkeit. Computer tomographie bei der Stradieneinteilung primärer Lymphknotenneoplasien. ROFO Fortschr Geb Rontgenstr Nuklearmed 132:21–30

Loftus WK, Metreweli C (1998) Ultrasound assessment of mild splenomegaly: spleen/kidney ratio. Pediatr Radiol 28:98–100

Mathieson JR, Cooperberg PL (1998) The spleen. In: Rumack CM, Wilson SR, Charboneau JW (eds) Diagnostic ultrasound, 2nd edn. Mosby, St. Louis, pp 155–174

Messinezy M, Macdonald LM, Nunan TO, et al. (1997) Spleen sizing by ultrasound in polycythaemia and thrombocythaemia: comparison with SPECT. Br J Haematol 98:103–107

Michels NA (1942) The variational anatomy of the spleen and splenic artery. Am J Anat 70:21

Miles KA, McPherson SJ, Hayball MP (1995) Transient splenic inhomogeneity with contrast-enhanced CT: mechanism and effect of liver disease. Radiology 194:91–95

Mirowitz SA, Brown JJ, Lee JK, et al. (1991) Dynamic gadolinium-enhanced MR imaging of the spleen: normal enhancement patterns and evaluation of splenic lesions. Radiology 179:681–686

Mittelstaedt CA (1987) In: Mittelstaedt CA (ed) Abdominal ultrasound. Churchhill Livingstone, New York, pp 565–604

Prassopoulos P, Daskalogiannaki M, Raissaki M, et al. (1997) Determination of normal splenic volume on computed tomography in relation to age, gender, and body habitus. Eur Radiol 7:246–248

Rabushka LS, Kawashima A, Fishman EK (1994) Imaging of the spleen: CT with supplemental MR examination. Radiographics 14:307–332

Reuter SR, Redman HC, Cho K (1986) In: Gastrointestinal angiography, 3rd edn. Saunders, Philadelphia, pp 40–43

Rodrigues AJ Jr, Rodrigues CJ, Germano MA, et al. (1995) Sonographic assessment of normal spleen volume. Clin Anat 8:252–255

Rosenberg HK, Markowitz RI, Kolberg H, et al. (1991) Normal splenic size in infants and children: sonographic measurements. AJR Am J Roentgenol 157:119–121

Schlesinger AE, Edgar KA, Boxer LA (1993) Volume of the spleen in children as measured on CT scans: normal standards as function of body weight. AJR Am J Roentgenol 160:1107–1109

Semelka RC, Shoenut JP, Lawrence PH, et al. (1992) Spleen: dynamic enhancement patterns on gradient-echo MR images enhanced with gadopentetate dimeglumine. Radiology 185:479–482

Shirkhoda A, Konez O, Shetty AN, et al. (1998) Contrast-enhanced MR angiography of the mesenteric circulation: a pictorial essay. Radiographics 18:851–861

Strijk SP, Wagener DJ, Bogman MJ, et al. (1985) The spleen in Hodgkin disease: diagnostic value of CT. Radiology 154:753–757

Vibhakar SD, Bellon EM (1984) The bare area of the spleen: a constant CT feature of the ascitic abdomen. AJR Am J Roentgenol 142:953–955

Weissleder R, Hahn PF, Stark DD, et al. (1988) Superparamagnetic iron oxide: enhanced detection of focal splenic tumors with MR imaging. Radiology 169:399–403

Whitley JE, Maynard CD, Rhyne AL (1966) A computer approach to the prediction of spleen weight from routine films. Radiology 86:73–76

3 Congenital Disorders of the Spleen

D. VANBECKEVOORT, G. VERSWIJVEL, and L. VAN HOE

CONTENTS

3.1 Introduction

Recognition and correct identification of congenital variants and anomalies of the spleen is essential in abdominal imaging. In this chapter, we describe and discuss reliable imaging features of the most frequent and most essential congenital splenic variants and anomalies. Knowledge of these features and an increased awareness will increase the diagnostic skills of the radiologist confronted with a splenic congenital anomaly.

3.2 Normal Variants in Position and in Splenic Shape

As discussed above, a great variety exists in the normal shape and position of the spleen in the normal individual. These normal variations may cause difficulties in measuring the exact size of the spleen or interpreting splenic disease on different imaging modalities.

The long axis of the spleen lies in the plane of the tenth rib; the anterior border reaches the mid-axillary line, and the posterior border lies approximately 4 cm from the mid-dorsal line (WILLIAMS et al. 1989). Due to its soft and pliable consistency, adjacent congenital (or acquired) organ enlargement or absence of adjacent organs (agenesis of the left kidney) may cause considerable splenic displacement in the abdomen and deformity of the splenic shape. Depending on the size of the colonic impression, the general shape of the spleen may vary from a slightly or prominently curved wedge to a tetrahedral aspect (WILLIAMS et al. 1989). This illustrates that the shape of the normal spleen has only relative importance but is nonetheless typical.

A common pseudotumoral splenic formation is the existence of a prominent, congenital, splenic lobule that extends from the splenic contour. Most frequently, it extends medially from the posterior pole of the spleen. This lobule usually lies anterior to the upper pole of the left kidney and can simulate a renal or adrenal mass on plain images or on excretory urography (Fig. 3.1; PIEKARSKI et al. 1980; GOODING 1981). However, its splenic origin can easily be explained on other imaging modalities, such as ultrasound (US), computed tomography (CT; Fig. 3.2) and magnetic resonance (MR) imaging. Very occasionally, a splenic lobule of this type extends posteriorly to the left kidney and displaces it anteriorly (PIEKARSKI et al. 1980). A prominent splenic lobule

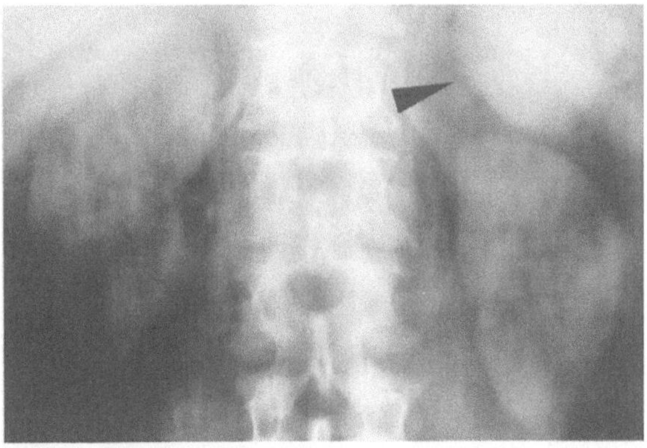

Fig. 3.1. Nephrotomography 1 min after intravenous contrast. A round mass representing a splenic nodule is seen adjacent to the upper pole of the left kidney (*arrowhead*)

D. VANBECKEVOORT, G. VERSWIJVEL, and L. VAN HOE; Department of Radiology, University Hospitals K. U. Leuven, Herestraat 49, B-3000 Leuven, Belgium

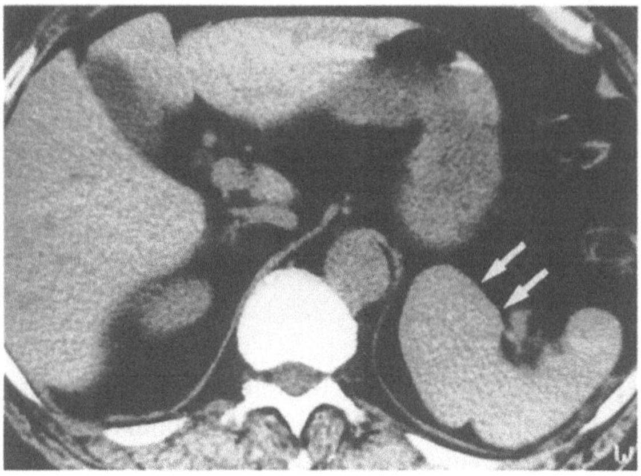

Fig. 3.2. A prominent splenic lobulation is shown (*arrows*)

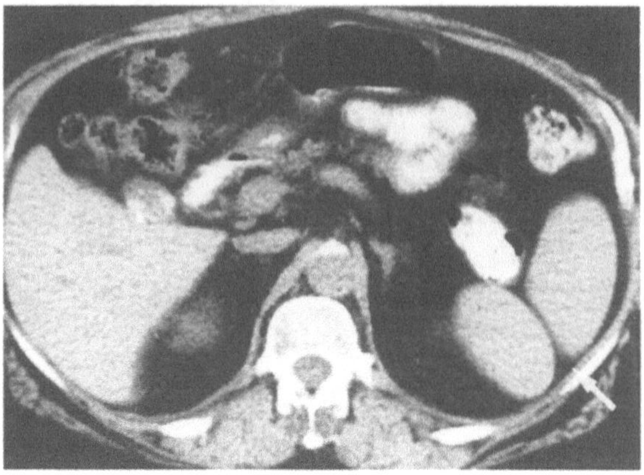

Fig. 3.4. A deep cleft (*arrow*) in a normal spleen

of this type may also be noted at the anterior or lateral margin of the spleen (Piekarski et al. 1980).

As described above, the spleen has a lobulated contour in the foetus. As a consequence, it may retain its foetal lobulated shape or may show deep notches or clefts in addition to those usually present on the superior margin (Fig. 3.3). These residual notches or clefts usually are sharp and can be prominent; they may be as deep as 2–3 cm (Fig. 3.4; Dodds et al. 1990). Often, they are present at the diaphragmatic or inferior border of the spleen. This may cause diagnostic problems in evaluating patients who had abdominal trauma, since this type of residual notching may mimic splenic lacerations. The absence of intra-abdominal or perisplenic free fluid and the normal texture of the splenic parenchyma on the different imaging modalities are keys used to differentiate an acute splenic laceration from a congenital lobulated spleen.

Under normal conditions, the splenic vessels traverse the posterior aspect of the body and tail of the pancreas to enter the splenic hilum, which is directed anteromedially in the abdomen. A rare variant is a splenic hilum that is directed superior to the left hemidiaphragm (Fig. 3.5). This usually occurs towards the medial portion of the diaphragm, but lateral orientations are reported. As a consequence, the convex surface of the spleen is directed towards the upper pole of the left kidney. This variant is called the "upside-down spleen" and can be mistaken for a left suprarenal mass on standard radiographs (Westcott and Krufky 1972; D'Altorio and Canno 1978). It is due to a developmental rotation of the spleen on its longitudinal anteroposterior axis, causing the splenic hilum to be directed cephaladly or laterally (D'Altorio and Canno 1978).

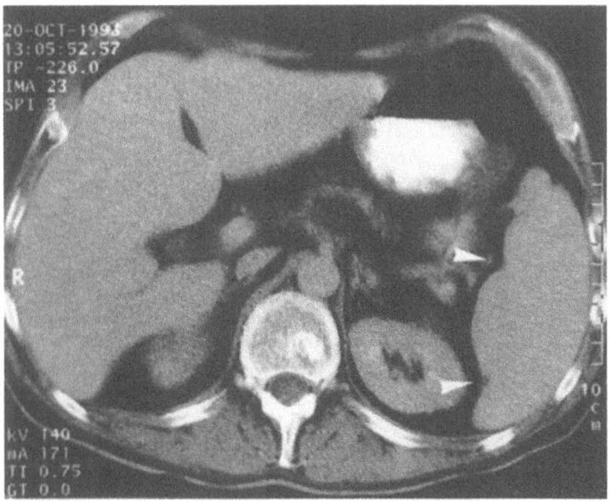

Fig. 3.3. Persistent foetal lobulated shape of the spleen, demonstrated by means of computed tomography (*arrowheads*)

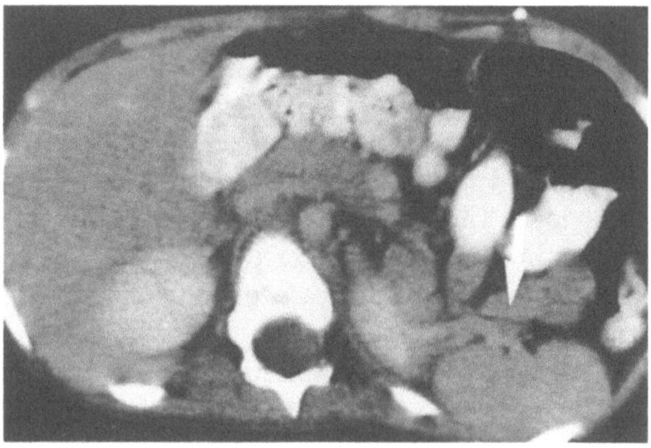

Fig. 3.5. Upside-down spleen; the splenic hilum (*arrow*) is directed superiorly to the left hemidiaphragm

When a deep peritoneal lateral recessus that is filled by the spleen or intestine persists, the spleen will have a pronounced posterior location behind the left kidney. This congenital anomalous location of the spleen is relatively common and is a very important feature when performing posterior percutaneous puncture of the left kidney (DODDS et al. 1990).

3.3 "Wandering" Spleen

In this entity (also called splenoptosis or ectopic, dystopic or "floating" spleen), laxity or absence of the supporting ligaments of the spleen allows the organ to move or migrate in or beyond the left upper quadrant. Fixation of the spleen in the abdomen originates from the synergistic work of the supporting splenic ligaments, which are the gastrosplenic, splenorenal, splenophrenic, splenocolic and splenopancreatic ligaments and the presplenic fold. All these ligaments are directly associated with the spleen. However, two others, which are indirectly associated with the spleen, are also important in splenic fixation: the pancreaticocolic and colophrenic ligaments (ALLEN et al. 1992). Absence or laxity of some of these ligaments or failure of fusion of the posterior mesogastrium results in increased splenic mobility (ALLEN et al. 1992). As described above, the splenic ligaments develop from the dorsal mesentery (or dorsal mesogastrium). In "abnormal" embryogenesis, they may be too long, too short, too wide, too narrow or abnormally fused, leading to increased splenic mobility and resulting in the "wandering" spleen (ALLEN et al. 1992). The most frequent locations of a wandering spleen are the upper and lower abdominal cavity and the pelvis (ALLEN et al. 1992).

This rare condition is more frequently found in women of childbearing age (GORDON et al. 1977; ALLEN et al.1992; BUEHNER and BAKER 1992); generally, it occurs in 0.2% of the overall population. There is great controversy in the literature about possible predisposing factors, such as pregnancy (associated with an increased ligamentary laxity on hormonal base) or splenomegaly. However, the aetiology is most likely multifactorial and cannot be explained as only induced by pregnancy or splenomegaly, since this entity also occurs in men, children and nulliparous women (ALLEN et al. 1992).

The clinical picture ranges from asymptomatic patients at one extreme to patients presenting with chronic abdominal pain – or, in the worst case, with an acute abdomen – at the other extreme. The latter is due to splenic infarction induced by torsion of the splenic vascular pedicle (GORDON et al. 1977; ALLEN et al. 1992; BUEHNER and BAKER 1992). Chronic splenic (sub-)torsion may lead to splenomegaly, hypersplenism and gastric varices (BUEHNER and BAKER 1992).

Abdominal plain films may show a large "mass" in conjunction with numerous gas-filled loops of bowel that occupy the empty splenic fossa in the left upper quadrant (BUEHNER and BAKER 1992). The shadow of the left kidney may be elevated (GORDON et al. 1977). The typical US or CT picture is that of absence of the spleen at its normal location, in combination with a "mass" with a "parenchymatous" aspect (representing the spleen) elsewhere in the abdomen (Fig. 3.6). The more "easy" cases are those where this abnormally located spleen has a characteristic shape and size, and cases where the splenic vasculature can be recognised (ALLEN et al. 1992). The presence of a "whirl appearance" of the splenic vessels and the surrounding fat, usually noted at the splenic hilum, is pathognomonic (RAISSAKI et al. 1998; Fig. 3.7). Torsion of the vascular pedicle may, of course, be associated with thrombosis, seen as spontaneous hyperdense splenic vessels on pre-contrast scans. The enhancement of the spleen itself is usually minimal (RAISSAKI et al. 1998). Due to the deficient splenic support structures, the splenic flexure of the colon may interpose itself posteriorly between the left hemidiaphragm and the dystopic spleen. In summary, the "typical" CT aspect of torsion of a wandering spleen is an enlarged, ectopic and minimally enhancing spleen with a whirled appearance of non-enhancing and occasionally spontaneous hyperdense splenic vessels (RAISSAKI et al. 1998).

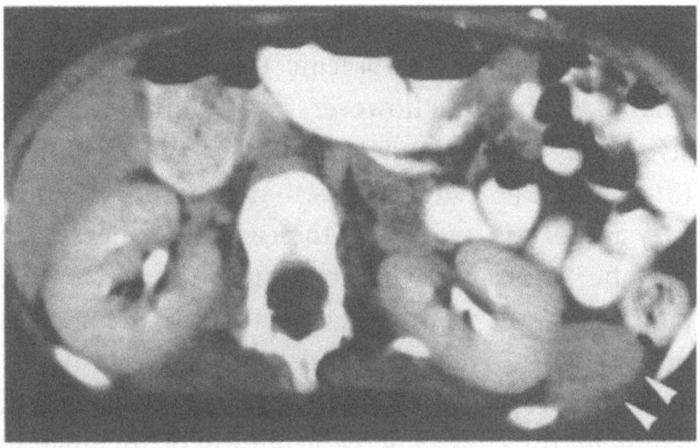

Fig. 3.6. Wandering spleen. Computed tomography scan showing an abnormal caudal displacement of the spleen (*arrowheads*) in apposition to the lower pole of the left kidney

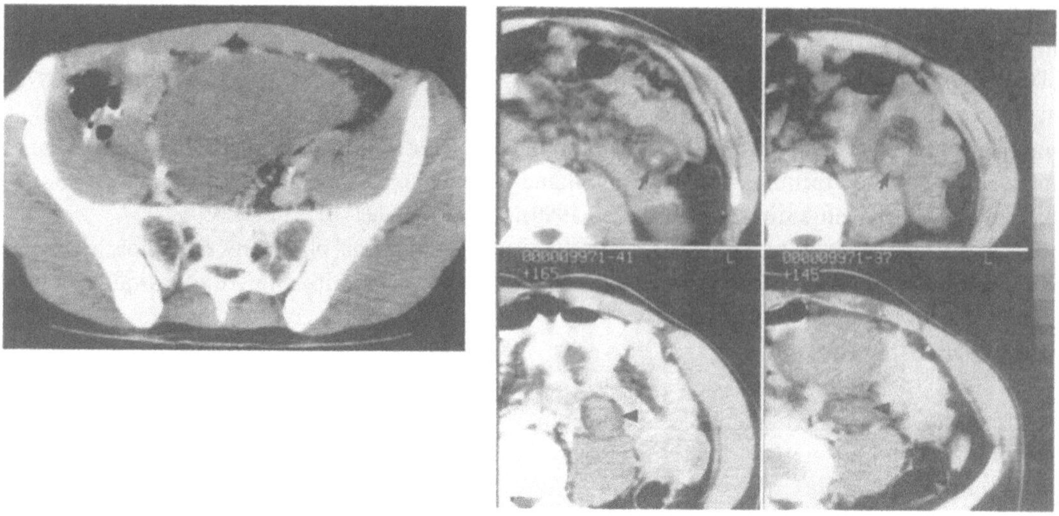

a b,c d,e

Fig. 3.7. A case of acute abdomen due to torsion of a wandering spleen. A post-contrast CT section through the pelvis. The torsioned spleen presents as a large pelvic mass without contrast enhancement. **b–e** The whirl sign, seen at different levels. **b, c** Non-enhanced upper-abdomen sections. The point of torsion is identified at a considerable distance from the spleen's hilum. The vessels within the pedicle appear hyperdense (*arrows*). **d, e** Post-contrast abdominal sections at a lower level, showing a non-enhancing pedicle surrounded by fat and a thick capsule, located in close contact to the upper margin of the spleen (*arrowheads*) (Raissaki et al. 1998)

However, sometimes a wandering spleen does not have "typical" characteristics, making the diagnosis more difficult. In these cases, MR imaging may help to detect signal intensities characteristic for splenic tissue; in addition, administration of superparamagnetic iron oxide may prove the reticuloendothelial background of the wandering spleen. If reduced splenic vascularisation or splenic infarction is present, the spleen will not show contrast enhancement on CT and MR imaging. Alternatively, radionuclide studies with ^{99m}Tc-sulfur colloid can be used to identify normal splenic tissue. However, if torsion with secondary splenic infarction is present, radionuclide imaging can yield a false negative signal; in these cases, CT and/or MR imaging seems more accurate (Allen et al. 1992; Buehner and Baker 1992). Angiography may also provide definitive evidence of splenic torsion and ectopic splenic localisation; however, this technique is invasive and is no longer indicated for diagnosis (Sheflin et al. 1984; Herman and Siegel 1991). A very important remark is that a wandering spleen may be associated with torsion of the tail of the pancreas. This can be explained by incomplete fusion of the embryonic posterior mesogastrium, with developmental failure of the splenorenal ligament; thus, the pancreatic tail will be included in the intraperitoneal splenic hilum (Sheflin et al. 1984). A "wandering" spleen associated with (oedematous) enlargement of the pancreatic tail should suggest an associated torsion of the pancreatic tail (Salomonowitz et al. 1984; Sheflin et al. 1984).

3.4 Congenital Cystic Lesions

Congenital cysts of the spleen are "true" cysts with an epithelial border. They are also called "epidermoid", "mesothelial" or "primary" cysts. Their true origin is not very clear; they may originate from infolding or entrapment of peritoneal mesothelial cells in the splenic parenchyma during embryogenesis (Dachman et al. 1986; Burrig 1988). Another explanation can be that they originate from normal lymphatic spaces (Dachman et al. 1986). They are usually discovered incidentally, are most frequently solitary and unilocular and are usually asymptomatic. An "acute abdomen" may occur when there is rupture or infection of the cyst. Rarely, reversible arterial hypertension due to renal artery compression by the cyst may be seen (Dachman et al. 1986). Compression of adjacent organs, such as the stomach, may of course also cause (nonspecific) abdominal symptoms.

Most frequently, cystic lesions are discovered incidentally in the second and third decades of life. A slight female predominance has been reported; familial clustering is very rare and is thought to be autosomal recessive (Gilmartin 1978; Ahlgren and Beardmore 1984; Ragozzino 1990).

Histopathologically, they are bordered with an epithelium and contain fluid. The wall of the cyst may show curvilinear or plaque-like calcifications. However, this is less common in "true" splenic cysts and is seen most frequently in post-traumatic cystic lesions (Dachman et al. 1986). Rapid or gradual increase in the size of the cyst may occur, most frequently due to secondary infection of the cyst, and may be the cause of abdominal pain.

Sonographically, they have all the characteristics of "simple" cysts: they are homogeneously anechoic, are characterised by "through transmission" and feature an imperceptible wall. CT shows a sharply demarcated lesion with "water density" and without contrast enhancement (Fig. 3.8). Often, they cannot be differentiated, using radiological imaging modalities, from intrasplenic pseudocysts, (old) post-traumatic cysts or degenerative cysts (secondary to splenic emboli and/or infarction). Only pathological examination can show the histology of the lining of the cyst wall to distinguish "true" from "false" cysts. Other differentials are intrasplenic abscesses, cystic neoplasms (like lymphangioma or hemangioma), hydatic cysts and cystic metastases (Dachman et al. 1986).

3.5 Accessory Spleen(s) (or Splenunculi)

The observation of an accessory spleen is a very frequent finding in radiological imaging modalities. It occurs in nearly 10–20% of individuals (Halpert and Gyorkey 1959; Wadham 1981). Their primary importance lies in the fact that they must be differentiated from other abdominal mass lesions.

Embryologically, they originate from splenic cells, which fail to fuse with the rest of the splenic onset, in the dorsal mesogastrium. Most frequently, a solitary accessory spleen is present. However, two or more accessory spleens have also been reported (Halpert and Gyorkey 1959; Wadham 1981). When multiple, they almost always occur together in a single location. They have only relative clinical importance: occasionally, they may mimic tumoral lesions and, in patients who have had a splenectomy for hypersplenism, they may grow and lead to relapse of the clinical symptoms. Therefore, it is important to identify this accessory splenic tissue, especially in haematology patients who may have a splenectomy.

Typically, accessory spleens are round or ovoid in shape and have smooth and sharp borders (Fig. 3.9). Their size varies from microscopic accessory splenic tissue to spleens 2–3 cm in diameter (in normal indi-

a

b

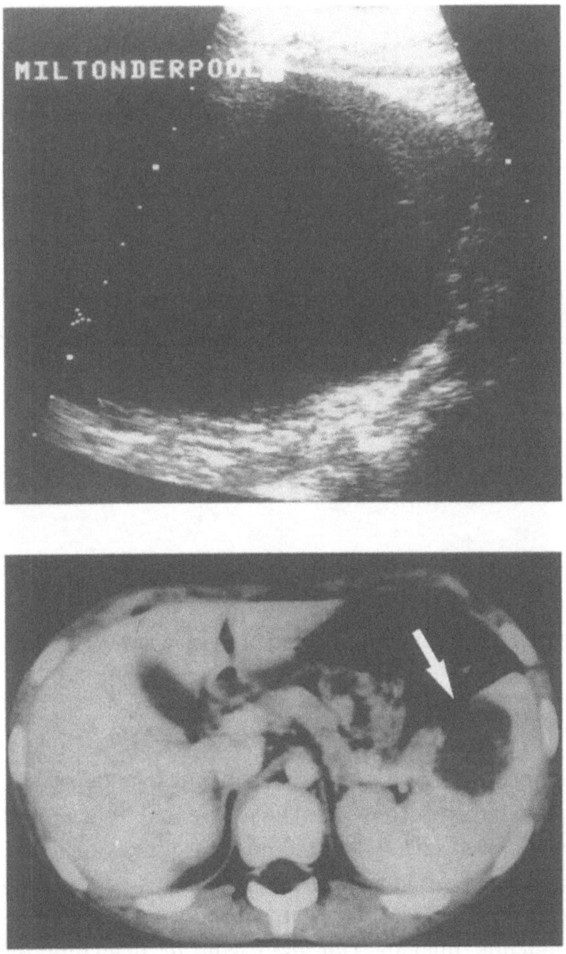

Fig. 3.8. Sonography (a) and computed tomography (b) showing a simple cyst of the spleen

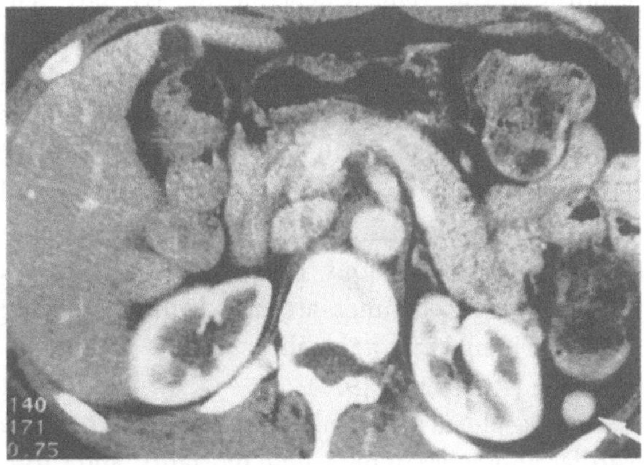

Fig. 3.9. A small accessory spleen (*arrow*)

viduals; Halpert and Gyorkey 1959; Beahrs and Stephens 1980). Most frequently, they occur at the hilum of the spleen, followed by the suspensory ligaments and the pancreatic tail. Only very rarely do they occur elsewhere in the abdomen (Halpert and Gyorkey 1959). Usually, an accessory spleen has its blood supply derived from the splenic artery (Subramanyam et al. 1984). The morphologic structure and function of the accessory splenic tissue is identical to that of the main spleen.

In all radiological imaging modalities, the normal accessory spleen has the same imaging characteristics as the normal spleen itself. Also, after contrast administration, they exhibit the same contrast-enhancement pattern (Halpert and Gyorkey 1959; Beahrs and Stephens 1980; Wadham 1981). When there is still doubt about the splenic origin of aberrant tissue in the abdomen, radionuclide studies can be useful (Beahrs and Stephens 1980; Hansen and Jarhult 1986). In post-splenectomy patients, the accessory splenic tissue may hypertrophy and can simulate tumoral lesions from adjacent organs. Therefore, to avoid hypertrophy of the accessory spleen, it is critical to correctly identify the presence of an accessory spleen in these patients. In these cases, the CT appearance will be that of a rounded mass of uniform soft-tissue density in the left upper quadrant. Again, the splenic nature can be confirmed by appropriate radionuclide imaging if there is any doubt (Beahrs and Stephens 1980).

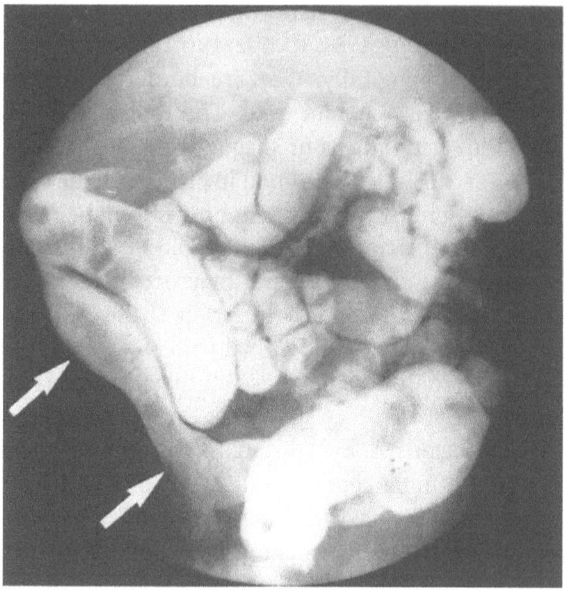

Fig. 3.10. Right isomerism (asplenia syndrome). Contrast study of the colon reveals congenital malposition with right-sided sigmoid and descending colon (*arrows*)

3.6 Asplenia

Absence of the spleen is usually associated with other congenital anomalies in the abdomen and the thorax. This entity is also called the "congenital asplenia syndrome" (or "right isomerism" or "Ivemark syndrome"; Rose et al. 1975). Abdominal heterotaxia or partial or complete *situs inversus* are frequently seen. Associated intestinal malrotation to varying degrees is also common (Fig. 3.10; Mishalany et al. 1982). Frequently, asplenia is associated with complex and severe cardiomyopathies (Fig. 3.11). Total anomalous pulmonary venous connection is the rule. Bilateral tri-lobed lungs are also common, as are genito-urinary tract anomalies, such as ambiguous genitalia (Rose et al. 1975).

Since asplenia frequently is associated with severe cardiac anomalies, it has a high mortality, and surgical correction is the rule. Sepsis, also frequently seen in association to asplenia, is another important factor contributing to the mortality rate in patients with Ivemark syndrome, which is estimated to be 80%.

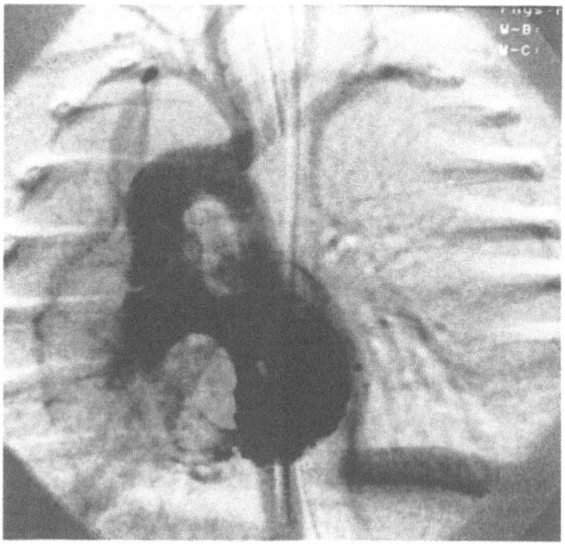

Fig. 3.11. Right isomerism. Aortic angiography. Dextrocardia is shown in the situs ambiguus

US, as well as CT or MR imaging, is essential in the diagnosis of asplenia and its possible associated conditions (Fig. 3.12; Tonkin and Tonkin 1982). Radionuclide imaging can be useful in depicting the intra-abdominal position of the liver and confirming the absence of the spleen (Fig. 3.13).

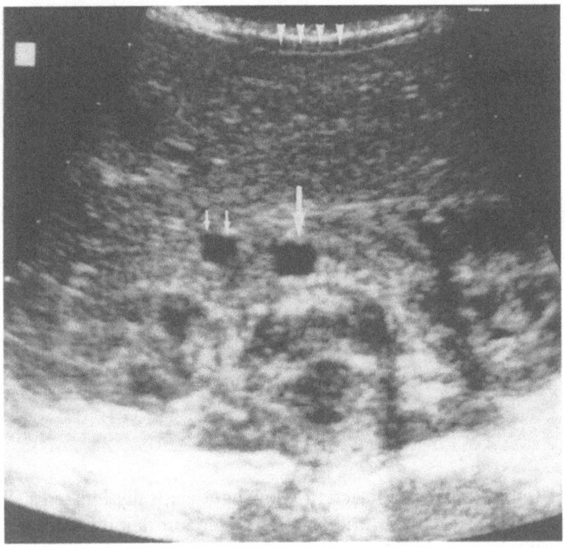

Fig. 3.12. Right isomerism. Transverse sonogram. Horizontal midline liver (*arrowheads*). The aorta (*large white arrow*) and the inferior vena cava (*small white arrows*) are in juxtaposition on the same side of the spine

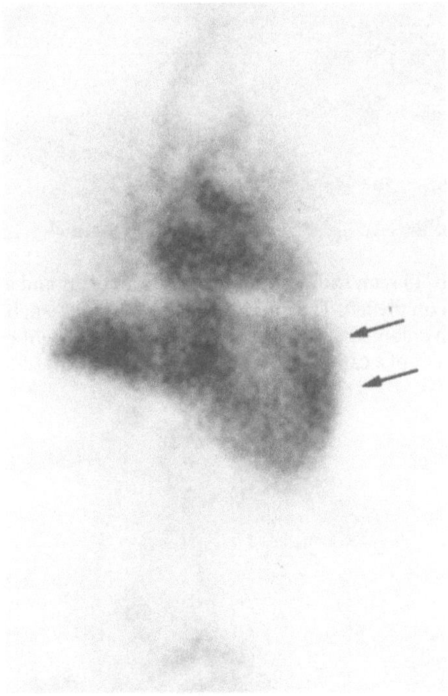

Fig. 3.13. Absence of the spleen on a ^{99m}Tc liver anteroposterior scan. Note the midline liver (*black arrows*)

3.7 Polysplenia

Polysplenia is another congenital syndrome characterised by the presence of multiple splenic formations and abdominal (situs), cardiovascular and pulmonary abnormalities. It occurs predominantly in males (Peoples et al. 1983; Winer-Muram et al. 1991).

Frequently, 2–16 splenic nodules of equal size can be found in the right or left upper quadrant (depending on the associated situs), ipsilateral to the greater curvature of the stomach, because the spleen develops in the dorsal gastric mesentery. Much less frequently, there is only a single bilobed spleen present, or there are only one or two larger spleens associated with multiple small splenic formations (Peoples et al. 1983). Malrotation of the intestinal tract and malposition of the mesentery are common associated findings (Vossen et al. 1987). In 50–85% of patients with polysplenia syndrome, absence of the hepatic segment of the inferior vena cava with azygos or hemiazygos continuation can be seen (Vossen et al. 1987; Fig. 3.14). Other reported anomalies are a short pancreas and venous anomalies, such as a preduodenal portal vein (Gayer et al. 1999)

Dextrocardia (42%), atrial septal defects (84%), ventricular septal defects (74%) and absence of the coronary sinus (42%) are the most common cardiac abnormalities in polysplenia syndrome (Vossen et al. 1987). Occasionally, the cardiac abnormalities are not significant and can even be normal, in contrast to the associated cardiac features in asplenia syndrome. As a consequence, polysplenia can be discovered incidentally on imaging studies (Peoples et al. 1983). Left isomerism with bilateral bilobed lungs is present in about 66% of cases (Vossen et al. 1987).

Plain films of the abdomen and chest (combined with abdominal sonography) are usually very helpful in the diagnosis of polysplenia (Sty and Conway 1985). Abdominal CT examination, even without intravenous contrast, can confirm the diagnosis of polysplenia in questionable or mixed situs anomalies. In these cases, multiple splenules, a midline liver and azygos or hemiazygos continuation of the inferior vena cava (with absence of the hepatic segment) can be seen. These are the major abdominal features of polysplenia syndrome (Fig. 3.15; Vossen et al. 1987; Winer-Muram and Tonkin 1989). MR imaging can demonstrate many of the abnormalities of the associated congenital heart diseases and the abdominal and vascular anomalies in polysplenia syndrome (Fig. 3.16). Also, radionuclide imaging can

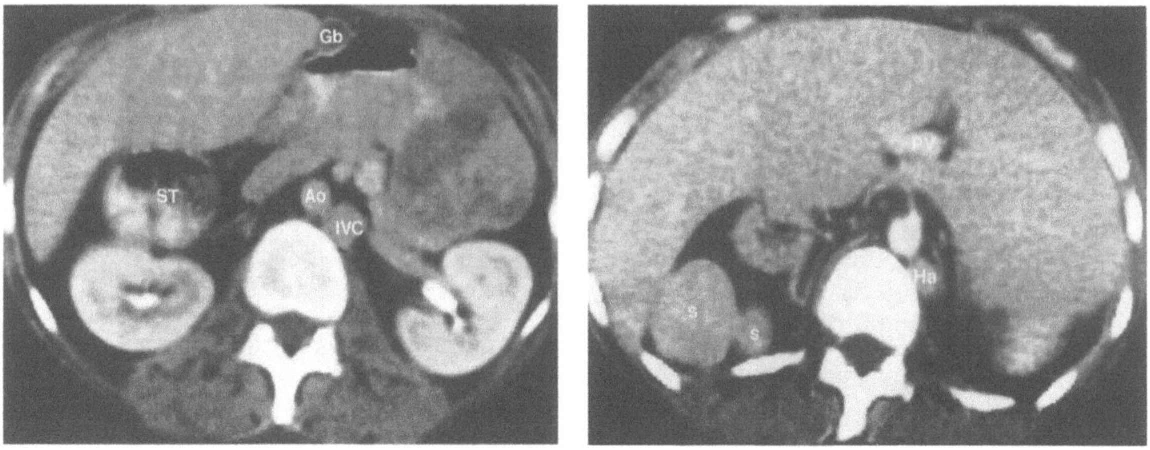

Fig. 3.14. Polysplenia Syndrome. **a.** Upper abdominal computed tomography (CT) section showing a centrally located gall bladder (*Gb*) and a right-sided stomach (*ST*). *Ao*, aorta; *IVC*; inferior vena cava. **b** Midhepatic CT section demonstrating a midline liver. *Ha*, hemiazygos vein; *PV*, portal vein; *s*, splenule (Vossen et al. 1987)

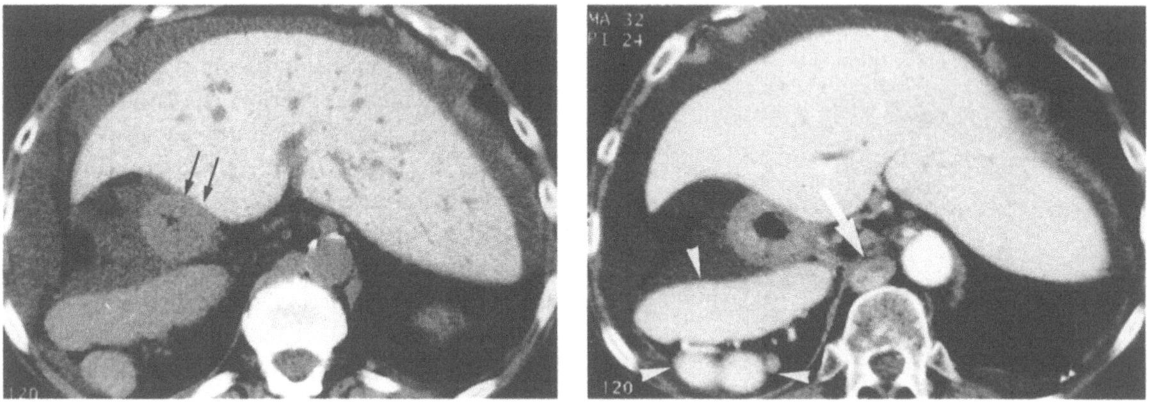

Fig. 3.15. A case of polysplenia. **a** A pre-contrast computed tomography (CT) scan shows abdominal situs inversus and a large midline liver. The stomach (*black arrows*) is located on the right, the aorta on the left. The inferior vena cava is not seen. **b** Post-contrast CT. Three right-sided spleens are demonstrated (*arrowheads*). An enlarged azygos vein is seen behind the right crus of the diaphragm (*white arrow*). The ascites was caused by peritoneal metastasis of a carcinoma of the ovary (not shown) (courtesy B. Op De Beeck)

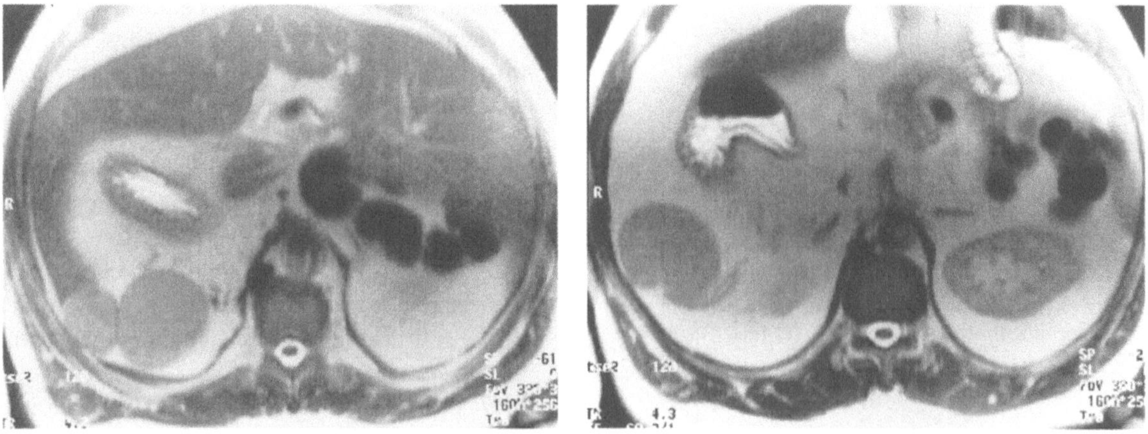

Fig. 3.16. Polysplenia syndrome. **a** Axial T2-W Haste magnetic-resonance image of the upper abdomen. Two spleens are seen within the right upper quadrant. The stomach is located on the right, while the liver is in midline position. The inferior vena cava is not seen, but the azygos vein is enlarged. **b** An axial slice at a slightly lower position shows a short pancreas

be useful in depicting the position of the liver and demonstrating the presence of multiple splenules (Sty and Conway 1985).

3.8 Splenogonadal Fusion

Splenogonadal fusion is a rare congenital malformation characterised by fusion of splenic tissue and a gonad. The left gonad is nearly always affected, and it is found predominantly in male patients. It is associated with orofacial and/or limb developmental abnormalities (Bearss 1980).

Embryologically, adhesion occurs between the gonadal primordial tissue and the developing spleen. As the gonad descends, it takes along this "extra" splenic tissue. Therefore, the splenic "pseudotumour", which histologically consists of normal splenic tissue, can be found in the tunica albuginea, in the epididymis or even in the spermatic cord. Usually, it appears as an encapsulated mass. Two types have been described: (a) the continuous type, in which a fibrous band, frequently containing additional splenic tissue, extends from the splenogonadal fusion site to the main spleen, and (b) the discontinuous type, if no connection is present. Undescended testis is reported in 15–20% of patients (Bearss 1980; Carragher 1990).

Clinically, these patients usually present with a longstanding, painless scrotal mass, virtually always on the left side, and cryptorchidism. Traumatic rupture or acute torsion of the ectopic splenic rests, bowel obstruction secondary to intraperitoneal bands (with the continuous type of encapsulated mass) or a painful scrotal swelling (secondary to mumps, malaria, exercise, leukaemia or mononucleosis) are less common presentations (Cirillo et al. 1999).

US and/or MR are helpful in suggesting the disorder (Cirillo et al. 1999; Fig. 3.17). However, splenogonadal fusion may be misinterpreted as a primary malignant testicular tumour or as an adenomatoid tumour of the epididymis (Bearss 1980; Carragher 1990). Knowledge of this entity is important in order to preserve the testis during surgery, as prior imaging can prove the "splenic" background of the scrotal "mass". Radiocolloid spleen scintigraphy, preferably enhanced by single-photon echo CT, can correctly identify the splenic component in splenogonadal fusion and is, therefore, the modality of choice when splenogonadal fusion is suspected (Carragher 1990).

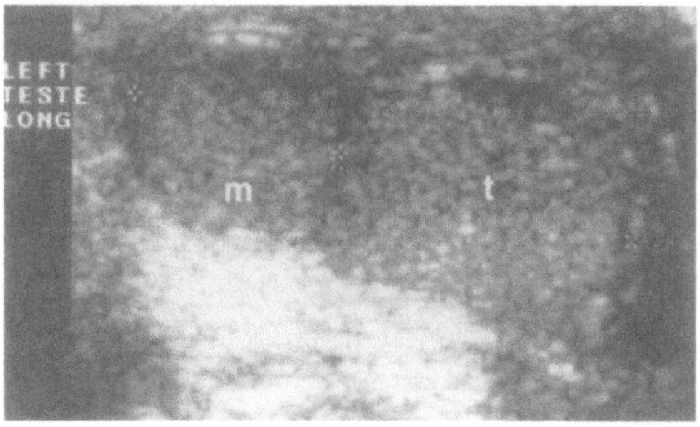

Fig. 3.17. Splenogonadal fusion of the discontinuous type. Scrotal sonogram. A homogeneous mass (*m*) is seen adjacent to the upper pole of the left testis (*t*) (Cirillo et al. 1999)

References

Ahlgren LS, Beardmore HE (1984) Solitary epidermoid splenic cysts: occurrence in sibs. J Pediatr Surg 19:56–58

Allen KB, Gay BB, Skandalakis JE (1992) Wandering spleen: anatomic and radiologic considerations. South Med J 85:976–984

Beahrs JR, Stephens DH (1980) Enlarged accessory spleens: CT appearance in postsplenectomy patients. AJR Am J Roentgenol 135:483–486

Bearss RW (1980) Splenogonadal fusion. Urology 16:277–279

Buehner M, Baker MS (1992) Wandering spleen. Surg Gynecol Obstet 175:373–387

Burrig KF (1988) Epithelial (true) splenic cysts. Pathogenesis of the mesothelial and so called epidermoid cyst of the spleen. Am J Surg Pathol 12:257–281

Carragher AM (1990) One hundred years of splenogonadal fusion. Urology 35:471–475

Cirillo RL, Coley BD, Binkovitz LA, et al. (1999) Sonographic findings in splenogonadal fusion. Pediatr Radiol 29:73–75

D'Altorio RA, Canno JY (1978) Upside down spleen as cause of suprarenal mass. Urology 11:422–424

Dachman AH, Ros PR, Marari PJ, et al. (1986) Nonparasitic splenic cysts: a report of 52 cases with radiologic-pathologic correlation. AJR Am J Roentgenol 147:537–542

Dodds WJ, Taylor AJ, Erickson SJ, et al. (1990) Radiologic imaging of splenic anomalies. AJR Am J Roentgenol 155:805–810

Gayer G, Apter S, Jonas T, et al. (1999) Polysplenia syndrome detected in adulthood: report of eight cases and review of the literature. Abdom Imaging 24:178–184

Gilmartin D (1978) Familial multiple epidermoid cysts of the spleen. Conn Med 42:297–300

Gooding GAW (1978) The ultrasonic and computed tomography appearance of splenic lobulations: a consideration in ultrasonic differential of masses adjacent to the left kidney. Radiology 126:719–720

Gordon DH, Burrell MI, Levin DC, et al. (1977) Wandering spleen – the radiological and clinical spectrum. Radiology 125:39–46

Halpert B, Gyorkey F (1959) Lesions observed in accessory spleens of 311 patients. Am J Clin Pathol 31:165–168

Hansen S, Jarhult J (1986) Accessory spleen imaging: radionuclide, ultrasound and CT investigations in a patient with thrombocytopenia 25 years after splenectomy for ITP. Scand J Haematol 37:74–77

Herman TE, Siegel MJ (1991) CT of acute spleen torsion in children with wandering spleen. AJR Am J Roentgenol 156:151–153
Mishalany H, Mahnovski V, Woolley M (1982) Congenital asplenia and anomalies of the gastrointestinal tract. Surgery 91:38–41
Peoples WM, Moller JH, Edwards JE (1983) Polysplenia: a review of 146 cases. Pediatr Cardiol 4:129–137
Piekarski J, Federle MP, Moss AA, et al. (1980) CT of the spleen. Radiology 135:683–689
Ragozzino MW, Singletary H, Patrick R (1990) Familial splenic epidermoid cyst. AJR Am J Roentgenol 155:1233–1234
Raissaki M, Prassopoulos P, Daskalogiannaki M, et al. (1998) Acute abdomen due to torsion of wandering spleen: CT diagnosis. Eur Radiol 8:1409–1412
Rose V, Izukawa T, Moes CAF (1975) Syndromes of asplenia and polysplenia: a review of 60 cases with special reference to diagnosis and prognosis. Br Heart J 37: 840–852
Salomonowitz E, Frick MP, Lund G (1984) Radiologic diagnosis of wandering spleen complicated by splenic volvulus and infarction. Gastrointest Radiol 9:57–59
Sheflin JR, Lee CM, Kretchmar KA (1984) Torsion of wandering spleen and distal pancreas. AJR Am J Roentgenol 142:100–101
Sty JR, Conway JJ (1985) The spleen: development and functional evaluation. Semin Nucl Med 15:276–298
Subramanyam BR, Balthazar EJ, Horii SC (1984) Sonography of the accessory spleen. AJR Am J Roentgenol 143:47–49
Tonkin IL, Tonkin AK (1982) Visceroatrial situs abnormalities: sonographic and computed tomographic appearance. AJR Am J Roentgenol 138:509–515
Vossen PG, Van Hedent EF, Degryse HR, De Schepper AM (1987) Computed tomography of the polysplenia syndrome in the adult. Gastrointest Radiol 12:209–211
Wadham BM, Adams PB, Johnson NA (1981) Incidence and location of accessory spleens. N Engl J Med 304:111
Westcott JL, Krufky EL (1972) The upside-down spleen. Radiology 105:517–521
Williams PL, Warwick R, Dyson M, et al. (1989) The spleen. In: Williams PL, Warwick R (eds) Gray's anatomy. Churchill Livingstone, Edinburgh, pp 827–832
Winer-Muram HT, Tonkin IL (1989) The spectrum of heterotaxic syndromes. Radiol Clin North Am 27:1147–1170
Winer-Muram HT, Tonkin IL, Gold RE (1991) Polysplenia syndrome in the asymptomatic adult: computed tomography evalutation. J Thorac Imaging 6:69–71

4 Splenosis

A.I. De Backer and A.M. De Schepper

CONTENTS

4.1 Definition and Location

Splenosis represents the heterotopic autotransplantation of splenic tissue that usually follows traumatic rupture of the splenic capsule. More rarely, splenosis occurs after an iatrogenic seeding of splenic tissue during splenectomy. The splenic remnants implant on the serosal surfaces of the abdomen and chest, derive their blood supply from surrounding tissue and grow into mature splenic tissue that is histologically indistinguishable from normal spleen (Fleming et al. 1976; Mathurin and Lallemand 1990; Storm et al. 1992; Normand et al. 1993). Splenosis is usually found intraperitoneally in the following sites (in order of frequency): serosal surface of the small bowel (Fig. 4.1), greater omentum, parietal peritoneum, serosal surface of the large intestine, mesentery and undersurface of the diaphragm. Implantation of splenic tissue takes place in these sites because they are close to the native spleen or the splenic fossa. Less frequently, extraperitoneal locations have been reported, such as the pleural space, pericardium, retroperitoneum and subcutaneous tissue (Fig. 4.2; Cohen 1954; Ovnatanian 1966; Dalton et al. 1971; Brewster 1973; Grantham 1990; Bock et al. 1991; Yoshimitsu et al. 1993; Arzoumanian and Rosenthall 1995; Hibbeln 1995; Gruen and Gollub 1996; Kiser et al. 1996; Katranci et al. 1998). In all of these cases, trauma or surgery may have created pathways through which splenic tissue can escape from the confines of the peritoneum. Post-traumatic thoracic or pericardiac splenosis occurs when splenic tissue crosses an injured diaphragm and proliferates at the serous surface in the thoracic cavity or the pericardium (Figs. 4.3, 4.4; Ovnatanian 1966; Katranci et al. 1998). Splenuli may be inseparable

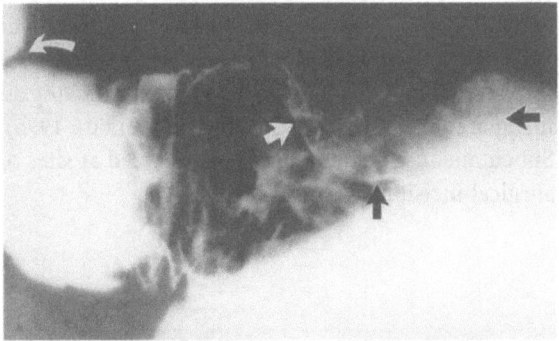

a

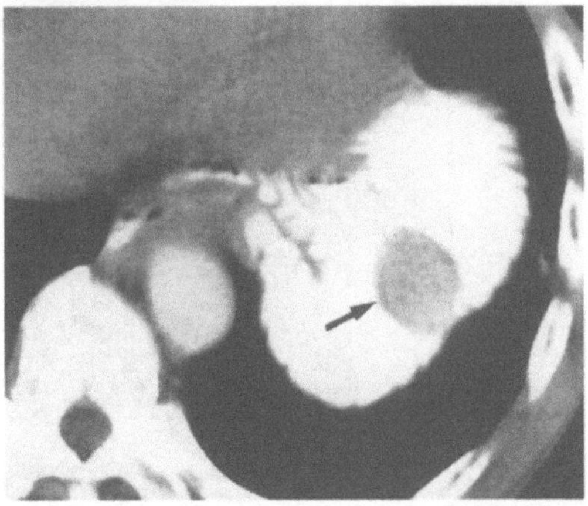

b

Fig. 4.1. **a** Splenic implant in the jejunum. Barium follow through shows a smooth, 4-cm intramural mass (*straight arrows*) on the superior border of the proximal jejunum near the esophagojejunal anastomosis (*curved arrow*). **b** A computed tomography scan shows a round, homogeneous soft-tissue mass (*arrow*) in the proximal jejunum (Marchant et al. 1995)

A.I. De Backer, A.M. De Schepper; Department of Radiology, University Hospital Antwerp, Wilrijkstraat 10, B-2650 Edegem, Belgium

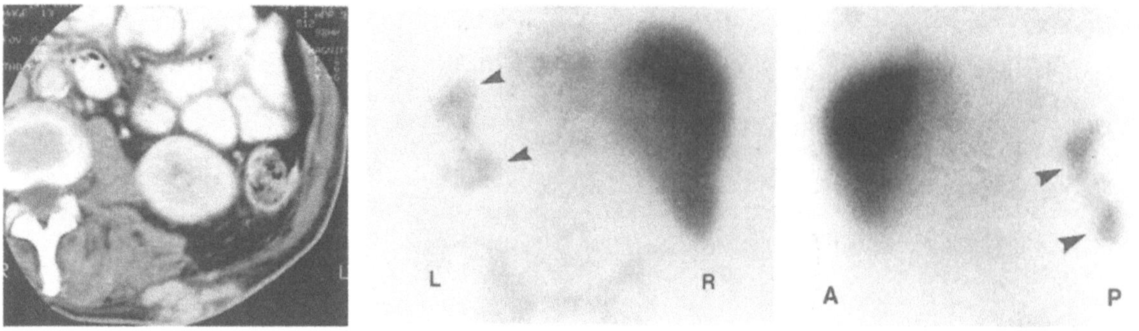

a,b c

Fig. 4.2. **a** Subcutaneous splenosis. A computed tomography scan shows multiple, small, confluent nodules in the subcutaneous fat, representing heterotopic splenic tissue. **b** ^{99m}Tc liver–spleen scintigraphy findings. A posterior planar image shows absence of a normal spleen and an area of lobulated uptake in the left upper abdominal quadrant (*arrowhead*). **c** A left lateral planar image shows far posterior location of tracer uptake (*arrowhead*) (Hibbeln et al. 1995)

from the kidney or liver (Bock et al. 1991; Yoshimitsu et al. 1993; Kiser et al. 1996). Intrahepatic splenosis has been reported to occur at the site of a hepatic biopsy performed during a previous elective splenectomy (Yoshimitsu et al. 1993). Splenosis may indent the surface of the liver (Arzoumanian and Rosenthall 1995) or may implant within the falciform ligament, mimicking an intraparenchymal mass (Gruen and Gollub 1996). Subcutaneous splenosis has been reported at sites of surgical incision (Grantham 1990).

4.2 Incidence

The true incidence of splenosis in the splenectomized population remains unknown, mainly because splenosis frequently remains asymptomatic. Studies show a variable frequency of splenosis after splenectomies performed following trauma, with a reported incidence ranging from 26% to 67% (Pearson et al. 1978; Kiroff et al. 1983; Livingston et al. 1983). The time delay from splenic rupture to splenectomy and the amount of blood described in the peritoneal cavity at surgery are not

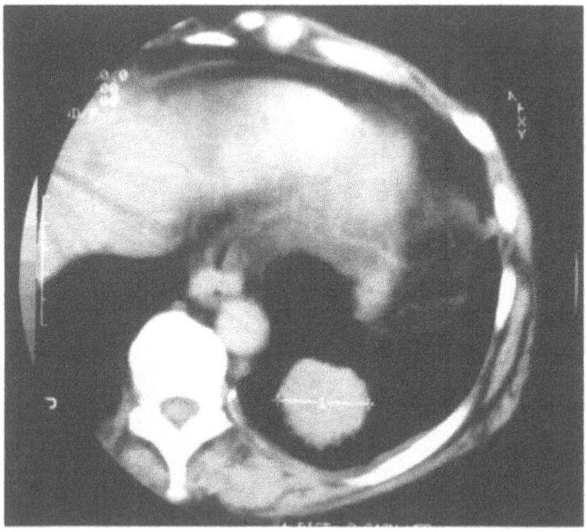

a

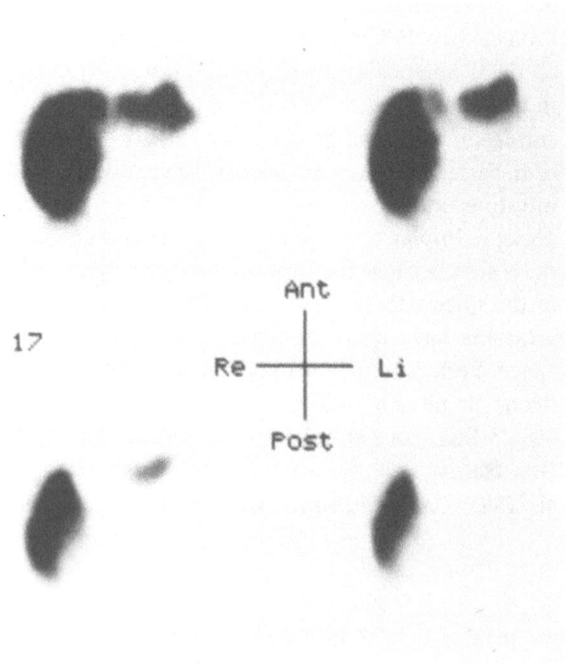

b

Fig. 4.3. **a** Thoracic splenosis. After intravenous contrast administration, a chest computed tomography (CT) scan shows a soft-tissue mass involving the posterior basal segment of the right lower lobe. **b** A liver–spleen scintiphotograph shows that the spleen is absent. The abnormal accumulation of radiocolloid in the left lower chest corresponds to the mass seen on the CT scan

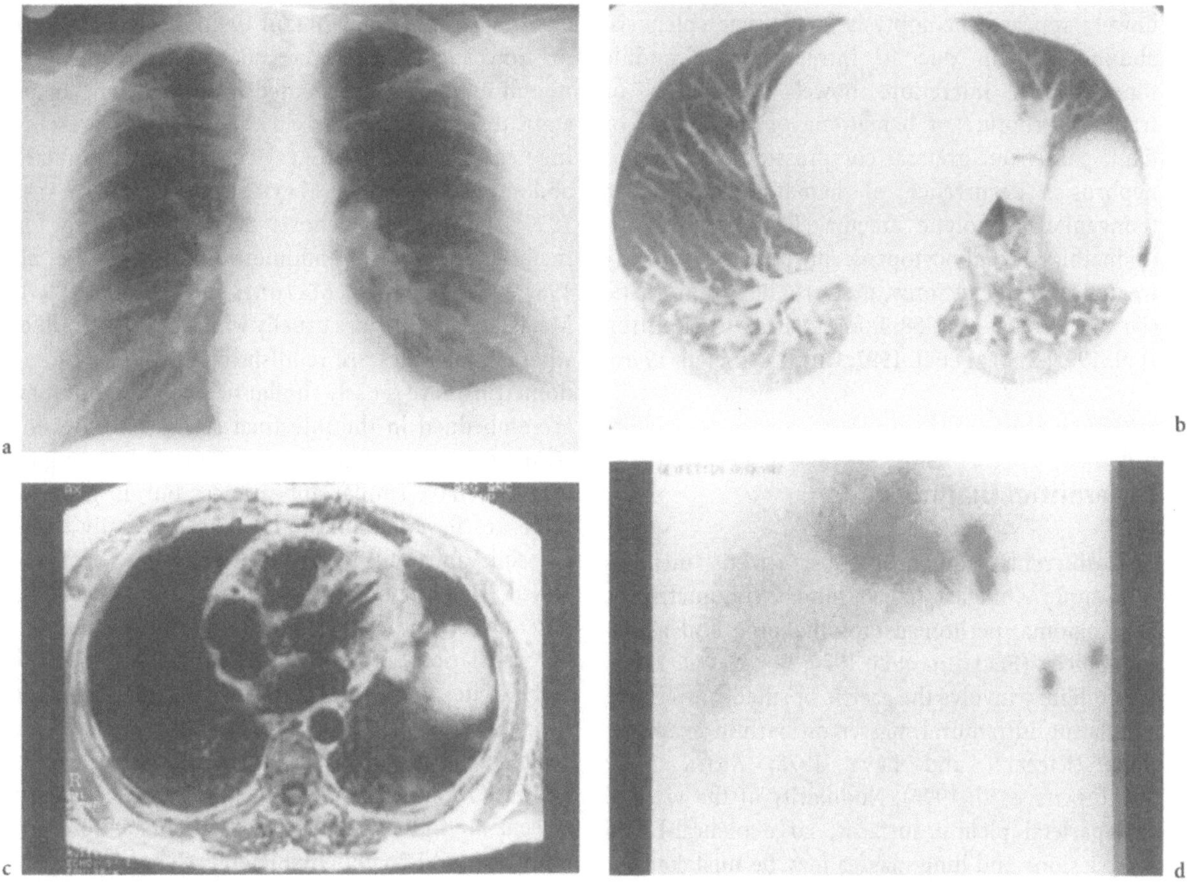

Fig. 4.4. **a** Intrathoracic splenosis following a thoracoabdominal stab wound. A chest radiograph shows nodules at the left paracardiac region near the pericardiophrenic angle. **b** Computed tomography scan. Three noncalcified nodules in the left hemithorax are seen; two of them are located in the left paracardiac region and the other one is lateral to the left hemidiaphragm. **c** A T1-weighted magnetic resonance image (repetition time/echo time = 882/20) shows the pericardiopleural-based mass with a signal intensity similar to that of the normal spleen. **d** Anterior scintigram with ^{99m}Tc-heat-damaged red blood cells. Increased radiopharmaceutical activity in the nodules in the left hemithorax and in the left upper quadrant of the abdomen is consistent with splenosis (Katranci et al. 1998)

related to the incidence of splenosis. The time interval between rupture and the diagnosis of splenosis varies from a few months to 32 years (Fleming et al. 1976).

Recurrent disease after splenectomy for hematologic diseases is mostly due to the presence of accessory spleens and is rarely reported as a consequence of splenosis (Fleming et al. 1976). The occurrence of splenosis seems to be highest in males less than 30 years old. This may reflect the increased ability of young splenic cells to implant, although most believe it simply represents the increased incidence of young males who sustain splenic injury (Turk et al. 1988).

The disrupted splenic pulp implants appear as multiple reddish-blue nodules and may be sessile or pedunculated. Their numbers vary from only a few to 400, and their sizes range from a few millimeters to 7 cm. Because the blood supply to the nodules is carried by small arteries penetrating the capsule and not by a major hilar artery, the nodules may outgrow their blood supply. This may be the reason that implants rarely have a diameter greater than 3 cm (Fleming et al. 1976).

4.3 Clinical Features

Splenosis rarely causes symptoms and is often incidentally found at surgery for unrelated problems or post-splenectomy adhesions, at autopsy, or during diagnostic imaging tests (Agha 1984; Delamarre et al. 1988). Symptoms associated with splenosis vary and include: gastrointestinal hemorrhage (when tissue implantation occurs in the stomach or small bowel); repeated hemoptysis in thoracic splenosis; abdominal pain due to intraperitoneal nodule torsion with infarction, bowel obstruction or traumatic rupture or hematoma of a splenule; or flank pain from ureteral compression and hydronephrosis. Recurrence of hematologic diseases (congenital hemolytic anemia, Felty's syndrome, idiopathic thrombocytopenic purpura), previously treated with splenectomy, may also be symptomatic (DELAMARRE et al. 1988; BOCK et al. 1991; CORDIER et al. 1992; STORM et al. 1992; CHIARUGI et al. 1996).

4.4 Differential Diagnosis

The differential diagnosis of splenosis includes solid tumors, metastatic carcinoma, endometriosis, hemangioma, peritoneal mesothelioma and accessory spleen (FLEMING et al. 1976; BOCK et al. 1991). Splenuli may involve the gastric or small-bowel wall, simulating intramural masses on barium examinations (KUTZEN and LEVY 1978; AGHA 1984; MARCHANT et al. 1995). Nodularity of the visceral and parietal pleural surfaces, large pleural-based mass lesions and lung masses may be mistaken for pleural or pulmonary neoplastic lesions (NORMAND et al. 1993; BORDLEE et al. 1995). Splenosis nodules that enlarged on serial roentgenograms of the chest have been described (DALTON et al. 1971). Nearly all patients with thoracic splenosis have a documented history of trauma, most commonly a gunshot or shrapnel wound (WHITE and MEYER 1998). Splenuli may be inseparable from the kidney and may simulate a solid renal neoplasm (TURK et al. 1988; BOCK et al. 1991; KISER et al. 1996). Intrahepatic splenic implants may mimic hepatic adenoma (YOSHIMITSU et al. 1993; GRUEN and GOLLUB 1996). In patients with previous surgery for cancer, subcutaneous splenotic noduli must be differentiated from recurrent metastatic disease (GRANTHAM 1990). Splenosis presenting as an intraperitoneal mass may simulate abdominal lymphoma (MATHURIN and LALLEMAND 1990). Peritoneal splenosis may be mistaken for metastatic disease or endometriosis (WATSON et al. 1982; BOCK et al. 1991; MATONIS and LUCIANO 1995). Metastatic nodules are usually white and plaque-like, whereas splenules are reddish blue. Nodules of endometriosis are grossly similar to splenules, but they are embedded in the intestinal serosa and are not sessile or pedunculated as in splenosis. Hemangiomas may have similar appearances but, in general, there are fewer nodules, and they are easily compressible and refill after the pressure has been released. Hemangiomas show marked enhancement on contrast studies. Peritoneal mesotheliomas have no association with splenic trauma, are associated with ascites and show no contrast enhancement (BOCK et al. 1991).

Splenosis and accessory spleens are two distinct entities (Table 4.1; SERVADIO et al. 1994). Accessory spleens are found in 10–44% of patients at autopsy, rarely exceed 1.5 cm in diameter, are usually solitary and rarely exceed six in number. Accessory spleens arise from the left side of the dorsal mesogastrium during the embryologic period of development and are most commonly located in the region of the splenopancreatic or gastrosplenic ligaments. Histologically, accessory spleens resemble the normal spleen and contain a hilus, parenchyma with normal pulp and a capsule. An accessory spleen always receives its blood supply from a branch of the splenic artery (FLEMING et al. 1976; GRUEN and GOLLUB

Table 4.1. Characteristics of accessory spleen and splenosis nodules

	Accessory spleen	Splenosis
Incidence	10–44% of all autopsies	Reported incidence ranging from 26% to 67%
Etiology	Embryologic development anomaly	Acquired; previous history of splenic trauma is almost always present
Number	Few, usually less than six	Vary from only a few to 400
Location	In the region of the splenopancreatic or gastrosplenic ligaments	Intra- or extraperitoneal location
Blood supply	Branches of the splenic artery via the hilum	Several small arteries penetrating the capsule
Structure	Resembles a spleen with a hilum	No characteristic shape, no hilum
Capsule	Elastic muscular capsule	Thick, fibrous tissue; no smooth-muscle component
Appearance	Usually pedunculated	Usually sessile, sometimes pedunculated
Size	May become as large as the original spleen following splenectomy	Usually small (rarely greater than 3 cm)

1996). Conversely, splenosis implants can be located anywhere, have no characteristic shape and have no hilus, and their blood flow is supplied by several small arteries penetrating the capsula. The capsular tissue of splenotic implants generally lacks a smooth-muscle component, while an accessory spleen has an elastic muscular capsule. Splenuli are usually multiple and measure from several millimeters to 7 cm in diameter. Lesions as large as 12 cm (along their greatest dimension) have been described (GRUEN and GOLLUB 1996).

4.5 Diagnosis and Management

The radiological diagnosis of splenosis requires awareness of both the condition and a patient's history of splenic trauma. Radionuclide scintigraphy plays a pivotal role in diagnosis. This technique, however, does not distinguish splenosis from accessory spleen, which has no clinical implication. Splenic node localization may differentiate splenosis from accessory spleens, with the latter located more often at the splenic hilus, around the pancreatic tail or at the stomach's greater curvature. Accessory spleens are also rarer than splenosis (MATHURIN and LALLEMAND 1990). ^{99m}Tc-sulfur colloid scintigraphy is able to reveal a nodule of splenic tissue 2-cm or larger. Because the normal liver takes up most of the sulfur colloid (whereas the spleen receives only 10% of this radiotracer), small splenosis nodules in the upper abdomen may be obscured by normal hepatic uptake of the sulfur colloid. However, because functioning splenic tissue will trap approximately 90% of damaged erythrocytes, ^{99m}Tc-labeled heat-damaged erythrocytes are reported to be more sensitive and specific than sulfur colloid in the identification of splenosis. Additionally, single-positron-emission computed tomography (CT) allows for direct correlation with other imaging techniques. Labeled red cell studies may be particularly useful in the settings of minimal splenic tissue, poor splenic uptake or overlap of the liver and spleen on sulfur-colloid imaging (GUNES et al. 1994; GRUEN and GOLLUB 1996).

Radiological examinations, such as chest radiographs, intravenous (IV) pyelogram, barium follow through, barium enema or arteriography may demonstrate masses but cannot reveal their splenic origin (DELAMARRE et al. 1988). Sonographic and CT findings are not specific for splenosis and show one or several homogeneous, solid, well-circumscribed, non-calcified soft-tissue nodules (Fig. 4.5). Splenules may have a variable shape; they can be oval, round, crescent or irregular. Coalescence of numerous small implants, forming sheet-like masses, is common. Since the splenules must be implanted into a structure to receive a vascular supply, they show poor margination and close adherence to

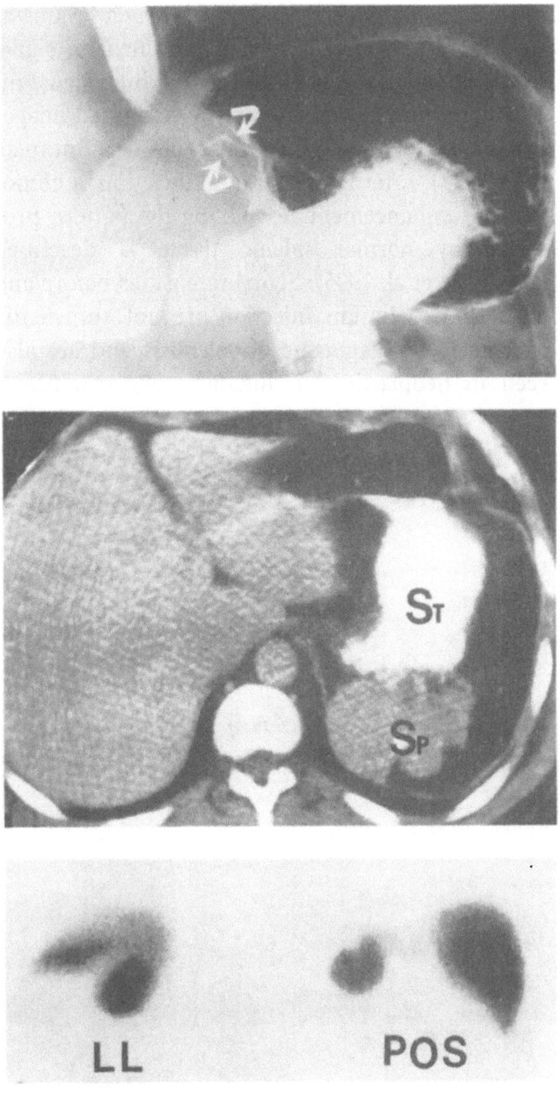

a b c

Fig. 4.5. **a** Splenosis masquerading as a gastric fundic mass. Barium follow-through shows distortion of gastric fundus by a mass lesion with overlying linear ulceration (*arrows*). The sharp margins of the mass lesion suggest an intramural, extramucosal location. **b** A computed tomography scan at the level of the fundus of the stomach shows a lobulated homogeneous mass indenting the gastric fundus from behind and medially. Note the absence of the spleen because of a previous splenectomy. The mass is regenerated splenosis. *Sp*, regenerated spleen; *ST*, stomach. **c** Radionuclide liver–spleen scan using a ^{99m}Tc-sulfur colloid confirms that the mass indenting the gastric fundus represents splenic tissue. *LL*, left lateral; *POS*, posterior (AGHA 1984) the tissue at the attachment site, resulting in location close to the abdominal or thoracic wall in contact with adjacent organs (Gentry et al. 1982; Mathurin and Lallemand 1990; Gunes et al. 1994). On CT scan, the lesions are usually hypodense or isodense to the liver and show a homogeneous enhancement after IV contrast injection (Gruen and Gollub 1996). On magnetic resonance imaging (MRI), the appearance of splenosis is limited to anecdotal cases, which have described such lesions as showing homogeneous low to intermediate signal intensity on T1-weighted images and high signal intensity on proton density- and T2-weighted images (Storm et al. 1992; Yoshimitsu et al. 1993; Bordlee et al. 1995). After IV gadolinium injection, a homogeneous enhancement resembling the pattern produced by normal splenic tissue is described (Bordlee et al. 1995). Signal intensities before and after IV gadolinium injection are not sufficiently specific to be diagnostic of splenosis and are also seen in neoplastic and inflammatory conditions. Superparamagnetic iron-oxide particles (Feridex) are distributed to phagocytic reticuloendothelial elements of liver and spleen in a tissue-specific way after IV injection (Fig. 4.6). Because splenules have reticuloendothelial cells, IV administration results in a decrease in the signal intensities of splenules on all pulse sequences; this decrease is similar to that seen in the liver (Storm et al. 1992). This decrease of signal intensity has been reported to be most pronounced on heavily T2-weighted images (Storm et al. 1992). Although nuclear medicine is the mainstay in the diagnosis of splenosis, MRI with superparamagnetic iron oxide combines a physiologic test of reticuloendothelial cell uptake with the anatomic detail of MRI. Moreover, superior contrast resolution and multiplanar imaging offered by MRI may be a major advantage over CT scan. The potential for misdiagnosis will always be present without adequate patient history. Surgery should be avoided, since the splenic implant may represent the only functional splenic tissue in the splenectomized

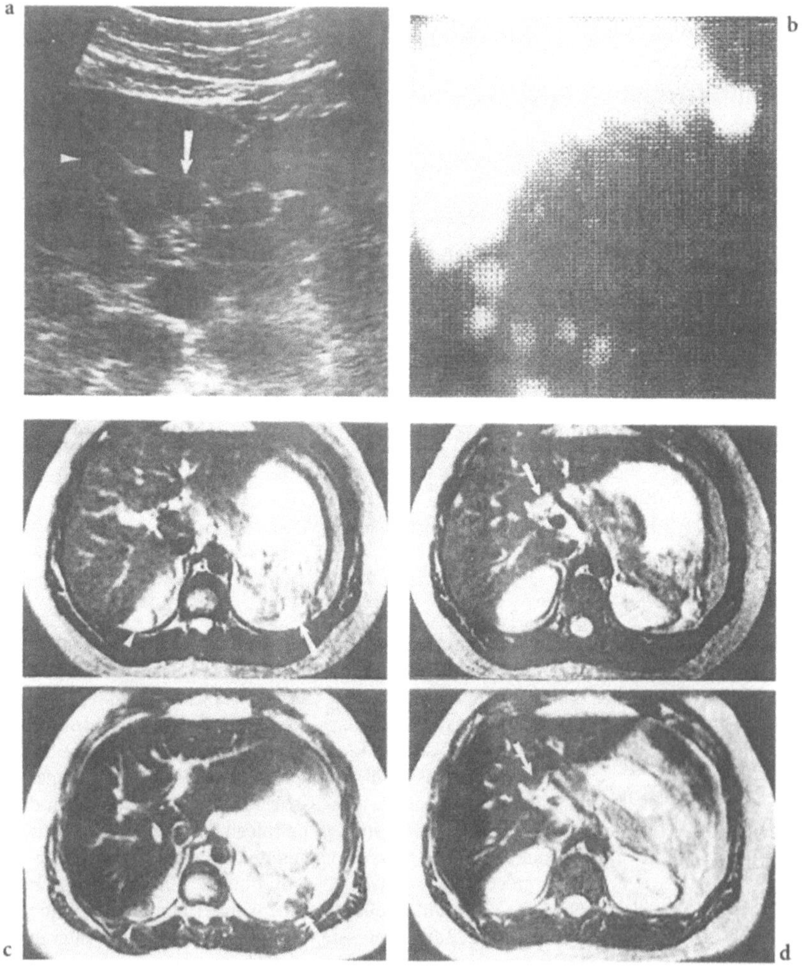

Fig. 4.6. a Splenosis in a 28-year-old woman. A sonogram shows multiple hypoechoic masses in the periportal region (*arrow*). The gall bladder (*arrowhead*) is visible. **b** A ^{99m}Tc-labeled red blood cell scintigram shows uptake of labeled cells in the splenic bed, subhepatic region, and lower right paracolic gutter, consistent with splenosis of the abdomen. **c, d** T2-weighted (2000/90) magnetic resonance images obtained before (*top*) and after (*bottom*) intravenous administration of superparamagnetic iron oxide show the T2-shortening effect of this contrast agent on the liver and on masses within the splenic bed (*arrows* in c) and right perirenal region (*arrowheads* in c). A periportal mass (*arrows* in d), which was not easily seen on computed tomography, shows decreased signal intensity after addition of superparamagnetic iron oxide (Storm et al. 1992)

patient. Percutaneous transthoracic tru-cut needle biopsy has been reported to be successful in diagnosis of thoracic splenosis (Gaines et al. 1986).

Because splenosis is not a pathologic process and is usually innocuous, it should not be electively removed. Removal of the splenic tissue may deny the patient potential splenic function. The splenic implants may be found during surgery or during unrelated diagnostic imaging. Its recognition in the preoperative evaluation would obviate unnecessary surgery. Surgery may be necessary when complications develop, such as: acute abdominal pain with torsion of the splenic implant or bowel obstruction; invasion of the bowel wall resulting in either intraperitoneal or gastrointestinal hemorrhage; and recurrent disease in cases of splenectomy for hematologic disorder (Brewster 1973; Fleming et al. 1976; Gruen and Gollub 1996). Absence of the spleen is associated with increased susceptibility to severe bacterial sepsis and meningitis, usually caused by *Streptococcus pneumoniae* and *Haemophilus influenzae* type B. This syndrome occurs most frequently in infants and young children and in children who have had splenectomies due to systemic conditions in which host defense mechanisms are altered. Residual splenic tissue is immunologically functional and may be beneficial in preventing these infections (Dalton et al. 1971). Return of splenic function has been documented 1–3 months after implantation of autologous splenic tissue following splenectomy for trauma (Neilsen et al. 1982). However, 20–30 cm^3 of regenerated splenic tissue is required to provide adequate function (Corazza et al. 1984). When splenectomy is required because of serious traumatic injury, autotransplantation of splenic tissue in the form of an omental pouch is performed intentionally by some surgeons to produce splenosis. The assumption is that this will afford protection from post-splenectomy infection (Patel et al. 1981; Gruen and Gollub 1996). In the setting of splenosis, damaged or nonfunctioning erythrocytes, including Howel-Jolly bodies, Heinz bodies and pitted cells, which are normally present in the peripheral circulation following splenectomy, are not seen or are rarer than normally expected following splenectomy (Scully et al. 1995). Furthermore, in patients who have undergone elective splenectomy for hematologic disorders, such as hemolytic anemia, idiopathic thrombocytopenic purpura or Felty's syndrome, the return of the hematologic disorder may indicate the development of splenosis (Scully et al. 1995; Gruen and Gollub 1996).

4.6 Conclusion

Splenosis is rarely symptomatic; however, occasionally it may gain clinical significance due to four factors: abdominal pain, hemorrhage, mimicking of a tumor and retained splenic function. A peripheral blood smear may show evidence of functioning splenic tissue. The diagnosis of splenosis is best established by a radionuclide-scintigraphic study of the liver and spleen with ^{99m}Tc-labeled heat-damaged erythrocytes or a less sensitive ^{99m}Tc–sulfur-colloid liver–spleen radionuclide scan. Detection of equivocal masses on CT scan, ultrasonography or other imaging studies in a post-splenectomy patient should lead to a search for splenosis using radionuclide scans, thus avoiding invasive procedures, such as guided biopsy or surgery. MRI, CT scan and ultrasonography may be useful in symptomatic patients to detect complications of splenosis, such as implant infarction or traumatic hematoma.

References

Agha FP (1984) Regenerated splenosis masquerading as gastric fundic mass. Am J Gastroenterol 79:576–578

Arzoumanian A, Rosenthall L (1995) Splenosis. Clin Nucl Med 20:730–733

Bock DB, King BF, Hezmall HP, et al. (1991) Splenosis presenting as a left renal mass indistinguishable from renal cell carcinoma. J Urol 146:152–154

Bordlee RP, Eshaghi N, Oz O (1995) Thoracic splenosis: MR demonstration. J Thorac Imaging 10:146–149

Brewster DC (1973) Splenosis. Report of two cases and review of the literature. Am J Surg 126:14–19

Chiarugi M, Martino MC, Buccianti P, et al. (1996) Bleeding gastric ulcer complicating splenosis in type-1 Gaucher's disease. Eur J Surg 162:63–65

Cohen EA (1954) Splenosis: review and report of subcutaneous splenic implant. Arch Surg 69:777–784

Corazza GR, Tarozzi C, Vaira D, et al. (1984) Return of splenic function after splenectomy: how much tissue is needed? BMJ 289:861–864

Cordier JF, Gamondes JP, Marx P, et al. (1992) Thoracic splenosis presenting with hemoptysis. Chest 102:626–627

Dalton ML Jr, Strange WH, Downs EA (1971) Intrathoracic splenosis: case report and review of literature. Am Rev Respir Dis 103:827–830

Delamarre J, Capron JP, Drouard F, et al. (1988) Splenosis: ultrasound and CT findings in a case complicated by an intraperitoneal implant traumatic hematoma. Gastrointest Radiol 13:275–278

Fleming CR, Dickson ER, Harrison EG (1976) Splenosis: autotransplantation of splenic tissue. Am J Med 61:414–419

Gaines JJ, Crosby HJ, Vinayak KM (1986) Diagnosis of thoracic splenosis by tru-cut needle biopsy. Am Rev Respir Dis 133:1199–1201

Gentry LR, Brown JM, Lindgren RD (1982) Splenosis: CT demonstration of heterotopic autotransplantation of splenic tissue. J Comput Assist Tomogr 6:1184–1187
Grantham JR (1990) Subcutaneous splenosis. AJR Am J Roentgenol 154:655
Gruen DR, Gollub MJ (1996) Intrahepatic splenosis mimicking hepatic adenoma AJR Am J Roentgenol 168:725–726
Gunes I, Yilmazlar T, Sarikaya I, et al. (1994) Scintigraphic detection of splenosis: superiority of tomographic selective spleen scintigraphy. Clin Radiol 49:115–117
Hibbeln JF, Wilbur AC, Schreiner VC, et al. (1995) Subcutaneous splenosis. Clin Nucl Med 20:591–593
Katranci N, Parildar M, Göksel T, et al. (1998) Quiz case of the month. Eur Radiol 8:151–152
Kiroff GK, Mangos A, Cohen R, et al. (1983) Splenic regeneration following splenectomy for traumatic rupture. Aust N Z J Surg 53:431–434
Kiser JW, Fagien M, Clore FF (1996) Splenosis mimicking a left renal mass. AJR Am J Roentgenol 167:1508–1509
Kutzen BM, Levy N (1978) Splenosis simulating an intramural gastric mass. Radiology 126:45–46
Livingston CD, Levine BA, Lecklitner ML, et al. (1983) Incidence and function of residual splenic tissue following splenectomy for trauma in adults. Arch Surg 118:617–620
Marchant LK, Levine MS, Furth EE (1995) Splenic implant in the jejunum: radiographic and pathologic findings. Abdom Imaging 20:518–520
Mathurin J, Lallemand D (1990) Splenosis simulating an abdominal lymphoma. Pediatr Radiol 21:69–70
Matonis LM, Luciano AA (1995) A case of splenosis masquerading as endometriosis. Am J Obstet Gynecol 173:971–973
Neilsen JL, Sorensen FH, Sakso P, et al. (1982) Implantation of autologous splenic tissue after splenectomy for trauma. Br J Surg 69:529–530
Normand JP, Rioux M, Dumont M, et al. (1993) Thoracic splenosis after blunt trauma: frequency and imaging findings. AJR Am J Roentgenol 161:739–741
Ovnatanian KT (1966) Splenosis of the pericardium. Vestn Khir Im I I Grek 97:59–62
Patel J, Williams JS, Shmigel B, et al. (1981) Preservation of splenic function by autotransplantation of traumatized spleen in man. Surgery 90:683–687
Pearson HA, Johnston D, Smith KA, et al. (1978) The born-again spleen. N Engl J Med 298:1389–1392
Scully RE, Mark EJ, McNeely WF, et al. (1995) Case records of the Massachusetts General Hospital. Weekly clinicopathologic exercises. Case 29-1995. N Engl J Med 333:784–791
Servadio Y, Leibovitch I, Apter S, et al. (1994) Symptomatic heterotopic splenic tissue in the left renal fossa. Eur Urol 25:174–176
Storm BL, Abbitt PL, Allen DA, et al. (1992) Splenosis: superparamagnetic iron oxide-enhanced MR imaging. AJR Am J Roentgenol 159:333–335
Turk CO, Lipson SB, Brandt TD (1988) Splenosis mimicking a renal mass. Urology 31:248–250
Watson WJ, Sundwall DA, Benson WL (1982) Splenosis mimicking endometriosis. Obstet Gynecol 59:51S–53S
White CS, Meyer CA (1998) General case of the day. Radiographics 18:255–257
Yoshimitsu K, Aibe H, Nobe T, et al. (1993) Intrahepatic splenosis mimicking a liver tumor. Abdom Imaging 18:156–158

5 The Spleen in Hematologic Disorders

K. Ito and D. G. Mitchell

CONTENTS

5.1 Introduction

Embryologically, the spleen develops from mesenchymal cells between the two mesothelial layers of the mesogastrium. These cells form the splenic pulp, the supporting connective tissue structures, and the capsule of the spleen. The primitive artery penetrates a lobulated embryonic spleen, and arterioles branch through the connective tissue into the splenic sinusoids. Continued growth and formation occurs during fusion of the splenic lobules.

The major functions of the spleen are the trapping and processing of blood cells (such as reticulocytes and morphologically abnormal cells), the filtration of abnormal particles, and the separation of plasma from red cells. As the spleen destroys aged red cells, it metabolizes their iron for reuse in hemoglobin. Additionally, the spleen has the capacity to produce red blood cells throughout adult life. The spleen's hematopoietic functions can be regained if chronic anemia develops or bone-marrow is lost. Although many of these functions have not been systematically observed under normal conditions, the response of the spleen to abnormal circumstances has provided evidence that such processes occur. Consequently, the spleen may be secondarily affected by and involved in the hematologic diseases, most of which cause diffuse microscopic changes that may be either undetectable by imaging modalities or reflected in changes in size or morphology. These hematologic disorders include sickle cell anemia, thalassemia, autoimmune hemolytic anemia, polycythemia vera, thrombocytopenic purpura, hypersplenism, and leukemia. In this chapter, we provide an overview of splenic abnormalities in several types of hematologic disorders, present characteristic features of these diseases in current imaging modalities, and discuss the management and clinical implications of these diseases.

5.2 Sickle Cell Disease

Sickle cell disease is a common hereditary disorder caused by a hemoglobinopathy. The erythrocytes in sickle cell disease tend to assume a rigid, sickled configuration, which is vulnerable to destruction by the spleen when the abnormal hemoglobin (HBS) is desaturated. In this situation, a vicious cycle of microthrombosis occurs in the microcirculation. Interruption of blood flow, local decrease in oxygen

K. Ito, D.G. Mitchell; Department of Radiology, Thomas Jefferson University Hospital, 132 South 10th Street, 1096 Main Building, Philadelphia, PA 19107, USA tension, and further sickling of more erythrocytes cause progressive infarction of the spleen (Fig. 5.1) and produce the characteristic periodic vaso-occlusive crises, leading to many complications of sickle cell disease.

5.2.1 Clinical Features

Splenomegaly appears in the first year and parallels the onset of declining splenic function. Patients with sickle cell anemia usually have repeated episodes of local splenic infarction and vascular occlusion that eventually result in a so-called autosplenectomy, consisting of a shrunken spleen containing diffuse, microscopic deposits of calcium and iron (Fishbone et al. 1977; Magid et al. 1984). Adults with homozygous sickle cell disease usually have small, densely calcified spleens, whereas those with heterozygous diseases often demonstrate splenomegaly with subcapsular calcification, sometimes with associated abscesses or iron deposition (Perlmutter et al. 1977; McCall et al. 1981; Adler et al. 1986). While the small and densely calcified spleen of homozygous sickle cell disease is a unique computed tomography (CT) finding, its clinical importance is minimal since, in the older child and young adult, the spleen has ceased to participate in active disease processes (Magid et al. 1984). However, in those with splenomegaly, large infarctions may necrose before they can fibrose, leaving the spleen mechanically weakened and at risk of rupture. Occasionally, splenic abscesses form within the parenchyma of an infarcted spleen, requiring drainage or splenectomy.

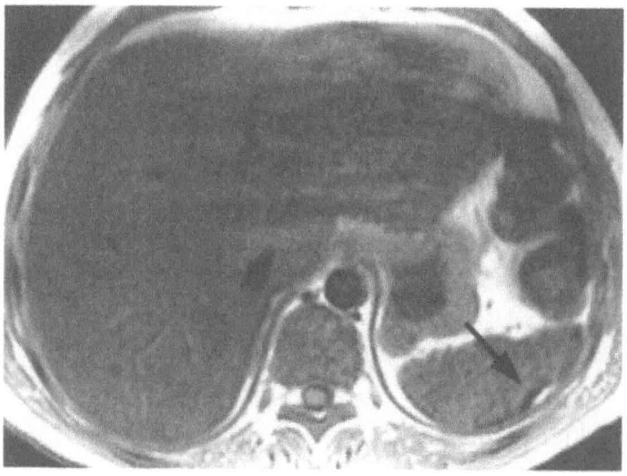

Fig. 5.1. Sickle cell disease in a 26-year-old man. A T1-weighted spin-echo axial magnetic resonance image (repetition time/echo time = 400/11) shows a small spleen with peripheral deformity (*arrow*) due to infarction. Note the diminished signal intensity (caused by iron deposition) of the liver and the spleen compared with that of the paraspinous muscle

5.2.2 Medical Imaging

The spleen in sickle cell disease shows low signal intensity on T2 and T2*-weighted magnetic resonance (MR) images in non-transfusion-dependent individuals as well as in transfusion-dependent ones (Siegelman et al. 1994; Fig. 5.2). Pathologically, the spleens of patients with sickle cell disease contain deposits of iron. The iron produces local field inhomogeneities and marked shortening of splenic T2, thus greatly reducing signal intensity. The reduction in signal intensity is thought to be a result of the heterogeneous distribution of ferritin and hemosiderin within the reticuloendothelial cells or splenic interstitial tissues. In patients with homozygous sickle cell anemia, small densely calcified spleens with microscopic perivascular and parenchymal calcification and iron deposition in the splenic tissue are seen (Fischer et al. 1977; Magid et al. 1984). Splenomegaly with subcapsular calcification can be identified in patients with heterozygous diseases. These calcifications can also contribute to the decreased signal intensity of the spleen (Fig. 5.3). Patients who underwent multiple transfusions may experience marked iron overload and deposition of excess iron in the spleen and liver.

5.2.3 Acute Splenic Sequestration

Acute splenic sequestration crisis is characterized by sudden massive splenic enlargement accompanied by an abrupt decline in hematocrit. Although the cause of acute splenic sequestration crisis is unknown, the triggering event may be acute obstruction to venous outflow from the spleen, leading to sequestration of red cells (mainly at the level of the smaller intrasplenic veins or within the sinusoids). CT demonstrates splenomegaly with multiple peripheral areas of low attenuation representing areas of subacute hemorrhage. These areas are seen as high-intensity signals on both T1 and T2-weighted MR images (Roshkow and Sanders 1990). Treatment of the acute episode requires immediate transfusion and correction of any underlying pathology. The response to transfusion is usually

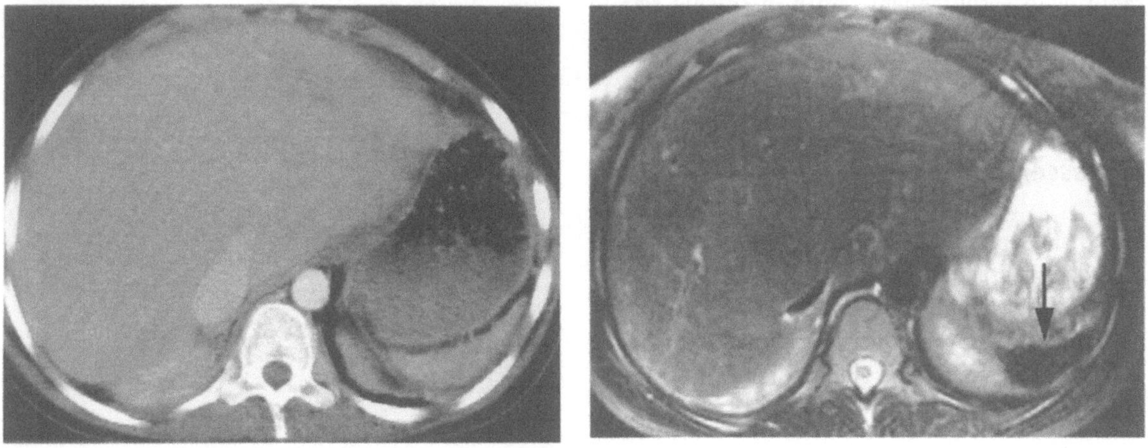

a b

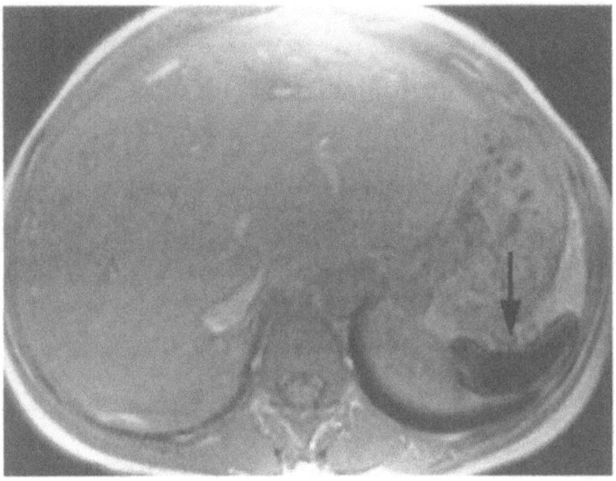

c

Fig. 5.2. Sickle cell disease in a 19-year-old woman. **a** A contrast-enhanced computed tomography scan shows a small spleen. However, abnormality of the splenic attenuation can not be seen. **b** A T2-weighted fast spin-echo (FSE) axial magnetic resonance (MR) image [repetition time/echo time (TR/TE) = 6666/100] demonstrates reduced signal intensity in the shrunken spleen due to iron deposition (*arrow*). **c** On the in-phase T1-weighted gradient-echo (GRE) axial MR image (TR/TE = 130/4.2), loss of the signal intensity in the spleen is more clearly seen (*arrow*), because GRE sequences are more sensitive to the paramagnetic effects of splenic iron than FSE sequences

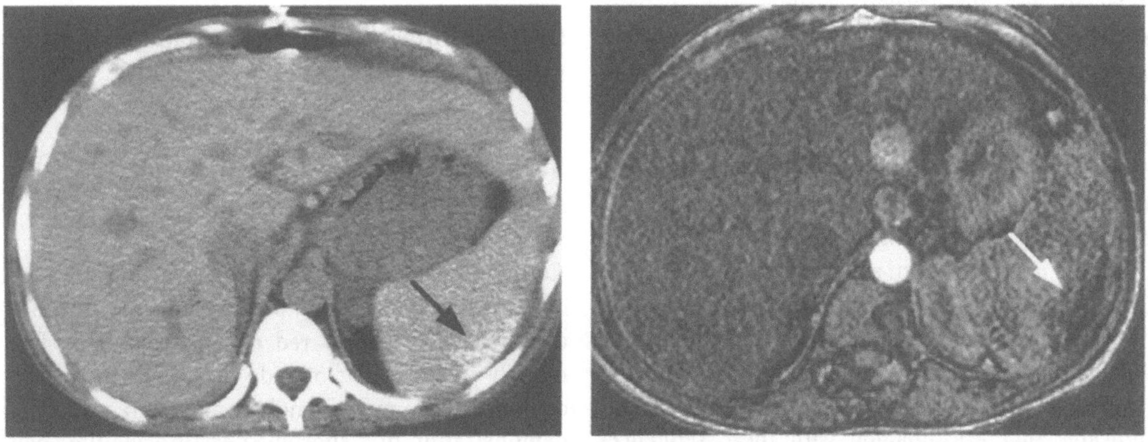

a b

Fig. 5.3. Sickle cell disease in a 27-year-old woman. **a** A non-enhanced computed tomography scan shows peripheral high attenuation areas in the spleen, indicating calcification (*arrow*). **b** An opposed-phase T1-weighted gradient-recalled-echo axial magnetic resonance image (repetition time/echo time = 120/2.4) shows calcification as an area of low signal intensity (*arrow*) rapid, with a subsequent return of splenic size to baseline.

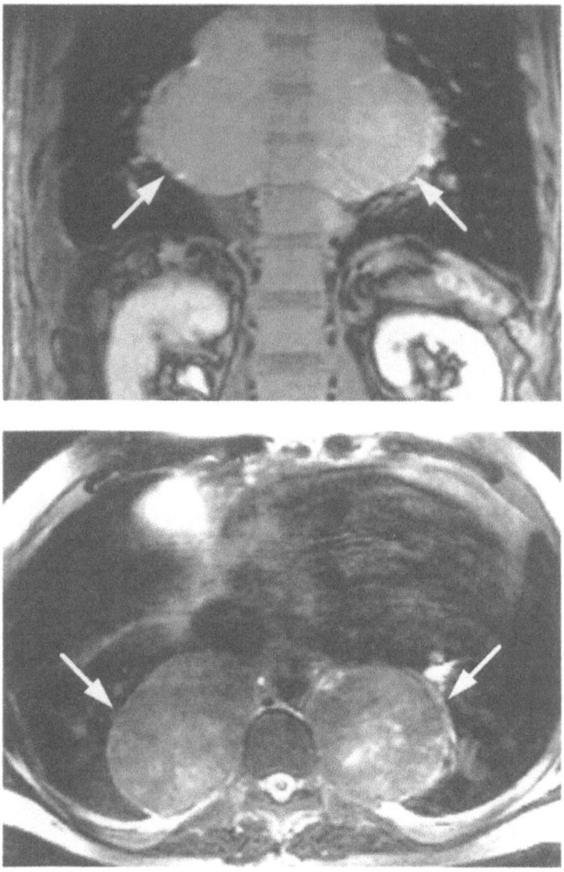

b

b

Fig. 5.4. β-Thalassemia in a 41-year-old man. **a** An opposed-phase T1-weighted gradient-recalled-echo coronal magnetic resonance (MR) image [repetition time/echo time (TR/TE) = 130/2.3] shows large, bilateral, paraspinal masses (*arrows*) in the thorax; these represent extramedullary hematopoieses. **b** On the T2-weighted fast spin-echo axial MR image (TR/TE = 4916/96), these masses show heterogeneous appearances (*arrows*)

5.3 Thalassemia

The thalassemias constitute a group of congenital disorders characterized by a defect in synthesis of one or more subunits of hemoglobin. The major abnormality is in the rate of synthesis of globin chains. This leads to ineffective globin-chain and red cell production, hemolysis, and anemia.

5.3.1 Clinical Features

Thalassemia can be subdivided into α and β-thalassemias. In β-thalassemia major, severe anemia is accompanied by hemolysis, systemic iron overload, and active erythropoiesis. Deposition of iron complexes into the reticulo-endothelial system of the spleen and other organs is demonstrable and, often, a predominant hemosiderosis results in parenchymal damage. In addition, patients suffering from thalassemia major usually need a large number of blood transfusions, exacerbating iron overload in the spleen and other organs throughout the body (Witzleben and Wyatt 1961; Ridson et al. 1975; Jacobs 1977).

5.3.2 Medical Imaging

Affected patients develop cardiomegaly, hepatosplenomegaly, and skeletal abnormalities due to the mass of the highly erythropoietic marrow (Fig. 5.4). CT can demonstrate iron deposition as increased attenuation of the spleen (Long et al. 1980; Mitnick et al. 1981). However, CT can not distinguish iron from copper. Also, CT is less sensitive for iron than MR imaging. MR imaging is a sensitive modality for detecting iron because of iron's paramagnetic effects (Fig. 5.5). A significant correlation has been shown between iron deposition (revealed by MR imaging with T2-weighted or T2*-weighted sequences) and iron concentration value (measured by biopsy). This indicates that MR imaging with these sequences can be used to accurately quantify the amount of iron (Gandon et al. 1994; Ernst et al. 1997). Therefore, MR imaging can be used to evaluate the severity of iron overload in the spleen in patients with thalassemias.

5.4 Acquired Hemolytic Anemia

Autoimmune hemolytic anemia is an acquired disorder which may be idiopathic or secondary to other disorders. The site of red cell destruction is frequently intravascular outside the spleen. In fact, a diagnosis of immune hemolytic anemia requires the demonstration of a shortened erythrocyte life span combined with the existence of erythrocyte-specific antibodies.

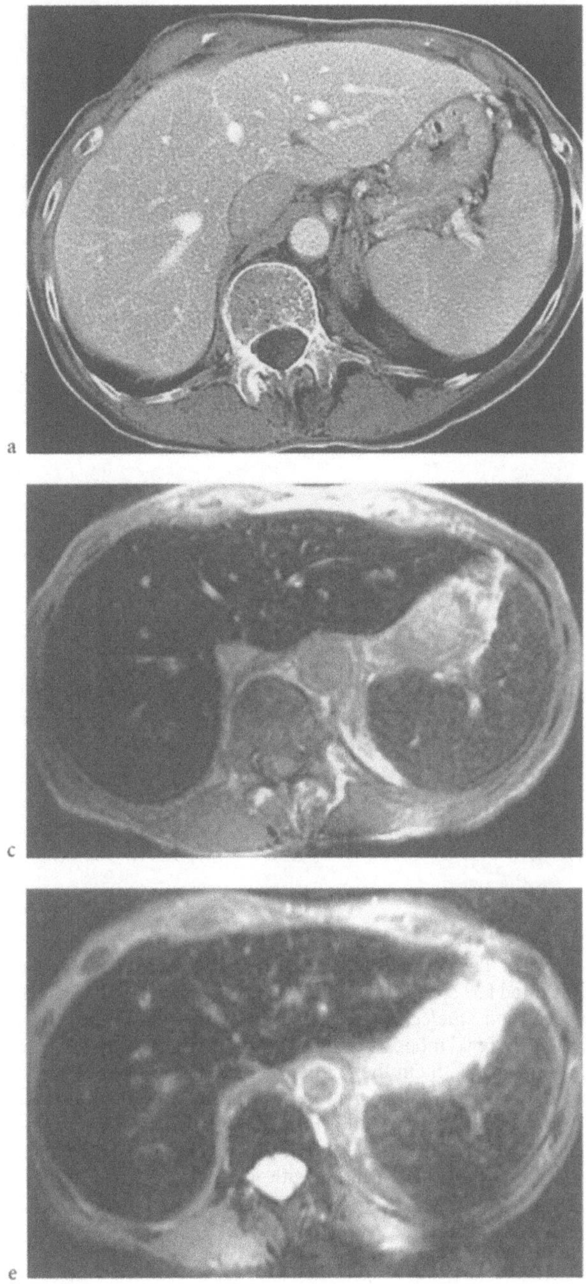

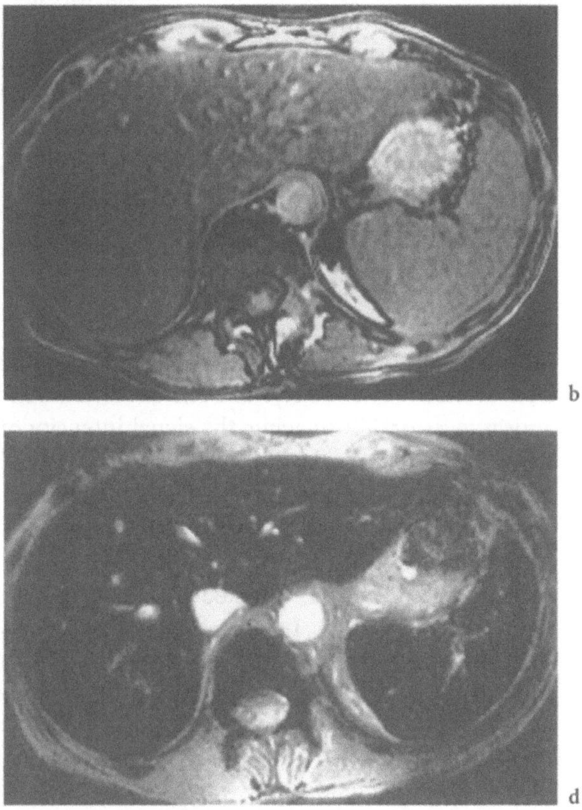

Fig. 5.5. Thalassemia minor in a 71-year-old woman. **a** A contrast-enhanced computed tomography (CT) scan shows a liver and spleen with normal appearances. **b** An opposed-phase T1-weighted gradient-recalled-echo (GRE) axial magnetic resonance (MR) image [repetition time/echo time (TR/TE) = 130/2.3] shows the spleen with a signal intensity similar to that of the paraspinous muscle. **c** An in-phase T1-weighted GRE axial MR image (TR/TE = 120/4.2) shows the spleen with low signal intensity, indicating the presence of iron in the spleen. Also note the signal loss in the liver. In-phase images were obtained with a longer TE (4.2) compared with opposed-phase images (TE = 2.3). **d** On GRE axial MR images (TR/TE = 43/15) with much longer TEs, dramatic loss of the signal in the spleen can be seen. GRE MR images with longer TEs are generally more sensitive to the detection of splenic iron compared with GRE images with shorter TEs. **e** A conventional T2-weighted spin-echo axial MR image (TR/TE = 2000/50) can also demonstrate iron deposition in the spleen and liver

5.4.1 Clinical Features

Death in this disease appeared to be related to profound anemia, gastrointestinal hemorrhage associated with thrombocytopenia, and infection but, in some patients, the cause remained undetermined. Autoimmune hemolytic anemia may complicate the course of lymphoproliferative disorders, including chronic lymphatic leukemia and Hodgkin's disease. Although splenomegaly is generally moderate, very large splenomegalies occur when lymphoproliferative diseases are accompanied by other abnormal conditions. In some instances, other cytopenias may be superimposed, and splenectomy may be required.

5.4.2 Paroxysmal Nocturnal Hemoglobinuria

Paroxysmal nocturnal hemoglobinuria (PNH), which is a subcategory of hemolytic anemia, is an acquired erythrocyte membrane disorder in which red cells become inordinately sensitive to complement. Affected patients may have chronic hemolysis with hemoglobinuria, iron-deficiency anemia, and venous thrombosis. PNH results in intravascular hemolysis with release of hemoglobin into the blood.

5.4.3 Imaging Findings of PNH

MR imaging is a useful modality for demonstrating iron overload. The kidneys in PNH show dramatic appearances on MR imaging; the signal intensity of the renal cortex is markedly reduced on T2-weighted or gradient-echo images, due to the deposition of hemosiderin within the renal cortex (ANONYMOUS 1997). Normal signal intensity of the spleen is similar to that of the liver on T1-weighted images and is high on T2-weighted images. In patients with PNH, iron is characteristically absent from the spleen, just as it is from the liver. However, diffuse low signal intensity of the spleen may occur if transfusional hemosiderosis is present. Tiny low-intensity nodules on T2- or T2*-weighted MR images may be seen (Fig. 5.6) when Budd-Chiari syndrome is present as a result of hepatic venous thrombosis (ANONYMOUS 1997). These nodules are called Gamna-Gandy bodies and correspond to organized hemorrhages in the spleen. This appearance is related to paramagnetic effects caused by the hemosiderin content of Gamna-Gandy bodies. The use of gradient-echo sequences, which are particularly sensitive to magnetic susceptibility, will also help to demonstrate these nodules more clearly.

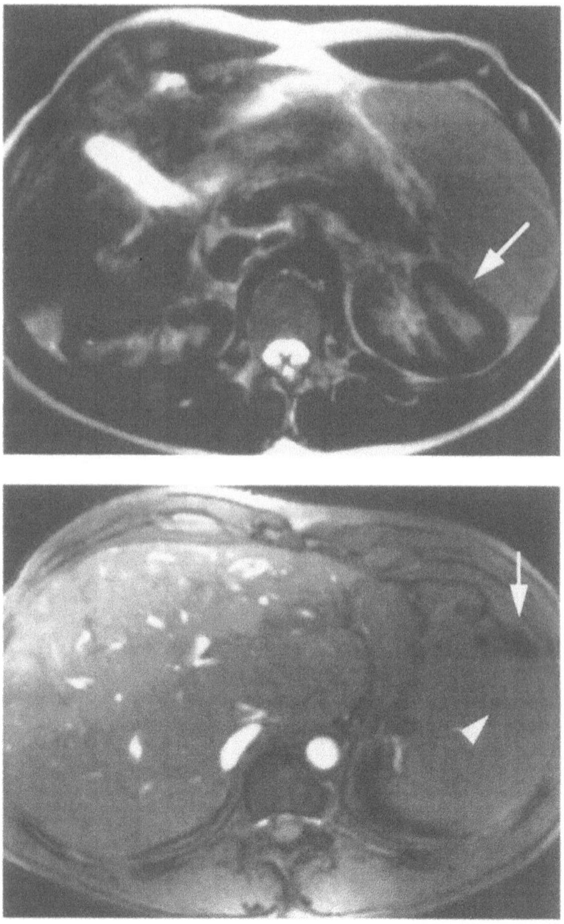

a

b

Fig. 5.6. Paroxysmal nocturnal hemoglobinuria. **a** A T2-weighted fast spin-echo axial magnetic resonance (MR) image [repetition time/echo time (TR/TE) = 6000/180] demonstrates reduced signal intensity in the renal cortices due to iron deposition (*arrow*). **b** On the gradient-recalled-echo axial MR images (TR/TE = 34/13), small low-signal-intensity regions are present in the spleen (*arrowhead*). The peripheral low-signal-intensity deformity of the spleen is compatible with a splenic infarct (*arrow*). (Reprinted with permission from Radiographics 17:263-265)

5.5 Idiopathic Thrombocytopenic Purpura

Idiopathic thrombocytopenic purpura (ITP) is a hemorrhagic disorder characterized by a decreased platelet count despite the presence of normal or increased megakaryocytes in the bone marrow. Another characteristic is that the platelet life span is greatly reduced owing to increased breakdown of the antibody-sensitized platelets in the spleen. Definitive diagnosis depends on ruling out other systemic illnesses and the ingestion of drugs capable of producing thrombocytopenia.

5.5.1 Clinical Features

ITP may occur in an acute, often post-infectious variety, especially in children and young adults. Over 80% of affected individuals recover spontaneously within 3–6 months. ITP may occur in intermittent and chronic varieties apparently unrelated to infection, predominantly in females aged from 20 years to 40 years (MUELLER-ECKHARDT 1977). The common symptom is bleeding from the vagina, gastrointestinal tract, or urinary tract. The antibody-coated platelets are removed by the spleen; platelet survival is markedly diminished, and platelet turnover is increased. Splenectomy is effective in ITP, not only because the spleen is the major site of platelet destruction but also because it is commonly the site of production of anti-platelet antibodies. Initial therapy of ITP consists of corticosteroid treatment for 6 weeks to 2 months. The doses administered to patients who respond to corticosteroids are subsequently tapered off. However, if drug therapy has a limited effect and/or must be extended over a lengthy period, splenectomy may be considered (Coon 1987). Histologically, the spleen in ITP frequently shows normal appearance even though its production of platelet antibodies may be considerable.

5.5.2
Medical Imaging

Splenomegaly is usually not identified in most patients with ITP. This is a unique characteristic of ITP, because all other diseases involving the spleen, functionally or structurally, are accompanied by splenomegaly. However, splenomegaly can be seen in 5% of all cases in ITP (Doan et al. 1960; Fig. 5.7).

Imaging modalities contribute little to the diagnosis of ITP, as there are no characteristic imaging features of the spleen in ITP. However, imaging modalities may have an important role in the follow-up examinations of patients with remission of thrombocytopenia after splenic resection, because post-splenectomy thrombocytopenia is sometimes caused by the existence of accessory spleens. One report showed that the smallest accessory spleen identified by CT and scintigraphy with ^{99m}Tc-labeled sulfur colloid was 1 cm in patients with post-splenectomy thrombocytopenia (Ambriz et al. 1985).

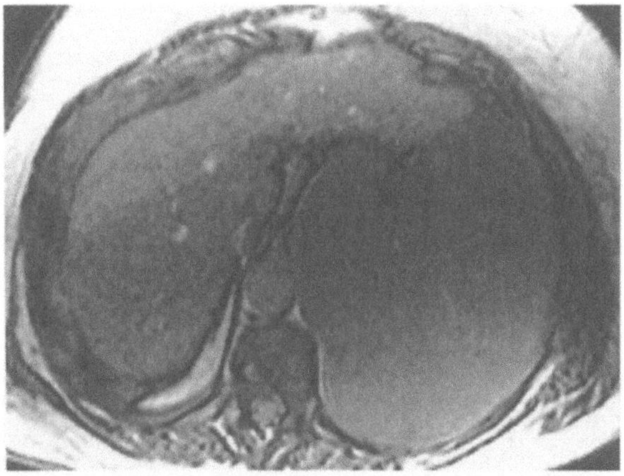

Fig. 5.7. Idiopathic thrombocytopenic purpura. An opposed-phase T1-weighted gradient-recalled-echo axial magnetic resonance image (repetition time/echo time = 120/2.1) shows marked splenomegaly

5.6
Polycythemia Vera

Polycythemia vera is characterized by a marked and persistent elevation in the total number of circulating red blood cells in association with ruddy cyanosis, leukocytosis, and thrombocytosis, although the etiology and pathogenesis of this disease are still unknown. There may be a variety of findings secondary to venous and arterial thrombosis. Ecchymoses and hematomas are not uncommon and are due to the unexpected bleeding tendency seen in polycythemia vera.

5.6.1
Clinical Features

Mild to moderate splenomegaly is seen in three-quarters of patients with polycythemia vera at the time of diagnosis (Corredoira et al. 1990). Some siderosis may be seen in the spleen, but it is not a prominent feature of this disease. Dense streaks of calcification are occasionally seen by several imaging modalities in the enlarged spleen. Although the cause of calcification is not clear, a possible explanation is that thrombosis of branches of the splenic artery leads to metastatic calcification of the infarcted splenic parenchyma (Srikanth et al. 1994). In the late stage of the disease, massive splenomegaly occurs, associated with splenic infarction and pressure effects on surrounding organs.

5.6.2
Medical Imaging

The typical appearance of peripheral, wedge-shaped splenic infarcts is well known, but some splenic infarcts may appear on CT as large hypodense lesions (Balcar et al. 1984). When massive splenic infarction is accompanied by liquefactive necrosis and intraparenchymal gas formation (Fig. 5.8), differentiation from an extensive splenic abscess may be difficult (Downer and Peterson 1993).

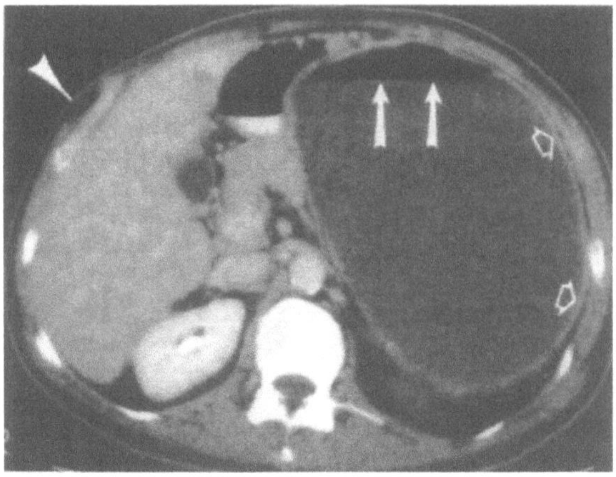

Fig. 5.8. Polycythemia vera. A contrast-enhanced computed tomography scan shows an enlarged, liquefied spleen containing an air-fluid level (*solid arrows*) and displacing the stomach and pancreas to the right of the midline. Contrast enhancement of splenic capsule is minimal (*open arrows*). Note an incidental lipoma within the chest wall on the right side (*arrowhead*). (Reprinted from DOWNER and PETERSON, 1993 AJR 161:79–80, with permission)

5.7 Myelogenous Leukemia

The spleen is often pathologically involved in patients with myelogenous leukemia. Splenomegaly, often of appreciable degree, is present in more than 90% of untreated cases.

5.7.1 Clinical Features

Clinically, the patients often present with a splenomegaly syndrome, such as a high basal metabolic rate, a tendency to sweat, weight loss and anemia. Leukemic spleens microscopically show diffuse and focal infiltration of leukemic cells. Numerous small infarcts may be seen throughout the splenic parenchyma. With progression of the disease, there is obliteration of the underlying architecture. The size of the spleen in myelogenous leukemia is variable during the course of the disease. Although the spleen is usually large in untreated phases, treatment with chemotherapy often reduces the size of the spleen, which may periodically return to normal. In chronic myelogenous leukemia, the splenic size is a sign of disease activity and is of the utmost importance to the clinician who is to follow patients through lengthy periods.

5.7.2 Medical Imaging

Cross-sectional imaging modalities, including ultrasound (US), CT, and MR imaging, can readily demonstrate both the enlarged spleen and the normal one (Fig. 5.9). Therefore, these modalities can play an important role in evaluating the size of the spleen and in assessing the severity of disease activity. On CT scans, the spleens of patients with chronic myelogenous leukemia maintain a homogeneous, normal attenuation value. However, splenomegaly associated with increased echogenicity on US similar to that resulting from benign processes has been reported (SILER et al. 1980). Although the cause of the increased echo pattern is unclear, diffuse infiltration of leukemic cells into the splenic parenchyma may be one possible explanation.

5.7.3 Rupture of the Leukemic Spleen

Spontaneous rupture of the leukemic spleen is known to occur. As in acute leukemia, a blast crisis is often accompanied by severe infections and by hemorrhagic diathesis as a result of thrombocytopenia. In this situation, diagnostic modalities are helpful in depicting focal infectious lesions (SHIRKHODA 1987). However, it should be noted that the underlying leukemia can have a similar appearance on CT and that 40% of the spleens display no focal abnormality on CT in patients with splenic fungal infections

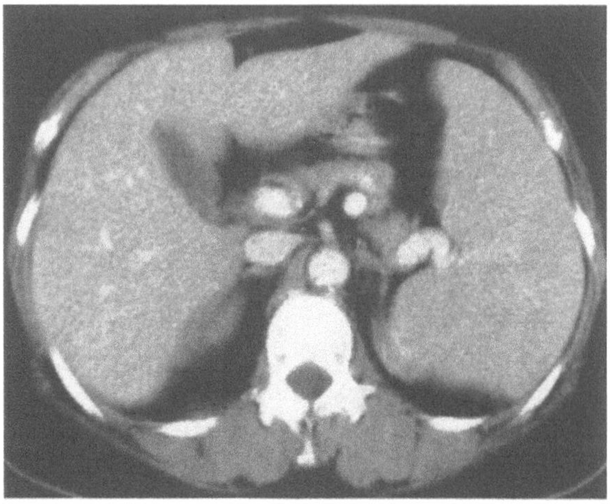

Fig. 5.9. Chronic myelogenous leukemia. A contrast-enhanced computed tomography scan shows splenomegaly with homogeneous appearances (courtesy of Dr. NOBUYUKI TANAKA)

(SHIRKHODA 1987). Therefore, when there are no focal defects and clinical diagnosis of splenic infection is likely, histologic confirmation may be necessary to initiate the appropriate therapy.

5.8 Myelofibrosis

Myelofibrosis is defined as a myeloproliferative state with defects of the bone-marrow matrix and myeloid metaplasia; it occurs primarily in the spleen and liver and occasionally in the lymph nodes and other tissues. Reticulosis and fibrosis of the bone marrow are typical of myelofibrosis, but such fibrosis can also occur in chronic myelogenous leukemia, aplastic anemia, and hemolytic anemia. Thus, fibrosis of the bone marrow may be interpreted as the ultimate histological stage of a number of different bone-marrow actions.

5.8.1 Clinical Features

Clinical manifestation of myelofibrosis is heterogeneous and dependent on the amount of normally functioning hematopoietic tissues remaining. The disease usually occurs in middle-aged or elderly individuals. Myelofibrosis can be clinically divided into three basic subgroups: (1) reactive myelofibrosis with marrow hyperplasia; (2) reactive myelofibrosis with marrow dysplasia; and (3) reactive myelofibrosis with aplastic or hypoproliferative bone marrow. In patients with marrow hyperplasia, splenomegaly is severe and progressive, resulting from fibrosclerotic obliteration of the bone-marrow space.

5.8.2 Medical Imaging

Cross-sectional imaging can demonstrate that the enlarged spleen retains its basic morphology without distortion (Fig. 5.10). Hemosiderosis resulting from repeated transfusion can sometimes be seen together with infarction of hemorrhage. On sonography, the affected spleen shows markedly increased echogenicity similar to that of the liver, probably attributed to the dominating red pulp, which is diffusely infiltrated by hematopoietic elements (HUNTER and HABER 1977).

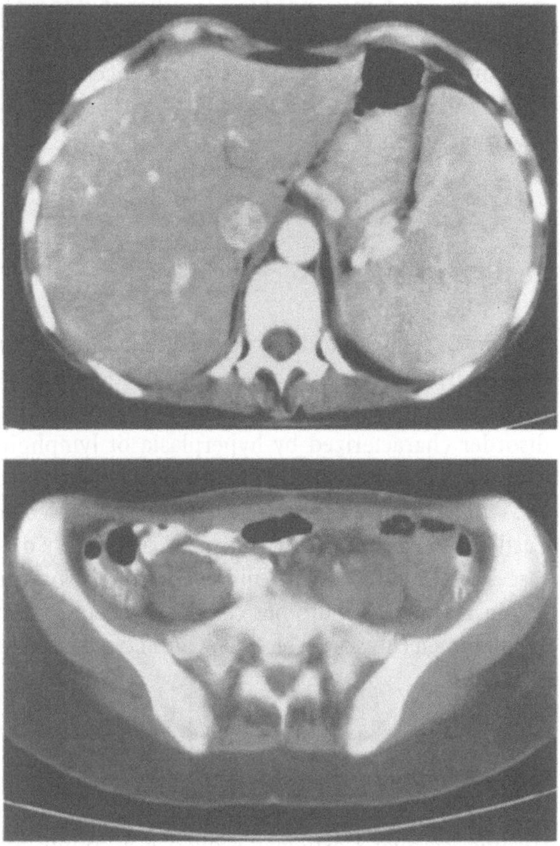

a

b

Fig. 5.10. Myelofibrosis. **a** A contrast-enhanced computed tomography (CT) scan obtained at the level of the splenic hilum shows splenomegaly with homogeneous enhancement. **b** A contrast-enhanced CT scan obtained at the level of the pelvis shows diffuse sclerosis of iliac bones

In myelofibrosis, surface radioactivity measurements after administration of ^{59}Fe demonstrate an uptake of iron by extramedullary foci (primarily in the spleen and occasionally in the liver). Accordingly, ^{59}Fe scanning may demonstrate iron uptake the spleen or the liver, while uptake in the bones is usually reduced.

5.8.3 Treatment

Splenectomy has been indicated for patients with repeated splenic infarction, clinical symptoms due to massive splenomegaly, and complications from hypersplenism. However, splenectomy is contraindicated for patients with enhanced megakaryocytopoiesis, since post-splenectomy thrombocythemia can pose serious thrombotic problems. Splenic irradiation provides only temporary control of symptoms and may produce significant pancytopenia. Transfusions are ineffective, as macrophages destroy both autologous and transfused cells. There has been recent success with allogeneic bone-marrow transfusion.

5.9 Castleman's Disease

Castleman's disease, also known as angiofollicular hyperplasia or benign giant lymph-node hyperplasia, is an uncommon benign lymphoproliferative disorder characterized by hyperplasia of lymphoid follicles (CASTLEMAN et al. 1956). There are two major histologic variants: hyaline-vascular Castleman's disease and plasma cell Castleman's disease. Castleman's disease more commonly occurs within the mediastinum but can rarely occur within the abdomen (LIBSON et al. 1988; CIRILLO et al. 1998).

5.9.1 Clinical Features

Hyaline-vascular Castleman's disease accounts for approximately 90% of cases and is usually encountered incidentally as a solitary mediastinal mass in asymptomatic patients. In contrast, plasma cell Castleman's disease is identified in 10% of cases and is usually associated with clinical manifestations including persistent fever, fatigue, weight loss, anemia, polyclonal hypergammaglobulinemia, and bone-marrow plasmacytosis.

Castleman's disease can present clinically as either a localized or a disseminated (multicentric) form. The localized form usually has a benign and indolent course confined to a single lymph-node region. The multicentric form is more aggressive, with involvement of multiple lymph-node regions and extranodal sites. Localized Castleman's disease requires surgical removal of the affected lymph nodes. Due to its aggressive course, multicentric Castleman's disease is treated with corticosteroids and anti-neoplastic chemotherapy.

5.9.2 Medical Imaging

CT findings in the multicentric form include splenomegaly, retroperitoneal and mesenteric lymphadenopathy, and ascites (Fig. 5.11). However, no CT finding is pathognomonic for multicentric Castleman's disease. Therefore, it is usually indistinguishable from other neoplastic disorders, such as lymphoma, thymoma, neurogenic disorders, and granulomatous diseases. The diagnosis of Castleman's disease can only be made on the basis of histologic examinations by observing its characteristic appearances and by excluding other diseases with similar histologic characteristics (thymoma and follicular lymphoma).

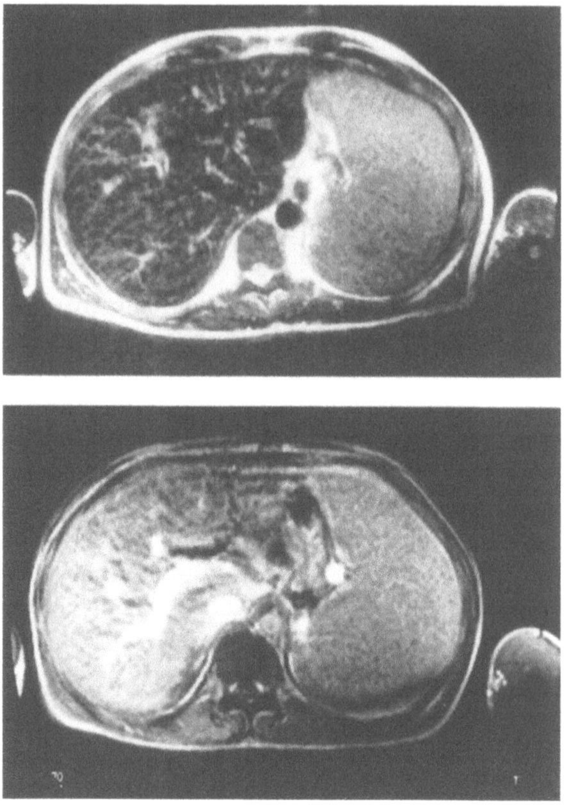

Fig. 5.11. Castleman disease. **a** T2-weighted magnetic resonance (MR) image. **b** Gradient-recalled-echo MR image. Marked splenomegaly with homogeneous appearance can be seen

References

Adler DD, Glazer GM, Aisen AM (1986) MRI of the spleen: normal appearance and findings in sickle-cell anemia. AJR Am J Roentgenol 147:843–845

Ambriz P, Munoz R, Quintanar E, et al. (1985) Accessory spleen compromising response to splenectomy for idiopathic thrombocytopenic purpura. Radiology 155:793–796

Anonymous (1997) Imaging interpretation session: 1996. Paroxysmal nocturnal hemoglobinuria (PNH). Radiographics 17:263–265

Balcar I, Seltzer SE, Davis S, et al. (1984) CT patterns of splenic

infarction: a clinical and experimental study. Radiology 151:723–729
Castleman B, Iverson L, Mecendez VP (1956) Localized mediastinal lymph node hyperplasia resembling thymoma. Cancer 9:822–830
Cirillo RL, Vitellas KM, Deyoung BR, et al. (1998) Castleman disease: mimicking a hepatic neoplasm. Clin Imaging 22:124–129
Coon WW (1987) Splenectomy for idiopathic thrombocytopenic purpura. Surg Gynecol Obstet 164:225–229
Corredoira JC, Gonzales M, Perez R, et al. (1990) A clinical and biological study of 33 cases of polycythemia vera. Rev Clin Esp 186:378–382
Doan CA, Bouroncle BA, Wiseman BK (1960) Idiopathic and secondary thrombocytopenic purpura: clinical study and evaluation of 381 cases over a period of 28 years. Ann Intern Med 53:861–876
Downer WR, Peterson MS (1993) Massive splenic infarction and liquefactive necrosis complicating polycythemia vera. AJR Am J Roentgenol 161:79–80
Ernst O, Sergent G, Bonvarlet P, et al. (1997) Hepatic iron overload: diagnosis and quantification with MR imaging. AJR Am J Roentgenol 168:1205–1208
Fischer KC, Shapiro S, Treves S (1977) Visualization of the spleen with a bone-seeking radionuclide in a child with sickle-cell anemia. Radiology 122:398
Fishbone G, Nunez D, Leon R, et al. (1977) Massive splenic infarction in sickle cell-hemoglobin C disease: angiographic findings. AJR Am J Roentgenol 129:927–928
Gandon Y, Guyader D, Heautot JF, et al. (1994) Hemochromatosis: diagnosis and quantification of liver iron with gradient-echo MR imaging. Radiology 193:533–538
Hunter TB, Haber K (1977) Unusual sonographic appearance of the spleen in a case of myelofibrosis. AJR Am J Roentgenol 128:138–139
Jacobs A (1977) Iron overload-clinical and pathologic aspects. Semin Hematol 14:89–113
Libson E, Fields S, Strauss S, et al. (1988) Widespread Castleman disease: CT and US findings. Radiology 166: 753–755
Long JA Jr, Doppman JL, Nienhus AW, et al. (1980) Computed tomographic analysis of b-thalassemic syndromes with hemochromatosis: pathologic findings with clinical and laboratory correlations. J Comput Assist Tomogr 4:159–165
Magid D, Fishman EK, Siegelman SS (1984) Computed tomography of the spleen and liver in sickle cell disease. AJR Am J Roentgenol 143:245–249
McCall IW, Vaidya S, Serjeant GR (1981) Splenic opacification in homozygous sickle cell disease. Clin Radiol 32:611–615
Mitnick JS, Bosniak MA, Megibow A, et al. (1981) CT in b-thalassemia: iron deposition in the liver, spleen, and lymph nodes. AJR Am J Roentgenol 136:1191–1194
Mueller-Eckhardt C (1977) Idiopathic thrombocytopenic purpura (ITP): clinical and immunologic considerations. Semin Thromb Hemost 3:125–159
Perlmutter S, Jacobstein JG, Kazam E (1977) Splenic uptake of Tc-99m-diphosphonate in sickle cell disease associated with increased splenic density on computerized transaxial tomography. Gastrointest Radiol 2:77–79
Ridson RA, Barry M, Flynn DM (1975) Transfusional iron overload: the relationship between tissue iron concentration and hepatic fibrosis in thalassemia. J Pathol 116:83–95
Roshkow JE, Sanders LM (1990) Acute splenic sequestration crisis in two adults with sickle cell disease: US, CT and MR imaging findings. Radiology 177:723–725
Shirkhoda A (1987) CT findings in hepatosplenic and renal candidiasis. J Comput Assist Tomogr 11:795–798
Siegelman ES, Outwater E, Hanau CA, et al. (1994) Abdominal iron distribution in sickle cell disease: MR findings in transfusion and non-transfusion dependent patients. J Comput Assist Tomogr 18:63–67
Siler J, Hunter TB, Weiss J, et al. (1980) Increased echogenicity of the spleen in benign and malignant disease. AJR Am J Roentgenol 134:1011–1014
Srikanth M, Mohan VS, Reddy JJM (1994) Calcific splenomegaly in polycythemia vera. AJR Am J Roentgenol 163:747
Witzleben CL, Wyatt JP (1961) The effect of long survival on the pathology of thalassemia major. J Pathol 82:1–12

6 The Spleen in Systemic Disorders

F. VANHOENACKER and A.M. DE SCHEPPER

CONTENTS

6.1 Introduction

The spleen is a lymphoreticular organ that is schematically arranged as a two-unit system consisting of the *white pulp* surrounded by areas of *red pulp*. The white pulp acts as a *lymph node*, whereas the red pulp is the site of the *reticuloendothelial system*, acting as a filtration system to remove normal and abnormal blood cells, microorganisms and particles. Splenic function is complex, and a variety of diseases, mainly affecting other organ systems, can interfere with splenic function and structure. For didactic reasons and because of the uncertain etiology of many of these disease entities, systemic diseases with splenic involvement will be classified into three different groups, depending on their site of action in the two-unit system of the spleen.

First, the classical *collagen vascular disorders*, which are associated with disordered immune regulation, are treated. The function and structure of the spleen, being an organ of the immune system, can be affected through lymphoid hyperplasia in the white-pulp area and through dysfunction of phagocytic red-pulp areas, which are responsible for the destruction of cells. This red-pulp dysfunction results from autoimmune cytopenias. Second, in the *storage diseases*, splenic dysfunction and anatomical distortion are the result of deposition of abnormal substances into the reticuloendothelial system (red-pulp area). Third, *multisystem diseases* that can't be classified into the first two groups will be treated as separate entities. Emphasis is placed on sarcoidosis, which is believed to be a granulomatous inflammation in white-pulp areas.

F. VANHOENACKER, A.M. DE SCHEPPER; Department of Radiology, University Hospital Antwerp, Wilrijkstraat 10, B-2650 Edegem, Belgium

6.2 Collagen Vascular Disease

6.2.1 Rheumatoid Arthritis and Felty's Syndrome

6.2.1.1 *Definition*

Rheumatoid arthritis (RA) is a chronic multisystem disease of unknown origin. In addition to the variable extra-articular manifestations, the characteristic feature of RA is persistent inflammatory synovitis involving peripheral joints in a symmetric distribution. Felty's syndrome consists of a triad of chronic RA, splenomegaly, neutropenia and, on occasion, anemia and thrombocytopenia (LIPSKY 1994). It occurs preferentially in the fifth to seventh decade of life and after a long-standing RA (of more than 10 years). Seventy percent of Felty's syndrome patients are female.

6.2.1.2 *Clinical Manifestations of Splenic Involvement*

Clinical features of articular and extrasplenic extra-articular disease are discussed elsewhere. RA has been associated in 5–10% of cases with clinically detectable splenomegaly, but radionuclide scanning may detect splenomegaly in up to 58% of patients with active RA. Splenomegaly is a characteristic feature of Felty's syndrome, but the splenic size does not correlate with the degree of hematologic abnormality (Fishman and Isenberg 1997). Spontaneous splenic rupture has been described in RA (Haskard et al. 1982). In Felty's syndrome, the patient is at risk of infection, splenic abscess formation and malignancies (especially lymphomas; Hofbauer et al. 1995). Reduced or absent splenic function has been documented in RA (Fishman and Isenberg 1997).

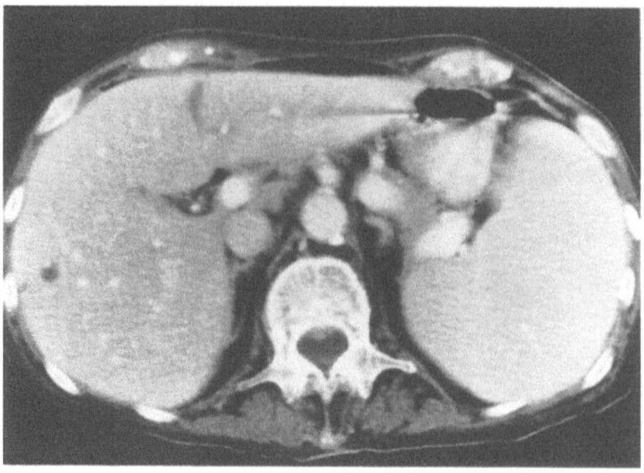

Fig. 6.1. Felty's syndrome. Contrast-enhanced computed tomography shows splenomegaly in a woman with known Felty's syndrome (courtesy of L. Declerck)

6.2.1.3 Histopathology of Splenic Involvement

The enlargement of the spleen in Felty's syndrome is due to expansion of the red pulp and sinuses, which contain many macrophages (Van Krieken et al. 1988).

6.2.1.4 Imaging

Splenomegaly (Fig. 6.1) may be assessed on different imaging modalities [ultrasound, computed-tomography (CT) scan, magnetic resonance imaging (MRI)]. Ultrasound and CT scans are excellent imaging tools for detection of complications such as splenic rupture or splenic abscesses. Rarely, splenic calcifications have been observed on plain film and CT scans in a patient with an overlap syndrome between RA and systemic lupus erythematosus (SLE; Van Linthoudt et al. 1990). A wandering spleen has erroneously been diagnosed as a pelvic malignancy in a patient with Felty's syndrome (Du Cret et al. 1991). ^{99m}Tc-labeled sulfur-colloid scans are used to evaluate splenic function. Impairment of the splenic reticuloendothelial function results in decreased or absent tracer uptake (Fishman and Isenberg 1997).

6.2.1.5 Treatment

Splenectomy has been advised by many authors in order to increase the number of circulating granulocytes in Felty's syndrome. Partial embolization is a valuable alternative to splenectomy, as it is less invasive and may allow preservation of greater immunocompetency than does splenectomy (Nakamura et al. 1994).

6.2.2 Systemic Lupus Erythematosus

6.2.2.1 Definition

SLE is a multisystemic disease of unknown cause in which tissues and cells are damaged by pathogenic autoantibodies and immune complexes. Ninety percent of cases are women, usually of childbearing age, but children, men and the elderly may also be affected. The prevalence is estimated to be 15–50 per 100,000 individuals (Hahn 1994).

6.2.2.2 Clinical Manifestations

The clinical manifestations depend on which organ is affected. The spleen is involved in 15–45% of patients. Splenomegaly and lymphadenopathy are the most commonly reported findings. Rare complications are splenic infarction, spontaneous splenic rupture (Tolaymat et al. 1995), functional asplenia and hyposplenia (due to atrophy or acute splenomegaly). Functional asplenia is defined as a failure of the spleen to accumulate radiocolloid. It is a potentially life-threatening complication that may be fatal due to overwhelming sepsis (Malleson et al. 1988).

The association between malignant lymphoma and SLE has been described and may be related to disturbance of immune regulation. Primary malignant lymphoma of the spleen in SLE is rare and has been described once (Buskila et al. 1989).

6.2.2.3 Histopathology of Splenic Involvement

On microscopic examination, large- and small-vessel necrotizing vasculitis with an onion-skin pattern is characteristic of SLE.

6.2.2.4 Imaging of Splenic Involvement

6.2.2.4.1

PLAIN X-RAY

SLE, RA and the overlap syndrome between RA and SLE are very rare causes of calcifications (Fig. 6.2) in the left upper quadrant (Van Linthoudt et al. 1990). Those calcifications are histologically centered on the small arteries and seem to be related to the process of vasculitis.

6.2.2.4.2

ULTRASOUND

Ultrasound is used to assess splenic size. Functional asplenia may be permanent due to an atrophic spleen (autosplenectomy) or transient due to an enlarged spleen during an acute lupus flare (Malleson et al. 1988).

6.2.2.4.3

SCINTIGRAPHY

The standard scintigraphic method of assessing splenic anatomic and especially functional integrity is ^{99m}Tc-labeled sulfur-colloid uptake. The tracer uptake correlates well with the splenic phagocytic function of the reticuloendothelial system. In cases of functional aplenia or hyposplenia, tracer uptake will be absent or decreased (Malleson et al. 1988).

6.2.2.4.4

COMPUTED TOMOGRAPHY

CT may be used to assess splenomegaly, splenic atrophy or splenic calcifications.

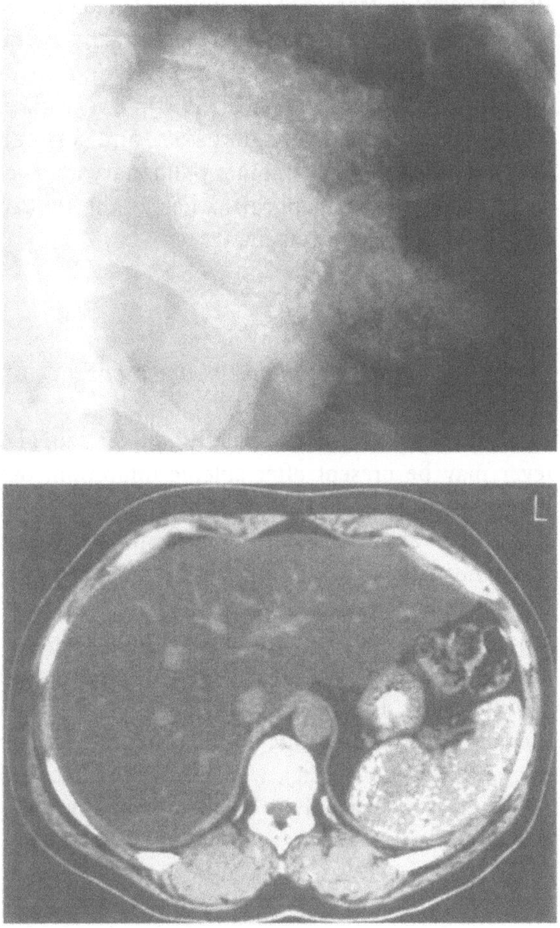

a
b

Fig. 6.2. Overlap syndrome with multiple calcifications of the spleen. **a** Abdominal plain X-ray. Numerous small opacities in the left hypochondrium. **b** Abdominal non-enhanced computed tomography. Multiple calcifications within the spleen, with predominant peripheral distribution. The fatty infiltration of the liver is due to long-term steroid use (Van Linthoudt et al. 1990)

6.2.3 Wegener's Granulomatosis

6.2.3.1 Definition

Wegener's granulomatosis is a systemic disease of unknown etiology. An aberrant hypersensitivity reaction to unknown antigens has been suggested (Kalaitzoglou et al. 1998). The criteria for the disease classification have been established by the American College of Rheumatology (Leavitt et al. 1990). It is characterized by a clinicopathologic complex of necrotizing granulomatous vasculitis of the upper and lower respiratory tract, glomerulonephritis and variable degrees of vasculitis of small arteries and veins. The disease can affect any organ system. Splenic involvement, however, generally is considered to be rare (Fonner et al. 1995). Two clinical forms are described (Armbruster and Vetter 1991): the *classic form* combines pulmonary involvement and glomerulonephritis, whereas the *limited form* lacks renal involvement.

6.2.3.2
Clinical Symptoms of Splenic Involvement

Left upper-quadrant pain and left shoulder pain and fever may be present after splenic infarction, but many patients have no abdominal symptomatology (Fonner et al. 1995). Acute abdominal pain due to spontaneous splenic rupture has been reported by Franssen et al. (1993). Nonspecific clinical presentation may be the reason for underestimation of the prevalence of splenic involvement of the disease (Fonner et al. 1995). Laboratory tests reveal a high titer of serum cytoplasmic antineutrophil cytoplasmic antibodies (cANCA), which is a sensitive and specific test for the activity of the disease (Leavitt et al. 1990).

6.2.3.3
Pathology of Splenic Involvement

On gross pathologic sections, a central area of infarction surrounded by a red peripheral zone of splenic parenchyma has been reported by Fonner et al. (1995). Microscopic examination reveals granulomatous vasculitis of small and medium-sized arteries and veins, which show thrombotic occlusion and hemorrhage, which causes infarction, because those small parenchymal arteries are end vessels that do not communicate with one another (Venbrux et al. 1993).

6.2.3.4
Imaging

Reports on imaging features of splenic involvement are rare. This may be due to the low prevalence of splenic involvement of Wegener's granulomatosis, but may also be due to clinical underestimation, as lack of specific abdominal symptomatology leads to infrequent examination with cross-sectional imaging.

Imaging features are the result of splenic infarction, which may be focal or diffuse. However, in most reported cases, a diffuse pattern predominates. Fonner et al. (1995) believed that the pattern of diffuse infarction is characteristic of splenic involvement of Wegener's granulomatosis, as panarteritis can explain massive infarction.

6.2.3.4.1
ULTRASOUND

Ultrasound may show a heterogeneous parenchymal architecture (Ruel et al. 1989; McHugh et al. 1991) or multiple hypoechoic intrasplenic nodules (Gregorini et al. 1990), with patency of the splenic artery and veins (McHugh et al. 1991). This reflects the histopathologic feature of medium- and small vessel vasculitis with sparing of the large splenic artery.

6.2.3.4.2
COMPUTED TOMOGRAPHY

A diffuse pattern of splenic infarction is reported by several authors. On contrast enhanced CT scans, a pattern of rim enhancement around a large central area of low attenuation is described (Fonner et al. 1995). The enhanced peripheral area presumably represents residual capsular blood flow (Cohen et al. 1984) originating as angiographically occult capsular vessels traversing the gastrosplenic and lienorenal ligaments. Some small central areas of enhancement within the necrotic low attenuation zone may be seen and have been attributed to viable tissue surrounding patent, small, penetrating vessels and their vasa vasorum. The differential diagnosis of the CT pattern should include abscess, tumor and hematoma.

6.2.3.4.3
MAGNETIC RESONANCE IMAGING

One report of MRI findings has been made so far (Kalaitzoglou et al. 1998). The appearance of diffuse low signal intensity on T1-weighted images and high signal intensity on T2-weighted images is consistent with necrosis, as seen in diffuse infarction (Fig. 6.3). This corresponds very well with the CT pattern of diffuse involvement.

6.2.3.4.4
SCINTIGRAPHY

The area of infarction has been reported by Morayati and Fink-Bennet (1986) to correspond to a photopenic area on ^{111}In leukocyte scans.

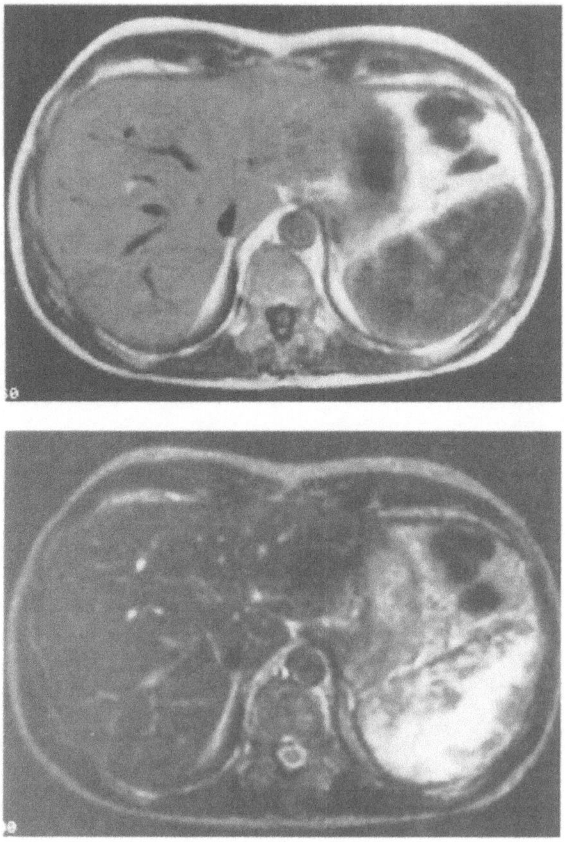

Fig. 6.3. Splenic infarction due to Wegener's granulomatosis. a Axial T1-weighted magnetic resonance (MR) image. Diffuse, inhomogeneous, low signal intensity of the spleen with a thin rim of enhancement and septa. b Axial T2-weighted MR image. Very high signal intensity of the central portion of the spleen, with an irregular peripheral area of mixed intermediate and high signal intensity (Kalaitzoglou et al. 1998)

6.2.4 Polyarteritis Nodosa

6.2.4.1 Definition

Polyarteritis nodosa (PAN) is a systemic inflammatory disease that causes a necrotizing vasculitis of medium-sized arteries; the disease is also characterized by aneurysm formation. The exact incidence of splenic involvement is unknown (Fishman and Isenberg 1997).

6.2.4.2 Clinical Manifestations

The most common visceral complication of PAN is mesenteric arteritis with bowel infarction and perforation. Rare splenic complications include splenic abscess formation and spontaneous splenic rupture (Fishman and Isenberg 1997). The mechanism leading to rupture is unclear. Rupture has been attributed to rupture of microaneurysms or to the process of vasculitis, which may lead to subcapsular infarction and rupture (Ford et al. 1986).

6.2.4.3 Imaging

Angiography may detect aneurysms of the splenic artery. Ultrasound and CT scans may be useful in the detection of splenic rupture or abscess formation.

6.2.5 Miscellaneous Rheumatic Diseases

Splenic involvement with splenomegaly has been reported in several other rheumatic disorders, such as juvenile chronic arthritis, Sjögren's syndrome, overlap syndromes, Churg-Strauss syndrome, leukocytoclastic vasculitis, eosinophilic fasciitis, Behçet's disease and Lyme disease (Fishman and Isenberg 1997).

6.3 Storage Disease

6.3.1 Lysosomal Storage Diseases

6.3.1.1 Gaucher's Disease

6.3.1.1.1

DEFINITION

Gaucher's disease is the most common lysosomal storage disease and is due to a deficiency in the enzyme glucocerebrosidase. This leads to the accumulation of glucocerebroside within the lysosomes of macrophages in different organ systems.

6.3.1.1.2

CLINICAL MANIFESTATIONS AND CLASSIFICATION

Clinical manifestations are related to organomegaly, especially splenomegaly, and to bone-marrow and splenic dysfunction (pancytopenia) (Rosenthal et al. 1992). The skeletal manifestations of the disease are well known, and a description is beyond the scope of this chapter. Gaucher's disease is classified into three types.

Type 1, the non-neuronopathic type or adult form, is the most frequent, accounting for 99% of all cases of Gaucher's disease (Taybi and Lachman 1996). The central nervous system is not involved. Clinical presentation can occur at any age and consists of pancytopenia, hepatosplenomegaly, skeletal damage and, occasionally, pulmonary and renal manifestations (Hill et al. 1992). The expected life span is nearly normal. *Type 2*, the acute neuronopathic type, is characterized by early onset of the disease, which consists of neurologic and visceral manifestations. Patients die within the first 2 years of age. *Type 3*, the subacute neuronopathic type or juvenile form, combines slow, progressive neurologic involvement and visceral and skeletal manifestations, but the onset of the disease is usually in childhood.

6.3.1.1.3
Imaging of Splenic Involvement and Histological Correlation

Splenomegaly is found in all patients and is seen on different imaging modalities. Some patients also have focal splenic parenchymal abnormalities on ultrasound, CT and MRI; these abnormalities consist of splenic nodules, splenic infarcts or both.

6.3.1.1.3.1
Ultrasound

Hill et al. (1986) correlated sonographic and histopathological findings of focal spleen lesions in 52 patients. Hypoechoic lesions (Fig. 4b) corresponded to clusters of Gaucher's cells, while hyperechoic lesions (Fig. 4a) were composed of Gaucher's cells, fibrosis or infarction. Aspestrand et al. (1996) reported a case with multiple hypoechoic lesions surrounded by hyperechoic rims (the "target" appearance). In accordance with Hill's observations, the authors state that the hypoechoic lesions represent an inner core of Gaucher's cells, while the hyperechoic rim consists of a mixture of Gaucher's cells, fibrosis and infarcted tissue. This hypothesis correlated very well with the CT and MRI characteristics of the focal lesions.

6.3.1.1.3.2
Computed Tomography

Reports are very rare. In the case, reported by Aspestrand et al. (1989), the lesions were hypodense and enhanced to a lesser degree than the surrounding splenic parenchyma on contrast-enhanced CT and on angiography. This may be due to the reduced vascularity of the focal Gaucher's cell deposits; it may also be the result of surrounding fibrosis or infarction.

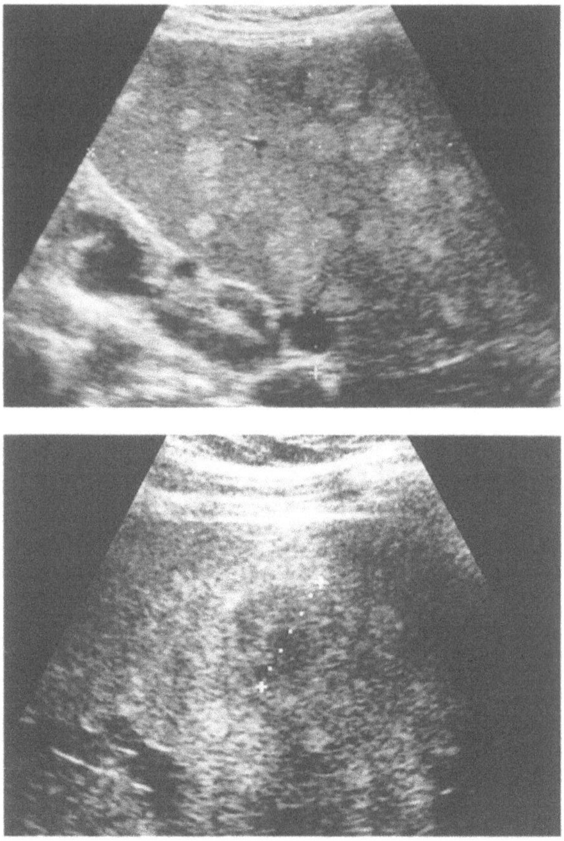

a

b

Fig. 6.4. Gaucher's disease. **a** Ultrasound of the spleen. Multiple hyperechoic lesions within an enlarged spleen. **b** Ultrasound of the spleen in another patient shows an inhomogeneous. enlarged spleen with a central target lesion consisting of a hypoechoic center surrounded by a iso- to hyperechoic rim (*arrow*) (courtesy of M. Maas and C.E. Hollak)

6.3.1.1.3.3
Magnetic Resonance Imaging

The splenic manifestations in a large number of patients on MRI have been described by Hill et al. (1992; 46 patients) and by Terk et al. (1995; 51 patients). All patients had hepatosplenomegaly. Focal splenic nodules with variable signal intensity and different sizes (5–40 mm) were found in 19% of the patients by Terk et al. Splenic nodules of variable signal intensity and different sizes (5–60 mm) were present in 30% of Hill's patient population, while 33% had splenic infarcts with or without associated subcapsular fluid collection, and 9% had both nodules and infarcts. Splenic infarction was more frequent in larger spleens. No adenopathy was found. Most splenic nodules were isointense on T1-

weighted images and hypointense on T2-weighted images (Fig. 6.5), while some lesions were hyperintense on T2-weighted images. A minority of lesions were hyperintense on the T1-weighted images. Target-like lesions were described on T1-weighted images (ASPESTRAND et al. 1989) and T2-weighted images (HILL et al. 1992). Blooming on gradient-recalled-echo images was seen in one case (TERK et al. 1995), suggesting that magnetic susceptibility may be related to the presence of iron (Fig. 6.6). The variable signal intensities in the splenic nodules seem to be related to the variable presence of Gaucher's cells, fibrosis, infarction, dilated sinusoids and blood degradation products in different lesions. However, pathologic correlation with MRI findings has been seen in a few patients so far, and further correlation studies are needed for better understanding of the imaging characteristics. It has been stated that, in target lesions, the peripheral hypointense rim on T1- and T2-weighted images may be due to fibrosis and infarcted tissue (ASPESTRAND et al. 1989). Hyperintense lesions on T2-weighted images may be due to the presence of blood-filled sinusoids, whereas low-signal-intensity lesions on T2-weighted images may correspond to clusters of Gaucher's cells (HILL et al. 1992).

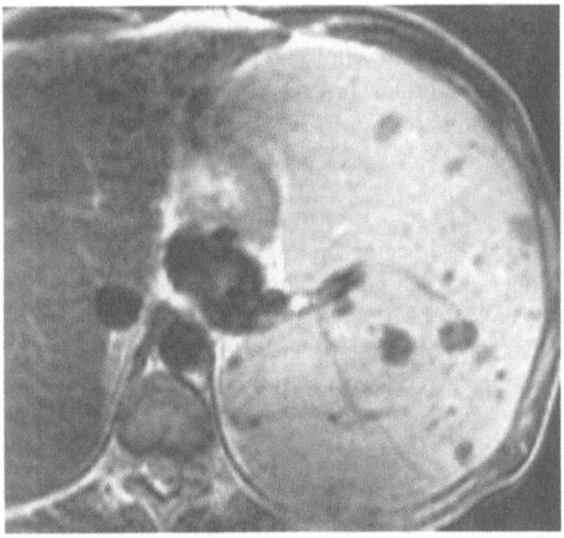

Fig. 6.5. Gaucher's disease. Axial T2-weighted magnetic resonance image. Splenomegaly, as well as multiple hypointense splenic nodules are seen within the splenic parenchyma (courtesy of P. HAHN)

6.3.1.1.4
THERAPY MONITORING

Enzyme replacement therapy using glucocerebrosidase will eliminate most of the clinical manifestations of Gaucher's disease, which consist of a depression of the central marrow activity, increase of the peripheral marrow activity, hepatosplenomegaly and increased reticuloendothelial activity in the lungs. Sequential ^{99m}Tc–sulfur-colloid scintigraphy is very helpful in monitoring the therapy response, as it can demonstrate the changes in bone-marrow and pulmonary uptake associated with improvement in hematological parameters and reduction of hepatosplenomegaly (LORBERBOYM et al. 1997). As splenomegaly is a good parameter for disease activity, CT and MR volumetry can also be used for therapy monitoring of visceral disease. Quantitative imaging methods (such as dual energy CT scan measuring spinal fat fraction, Xenon scanning and MR chemical shift imaging) to evaluate the response of skeletal manifestations to therapy correlate very well with CT and MR volumetry (ROSENTHAL et al. 1992).

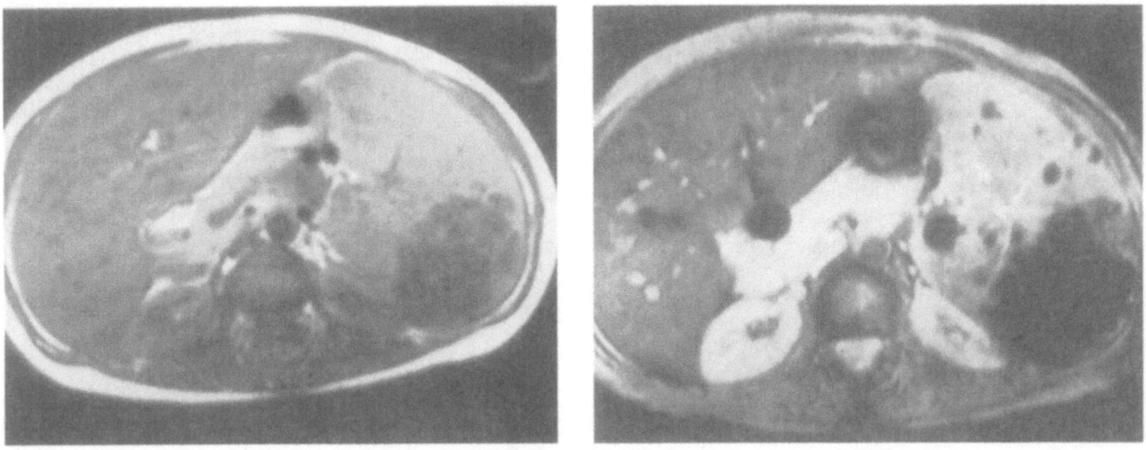

a b

Fig. 6.6. Gaucher's disease. **a** Axial T1-weighted magnetic resonance (MR) image shows coalesced lesions in the posterior part of the spleen. **b** Axial gradient-recalled-echo MR image. "Blooming" of low-signal-intensity lesions, suggesting magnetic susceptibility (TERK et al. 1995)

6.3.1.2
Niemann-Pick Disease

6.3.1.2.1
DEFINITION AND CLASSIFICATION

Niemann-Pick disease represents a group of recessive autosomal diseases that are clinically and biochemically heterogeneous (OMARINI et al. 1995). The basic defect is a disorder of sphingomyelin metabolism, leading to lipid deposition in certain organs (brain, liver, spleen). Four clinical forms of Niemann-Pick disease have been distinguished by SCHUBERT (1994) on the basis of differences in the age of onset and the presence of neurological symptoms.

Type A (NP-A), the neurovisceral form, begins shortly after birth and features neurologic impairment and hepatosplenomegaly. Retinal cherry-red spots may be seen. *Type B (NP-B)*, the visceral form, is mainly characterized by hepatosplenomegaly and pulmonary manifestations (interstitial fibrosis). There is no neurologic involvement. Type B is also called the adult type of Niemann-Pick disease. In *type C (NP-C)*, progressive neurologic deterioration in late infancy and childhood is at the forefront, but hepatosplenic involvement has also been described. Splenomegaly is more frequent than hepatomegaly. *Type D (NP-D)*, the Nova Scotian form, combines hepatosplenomegaly and neurological manifestations. However, the age of onset is later (early to middle childhood).

Two distinct biochemical disorders have recently been characterized. Types A and B are caused by a primary genetic deficiency of sphingomyelinase. Type C is due to a defect in intracellular cholesterol transport. The etiology of type D has not been established yet.

6.3.1.2.2
HISTOLOGY

The metabolic defect results in the storage of lipids (sphingomyelin and cholesterol) in the histiocytes. These multivacuolated, lipid-laden cells (or foam cells) are mainly found in the reticuloendothelial system of the spleen and liver, the lymph nodes, bone marrow and lungs. In types A, C and D, they are also found in the central nervous system. Some macrophages (the "sea-blue" histiocytes) are colored blue by the Giemsa stain.

6.3.1.2.3
CLINICAL MANIFESTATIONS

Depending on the clinical type of the disease, neurological symptoms and symptoms related to visceral infiltration are seen.

6.3.1.2.4
IMAGING OF SPLENIC INVOLVEMENT

Reports of imaging findings are rare. Apart from a moderate splenomegaly, multiple focal lesions in the spleen have been reported by several authors in type B (PASTOR SANTOVENA et al. 1993; SCHUBERT 1994) and type C (OMARINI et al. 1995).

6.3.1.2.4.1
Ultrasound

Nodular splenomegaly with multiple, well-defined hyperechogenic nodules within the spleen are found in types B and C. The hyperechogenicity of the nodules (Fig. 6.7a) has been attributed to their high lipid content by OMARINI et al. (1995).

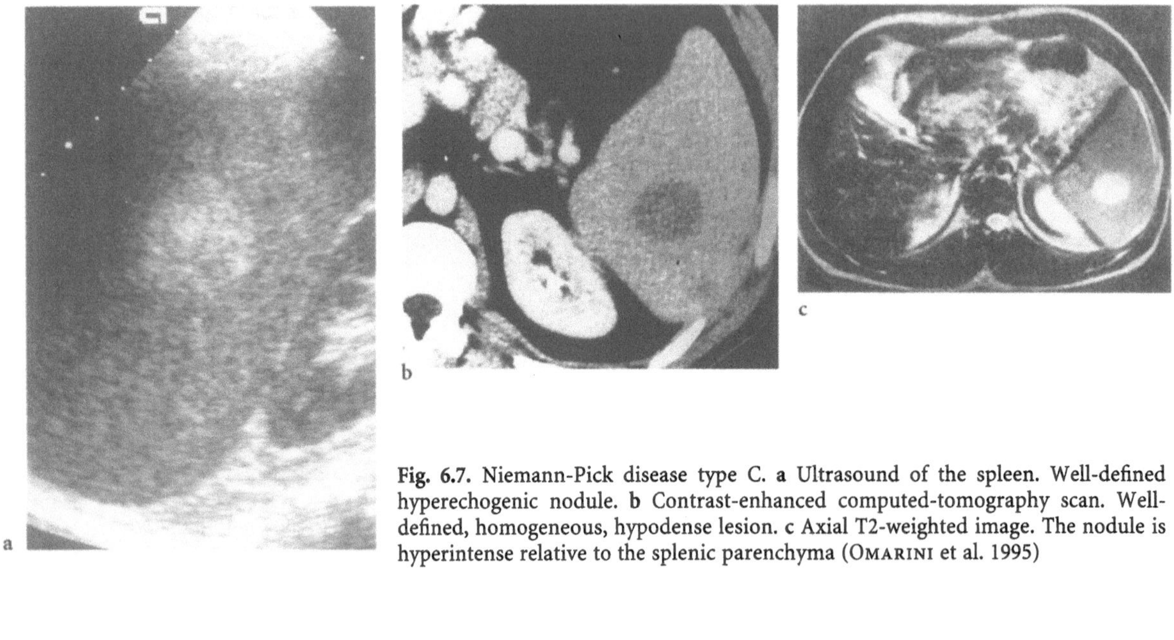

Fig. 6.7. Niemann-Pick disease type C. **a** Ultrasound of the spleen. Well-defined hyperechogenic nodule. **b** Contrast-enhanced computed-tomography scan. Well-defined, homogeneous, hypodense lesion. **c** Axial T2-weighted image. The nodule is hyperintense relative to the splenic parenchyma (OMARINI et al. 1995)

6.3.1.2.4.2
Computed Tomography
The nodular lesions are hypodense on a contrast-enhanced CT scan (Fig. 6.7b), probably a result of diminished blood flow and delayed wash-out of the contrast agent due to the presence of densely packed macrophages (OMARINI et al. 1995).

6.3.1.2.4.3
Magnetic Resonance Imaging
OMARINI et al. (1995) reported a case of type-C Niemann-Pick disease in which the signal intensity of the spleen was increased on T1-weighted and T2-weighted images in comparison with that of the normal volunteer. This probably results from the lipid infiltration of the splenic parenchyma and would suggest that MRI is an excellent tool for the diagnosis of fatty infiltration. The signal intensities of the nodular lesions within the spleen, however, were nonspecific (Fig. 6.7c); they were isointense on T1-weighted images and hyperintense on T2-weighted images, and there was progressive enhancement after gadolinium diethylenetriaminepentaacetic acid administration.

6.3.1.3 Other lysosomal Storage Diseases

Many lysosomal storage diseases are accompanied by some degree of splenic involvement (Table 6.1). Enlargement of the spleen usually occurs later in the course of the disease than hepatomegaly.

Clinical manifestations of splenic infiltration are nonspecific and are due to splenomegaly or hypersplenism. Imaging may reveal a nonspecific splenomegaly. EDELSTEIN et al. (1988) reported a case with massive, symptomatic splenomegaly and a splenic abscess in a patient with cholesteryl-ester storage disease. Tangier disease is a very rare autosomal co-dominant, inherited condition characterized by reduced total cholesterol, raised triglycerides, peripheral neuropathy and accumulation of cholesteryl esters in macrophages; it causes enlargement of the liver, spleen and tonsils (RUST et al. 1998).

6.3.2 Langerhans' Cell Histiocytosis

6.3.2.1 Definition

Langerhans'cell histiocytosis (LCH), previously known as histiocytosis X, is a rare disorder of the bone-marrow-derived histiocytes; it may present as a single-system disease (mainly affecting the bone) or as a multi-system disease. Bone, skin, bone marrow, liver, spleen, lungs, lymph nodes, pancreas, intestine, brain, pituitary gland and buccal involvements have been described. Splenic involvement is

Table 6.1. Lysosomal storage diseases affecting the liver and/or spleen (ISSELBACHER et al. 1994)

Disorder	Enzyme deficiency	Stored material	Genetics
G_{M1} gangliosidosis	β-Galactosidase	G_{M1} ganglioside, glycoproteins, keratan sulfate	AR
Niemann-Pick disease (types B and C)	Sphingomyelinase in types A and B, but not type C	Sphingomyelin, cholesterol	AR
Gaucher's disease	β-Glucocerebrosidase	Glucosylceramide	AR
Cholesteryl ester storage disease	Acid lipase	Cholesteryl ester triglyceride	AR
Fucosidosis	α-Fucosidase	Glycopeptides, glycolipids, oligosaccharides	AR
Mannosidosis	α-Mannosidase	Oligosaccharides	AR
Mucopolysaccharidosis I (Hurler and Scheie forms)	α-Iduronidase	Dermatan sulfate, heparan sulfate	AR
Mucopolysaccharidosis II (Hunter form)	Iduronosulfate sulfatase	Dermatan sulfate, heparan sulfate	X-linked
Mucopolysaccharidosis III types A, B, C, D (Sanfilippo form)	Variable according to different type	Heparan sulfate	AR
Mucopolysaccharidosis IV (Morquio form)	*N*-Acetylgalactosamine-6-sulfate sulfatase	Keratan sulfate	AR
Mucopolysaccharidosis VI (Maroteaux-Lamy form)	*N*-Acetylhexosamine-4-sulfate sulfatase (arylsulfatase B)	Dermatan sulfate	AR
Mucopolysaccharidosis VII (β-glucuronidase deficiency)	β-Glucuronidase	Dermatan sulfate, heparan sulfate (?)	AR
Multiple sulfatase deficiency	Arylsulfatases A, B, and C, other sulfatases	Sulfatides, mucopolysaccharides	AR
Sialidosis	Sialidase	Sialyloligosaccharides	AR
Galactosialidosis	Protective glycoprotein	Sialyloligosaccharides	AR

AR, autosomal recessive

usually part of multi-system disease, while isolated involvement of the spleen is exceptional (Lam et al. 1996). The etiology of the disease is still unclear, and it is still debated whether LCH is a reactive lesion or a true neoplastic lesion.

6.3.2.2
Clinical Manifestations

The symptomatology depends on the affected organ systems. Multi-system involvement is mainly found in children, and the prognosis depends on the age of onset. Early-onset of multi-system involvement (before 2 years of age) has a poor prognosis. Children with systemic involvement diagnosed after the age of 2 years have an intermediate prognosis. Multi-system involvement in adults is rare but has a better prognosis than in children (McLelland and Chu 1990). Single-system disease found in children and adults has a very good prognosis.

6.3.2.3
Pathology of Splenic Involvement

Splenic infiltration of systemic LCH is usually found at autopsy and is characterized by a diffuse splenic red-pulp infiltration by Langerhans' cells. Splenomegaly and splenic rupture have been described on gross findings, but a solitary nodular lesion is rare (Lam et al. 1996). Microscopic findings include the presence of Langerhans' cells, with the characteristic Birbeck granule within their cytoplasms on electron microscopic examination.

6.3.2.4
Imaging

Reports on imaging findings of LCH are very rare.

6.3.2.4.1
ULTRASOUND
Muwakkit et al. (1994) described a case of disseminated LCH in a 4-week-old infant with multiple, round, hypoechoic lesions of varying sizes in an enlarged spleen (Fig. 6.8). Apart from the splenic lesions, lesions were found in the lungs and the pancreas. A second case of a solitary hyperechoic lesion within the spleen was reported by Williams and Fairhurst (1995) in a child with LCH, but the exact nature of the splenic lesion was uncertain.

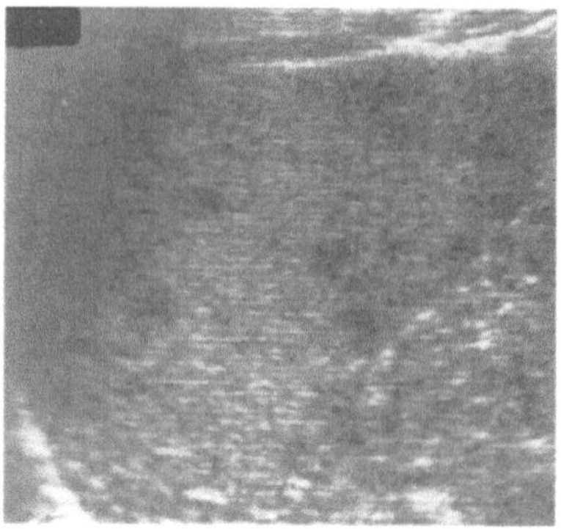

Fig. 6.8. Langerhans' cell histiocytosis. Sagittal ultrasound of the spleen. Multiple hypoechoic lesions of varying size within an enlarged spleen (Muwakkit et al. 1994)

6.3.2.4.2
COMPUTED TOMOGRAPHY
A rare case of LCH with hepatosplenic involvement in an adult was reported by Mampaey et al. (1999). On contrast-enhanced CT, multiple, well-defined, rounded or oval low-attenuation nodules with subtle ring enhancement were seen in the liver and the spleen (Fig. 6.9).

6.3.2.5
Differential Diagnosis

Malignant (aggressive) LCH must be distinguished from hemophagocytic syndrome, which consists of a generalized histiocytic proliferation and marked hemophagocytosis. Clinically, it presents as pancytopenia and hepatosplenomegaly. It may be complicated by spontaneous splenic rupture (Bell and Wright 1992).

6.3.3
Amyloidosis

6.3.3.1
Definition

Amyloidosis is the deposition of eosinophilic proteinaceous material (amyloid substance) in different organs. Generally, two clinical types of amyloidosis are distinguished. In *primary* amyloidosis, there is no evidence for co-existing disease whereas, in *secondary* amyloidosis, there is a well-known association with chronic infection, RA, multiple myeloma

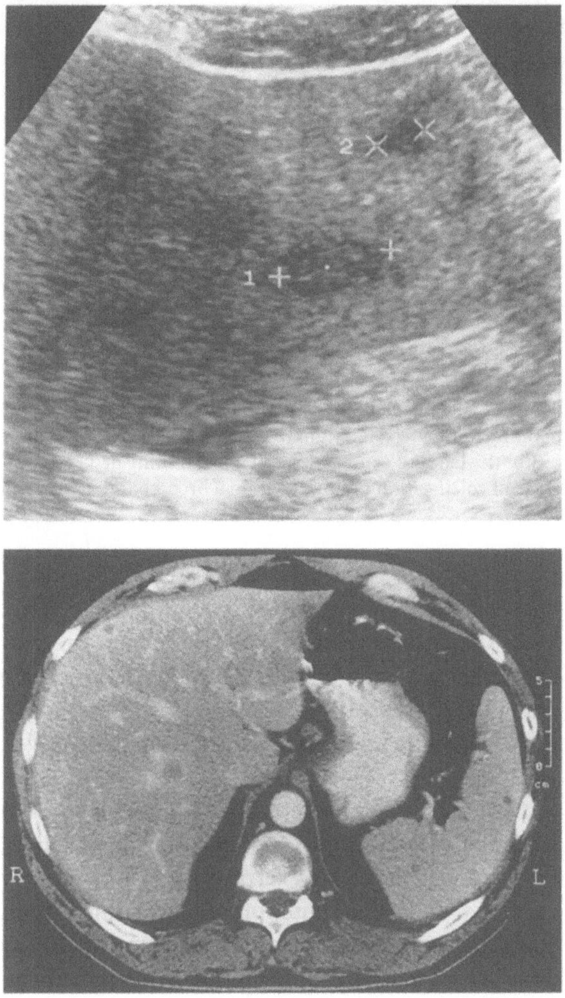

a

b

Fig. 6.9. Langerhans' cell histiocytosis. **a** Ultrasound of the liver. Multiple target lesions with a bull's-eye appearance within a slightly enlarged liver. **b** Contrast-enhanced computed-tomography scan. Multiple, well-circumscribed, hypodense lesions within the liver and the spleen. There is mild splenomegaly (MAMPAEY et al. 1999)

and long-standing hemodialysis. Splenic involvement in amyloidosis is common, as the cells of the reticuloendothelial system play a major role in the formation of amyloid (KOZICKY et al. 1987).

6.3.3.2
Clinical Manifestations of Splenic Involvement

Although splenic involvement of amyloidosis is frequent, most patients present without symptoms, or their symptoms are nonspecific. Clinical manifestations include fullness in the left upper quadrant due to splenomegaly, deficiency of factor-X coagulation factor, splenic rupture and, rarely, splenic infarction (KOZICKY et al. 1987). On physical examination, however, splenomegaly is only found in a minority of patients with known amyloidosis (WILSON and YAWN 1979). A rare life-threatening complication of amyloidosis of the spleen is spontaneous splenic rupture with resulting acute abdominal pain, hemoperitoneum and hypotension (RUSSELL and FERRERA 1998). Most of the reported cases are due to primary amyloidosis, and the splenic rupture was the initial sign of previously undiagnosed disease.

The mechanism for splenic rupture in amyloidosis remains unclear. KOZICKY et al. (1987) suggested that vascular fragility from amyloid deposition and factor-X deficiency may play a role in the pathogenesis of spontaneous splenic rupture.

6.3.3.3
Pathology of Splenic Involvement

Amyloid deposits are usually found in the splenic parenchyma and in the splenic vasculature (CUBO et al. 1997).

6.3.3.4
Imaging

Cross-sectional imaging is rarely performed in patients with amyloidosis of the spleen, because most patients have no clinical symptoms related to splenic amyloid infiltration. Apart from nonspecific features, such as organomegaly and heterogeneous attenuation, no characteristic features that distinguish amyloidosis from other infiltrative disorders have been reported. In exceptional cases, extensive visceral calcifications involving both the liver and the spleen are seen in primary amyloidosis (Fig. 6.10). According to JACOBS et al. (1997), the affinity of amyloid fibrils for calcium explains this association.

In cases of acute spontaneous splenic rupture and when the patient is hemodynamically stable, ultrasound and emergency CT of the abdomen are the procedures of choice to confirm hemoperitoneum and an enlarged inhomogeneous spleen. However, preoperative diagnosis remains difficult, as this condition mimics many abdominal emergency states (CUBO et al. 1997). Scintigraphic imaging and turnover studies with ^{131}I-labelled serum amyloid component P have been used successfully by HAWKINS et al. (1998) in diagnosis and therapy monitoring of systemic amyloidosis with spleen involvement.

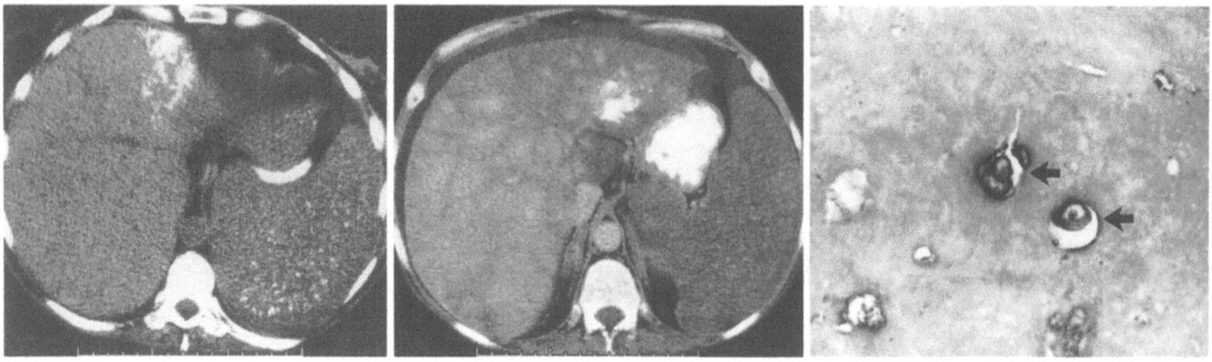

Fig. 6.10. Amyloidosis. **a** Unenhanced computed tomography (CT) scan. Hepatosplenomegaly with extensive left hepatic-lobe calcification and diffuse calcification of the splenic parenchyma. **b** Contrast-enhanced CT scan. Heterogeneous hepatic enhancement, with large regions of decreased parenchymal attenuation within the left and caudate lobes. Global diminished enhancement of the spleen. **c** A histopathologic section shows prevalent areas of calcification (*arrows*) within a broad band of amyloid (*H* and *E*; 400×) (Jacobs et al. 1997)

6.3.4 Iron-Overload Diseases

6.3.4.1 *Definition and Classification*

Iron-overload diseases can be separated into two different groups depending on the location of iron deposition (Dachman et al. 1993; Yoon et al. 1994). *Hemochromatosis* is the term used for abnormal *parenchymal* iron deposition, which occurs mainly in the hepatocyte but also in the pancreas, heart and synovium. Hemochromatosis can be idiopathic due to an inborn error of metabolism that leads to an inappropriate increase in intestinal iron absorption. The absorbed iron is bound to plasma transferrin and preferentially deposited (in the form of ferritin and hemosiderin) into parenchymal cells of the liver, pancreas, heart and other organs. Moreover, the reticuloendothelial cells in patients with hereditary hemochromatosis are also abnormal and are unable to store iron effectively. The consequence is that iron deposition in the spleen does not occur in hemochromatosis. Secondary hemochromatosis may occur in cases of intravascular hemolysis, congenital transferrin deficiency disorders, dietary iron ingestion, portacaval shunts or ineffective erythropoiesis in the bone marrow (erythropoietic hemochromatosis). In cases of intravascular hemolysis, red blood cells are destroyed within the circulation, and the resultant free hemoglobin is bound to plasma haptoglobin and taken up by the hepatocytes. If the haptoglobin system becomes saturated, the free hemoglobin is filtered by the kidney and stored in the real parenchyma. Erythropoietic hemochromatosis develops in patients with thalassemia major, sideroblastic anemia, megaloblastic anemia or, rarely, any chronic anemia. These patients hyperabsorb iron inappropriately, although the responsible mechanism is unknown (Yoon et al. 1994).

Hemosiderosis is the term used for iron deposition in the *reticuloendothelial system* of the liver, spleen, lymph nodes and bone marrow; it most commonly develops following multiple blood transfusions (transfusional iron overload). Rhabdomyolysis may be another cause of iron deposition in the reticuloendothelial system.

6.3.4.2 *Clinical Manifestations*

Distinction of hemochromatosis and hemosiderosis is clinically important, because parenchymal iron deposition may cause cellular damage and organ dysfunction, while iron deposition in the reticuloendothelial system is usually innocent. In severe disease, when the reticuloendothelial-system storage capacity of 10 g of iron becomes saturated, the iron begins to accumulate in parenchymal cells of different organs, and toxic effects may occur (Dachman et al. 1993). Clinical manifestations depend on the involvement of the different parenchymal organs in hemochromatosis. Hepatic involvement usually presents as hepatomegaly, with surprisingly normal liver function tests. Evolution to cirrhosis occurs. Hepatocellular carcinoma is a life-threatening complication that develops in about 30% of patients with cirrhosis. Splenomegaly is present in half of the symptomatic cases (POWELL and ISSELBACHER 1994). Diabetes mellitus occurs in 65% of patients and is due to combination of pancreatic involvement and a familial predisposition (POWELL and ISSELBACHER 1994). Cardiac involvement with cardiac arrhythmias and congestive heart failure, arthropathy, skin pigmentation and endocrine dysfunction are other well-known clinical features.

6.3.4.3 *Histopathology of Splenic Involvement*

Iron deposition occurs in the reticuloendothelial system of the spleen in hemosiderosis. Splenomegaly occurs in association with symptomatic liver involvement in hemochromatosis.

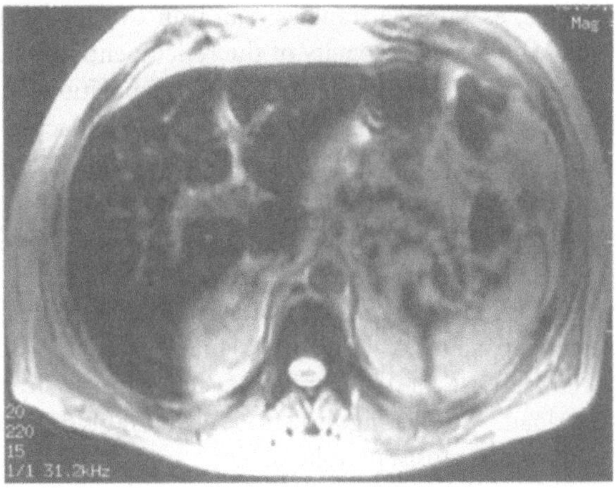

Fig. 6.11. Hemochromatosis. Axial gradient-echo T2*-weighted image. Low signal intensity of the liver (and pancreas) and a normal signal intensity of the spleen (courtesy of F. DECKERS)

6.3.4.4 *Imaging*

Plain film is very insensitive but may demonstrate, in very rare cases, a homogeneous increased hepatic radiopacity (DACHMAN et al. 1993). Ultrasound and scintigraphy are of little use in documenting non-complicated iron overload but may detect secondary cirrhosis and hepatocellular carcinoma (DACHMAN et al. 1993).

6.3.4.4.1 COMPUTED TOMOGRAPHY

In the past, non-contrast CT and dual-energy CT scans have been used for diagnosis and therapy monitoring of iron-overload diseases. Hemochromatosis causes elevated densities of the liver between 75 Hounsfield units and 130 Hounsfield units, and shows a contrast of the intrahepatic veins against the background of the hyperdense liver. However, these findings are not specific and are very insensitive for moderate degrees of iron deposition. CT cannot detect iron overload below four times the normal level and remains of limited clinical value, especially in cases of coexisting steatosis. Even dual-energy CT scans seem to be of little value (GUYADER et al. 1992). Complications like cirrhosis and hepatocellular carcinoma can be detected, however.

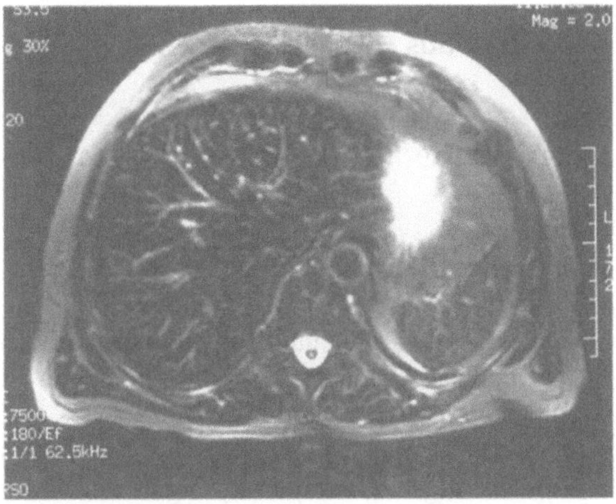

Fig. 6.12. Hemosiderosis. Axial fat-suppressed fast spin-echo T2-weighted image. Low signal intensity of the liver and the spleen (courtesy of F. DECKERS)

6.3.4.4.2 MAGNETIC RESONANCE IMAGING

MRI is a more sensitive and specific method than CT scans in detecting iron overload, due to the magnetic-susceptibility effect caused by the accumulated iron. A markedly decreased signal intensity (compared with that seen in skeletal muscle) is seen in involved organs on T2-weighted images, especially on T2*-weighted gradient-echo images (because of the greater sensitivity of gradient-echo sequences to susceptibility artifacts).

The pattern of iron distribution in different organs enables distinction of hemochromatosis from hemosiderosis. In hemochromatosis (Fig. 6.11), a low signal intensity on T2- and T2*-weighted images is found in the liver, pancreas, myocardium and endocrine glands, but the spleen remains normal (SIEGELMAN et al. 1991). In hemosiderosis (Fig. 6.12), iron deposition predominates in the liver, spleen and bone marrow but not in the pancreas. However, there is some overlap between the two groups, as massive transfusional iron overload beyond the storage capacity of the reticuloendothelial system can lead to parenchymal iron deposition, especially in the pancreas (Yoon et al. 1994). According to Yoon et al. (1994), however, the signal intensity of the spleen may allow distinction between transfusional iron overload and (erythropoetic) hemochromatosis. The distinction between the primary form of hemochromatosis and secondary hemochromatosis, however, remains difficult on MRI because of the similar mechanisms of iron overload. To distinguish these two subtypes of hemochromatosis, peripheral blood smears or bone-marrow biopsies are still necessary (Yoon et al. 1994).

6.4 Miscellaneous Diseases

6.4.1 Sarcoidosis

6.4.1.1 Definition

Sarcoidosis is a chronic multisystem disease of unknown etiology characterized by accumulation of T-cell lymphocytes, mononuclear phagocytes and formation of non-caseating epithelioid granulomas in different organs. Nearly every organ can be affected, but lung involvement is the most frequent, followed by the skin, eyes, lymph nodes, abdominal viscera, central nervous system and bones. Any age group can be affected, but most patients present between 20 years and 40 years of age. The prevalence is 10–40 per 100,000 individuals, and there is a large diversity among certain ethnic and racial groups (Crystal 1994).

6.4.1.2 Clinical Manifestations

The clinical manifestations depend on the affected organ system and may be generalized or focused on certain organs. Thoracic manifestations are well known and are discussed elsewhere in detail. Splenic involvement can accompany hepatic involvement, but isolated splenic or hepatic involvement has also been described (Scott et al. 1997). Splenomegaly is only noted in 5–10% of patients with sarcoidosis, while hepatomegaly and/or biochemical evidence of hepatocellular dysfunction is present in 20–30%. Hepatosplenic involvement can occur in association with or in the absence of intrathoracic disease. Splenic rupture is an unusual complication of splenic sarcoidosis (Albala et al. 1989). Abdominal manifestations are well correlated to disease activity but are not related to changes in chest radiographic stage or disease duration. Angiotensin-converting enzyme (ACE) is a very good parameter of disease activity and reflects the total body burden of the disease (Warshauwer et al. 1995). However, caution should be used in evaluation of ACE level in patients who receive systemic steroids. These drugs reduce ACE levels in patients with sarcoidosis.

6.4.1.3 Histopathology

Histologically, non-caseating epithelial granulomas are found within affected organs. There is a big discrepancy between the clinical or radiological evidence of hepatosplenic disease and the presence of liver granulomata on necropsy (70%) and splenic granulomata on fine needle aspiration (up to 59%) in patients with sarcoidosis. The exact incidence of hepatosplenic involvement is, therefore, uncertain (Scott et al. 1997).

6.4.1.4 Imaging of Splenic Involvement

The most common imaging features are nonspecific and consist of hepatosplenomegaly and retroperitoneal adenopathy, followed by focal hepatic and/or splenic nodules. Focal hepatic and splenic lesions were identified in 5% and 15% of cases of splenic sarcoidosis, respectively, by Warshauwer et al. (1994a). This nodular pattern seems to be more common in the first 5 years of the disease and is frequently accompanied by abdominal or systemic symptomatology and elevation of the level of ACE (Warshauwer et al. 1995). Rare complications of splenic sarcoidosis, such as splenic rupture, can be documented by cross-sectional imaging (Fig. 6.13).

6.4.1.4.1 Ultrasound

In a series of 17 patients with biopsy-proven sarcoidosis reported by Kessler et al. (1993), eight patients had a normal splenic echogenicity and a

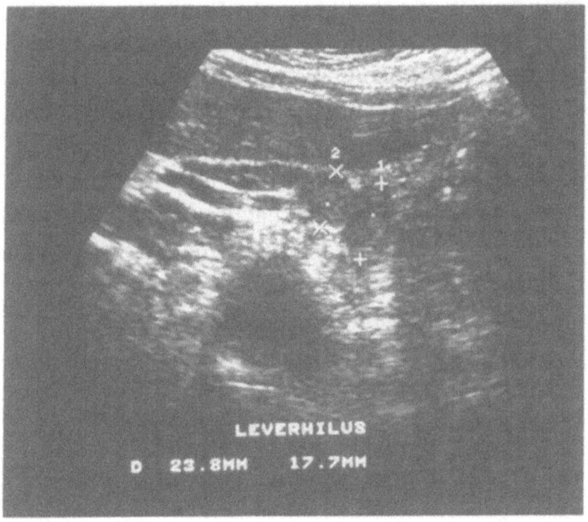

a

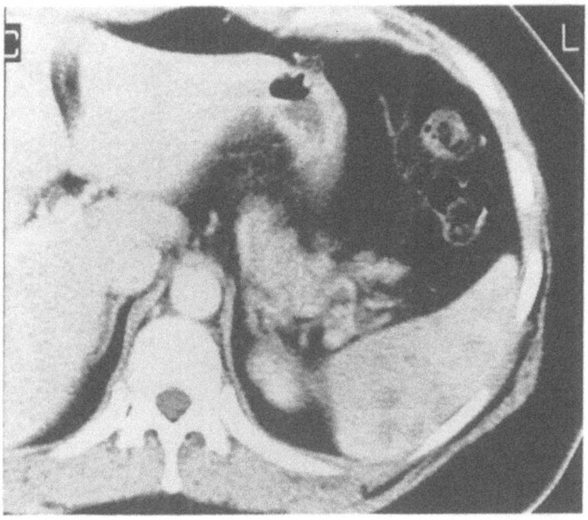

b

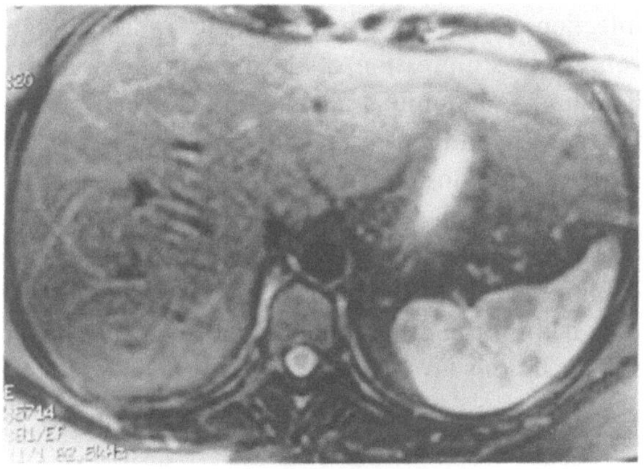

c

Fig. 6.13. Sarcoidosis. **a** Ultrasound of the spleen. Multiple round and oval, well-delineated hypoechoic nodules (lymph nodes) within the porta hepatis (periaortic and interaortocaval region). **b** Contrast-enhanced computed-tomography scan of the upper abdomen, in another patient. Multiple hypodense lesions within the spleen ("spotted spleen") (courtesy of S. Declerck). **c** Axial T2-weighted image of the upper abdomen. Multiple low-signal-intensity lesions throughout the spleen

normal spleen size, eight presented with a normal echogenicity in an enlarged spleen and one patient had discrete hypoechoic nodules within an enlarged spleen. Abdominal adenopathy (Fig. 14a) with periportal and peripancreatic distribution was demonstrated in three patients. On ultrasound, most patients (11 of 17) also displayed liver abnormalities, including hepatomegaly, homogeneous or heterogeneous increased echogenicity, irregular contour, focal hypoechoic nodules or calcifications.

6.4.1.4.2
Computed Tomography

Scott et al. (1997) reviewed 30 cases of splenic sarcoidosis with nodular patterns appearing as hypodense lesions on contrast-enhanced CT scans (Fig. 14b). Common to all cases was the multiplicity and variability in nodular lesions, which often ranged in size from 1 mm to 30 mm and were generally innumerable. CT detection of focal lesions in sarcoidosis is much less frequent than the incidence of granulomata on histology, but recent improvements in intravenous contrast delivery techniques, CT spatial resolution and rapid scanner times will probably improve the detection of hepatosplenic nodules in the future. According to Warshauwer et al. (1995), these nodules correspond to the coalescence of microscopic sarcoid granulomata. The cause of this aggregation is uncertain and may be related to an immunologic response. There is no strict correlation between organomegaly and the nodular pattern.

6.4.1.4.3
Magnetic Resonance Imaging

Kessler et al. (1993) reported MRI splenic abnormalities, including splenomegaly, contour irregularity, nodularity and heterogeneous low signal inten-sity, suggestive of iron overload. According to Warshauwer et al. (1994b), sarcoid lesions are small (<1 cm) and hypovascular. Due to their hypovascularity, the lesions are of low signal intensity on T1- and T2-weighted images and enhance on gadolinium-enhanced images in a delayed fashion.

a

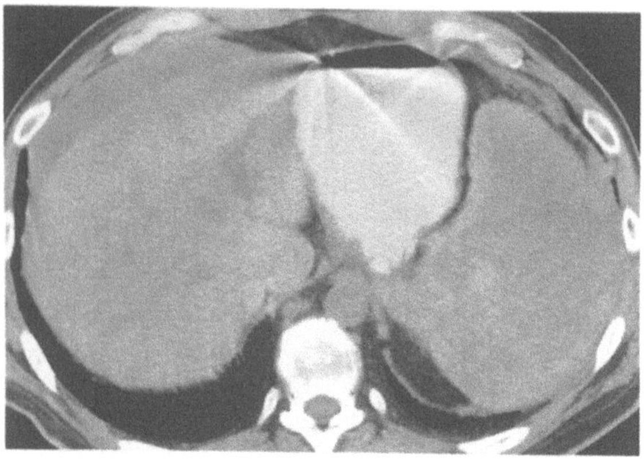

b

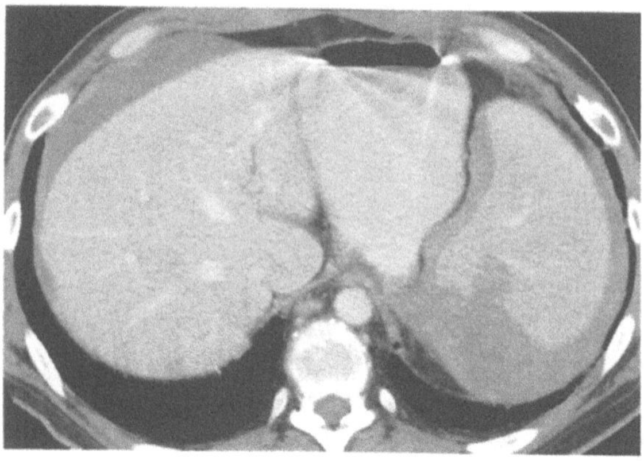

Fig. 6.14. Sarcoidosis. **a** Non contrast-enhanced computed-tomography (CT) scan of the upper abdomen. **b** Contrast-enhanced CT scan of the upper abdomen. Surgically proven splenic rupture due to sarcoid vasculitis. Note the enlarged spleen and the perisplenic and perihepatic free fluid, which is hyperdense around the spleen on the non contrast-enhanced images, suggesting acute splenic rupture (courtesy of P. Hahn)

Low signal intensity on T2-weighted images is a differential diagnostic characteristic used to distinguish between nodular sarcoid lesions and acute infections (Fig. 14c).

6.4.1.5 Differential Diagnosis

The differential diagnosis of the multinodular pattern includes lymphoma, leukemia, splenic metastases, infectious lesions and benign entities, such as hemangiomatosis and unknown clinical benign entities. Warshauwer et al. (1998) distinguished three categories of patients presenting with multiple focal splenic lesions, based on differences in symptomatology and the notion of known primary malignancy. In the symptomatic patient without known malignancy, one should mainly think of lymphoma, infection and sarcoid. In the asymptomatic patient without known malignancy, benign tumor, sarcoid, and non-lymphomatous metastatic disease should be considered whereas, in patients with known malignancy, multiple focal lesions may represent metastases. Good differential diagnostic parameters are lesion size on CT scan and low signal intensity of the lesions on T2-weighted MRI, in addition to clinical data and the distribution and size of associated lymphadenopathy. Although overlap exits among diagnostic groups, lymphoma tends to have larger, more variable nodules, whereas infection tends to occur with smaller, more uniform nodules. Sarcoid is intermediate in appearance (Warshauwer et al. 1998). The low signal intensity on the T2-weighted images may help in the differential diagnosis with infection. Moreover, infection usually appears in the context of suppression of the immune system. In lymphoma, abdominal adenopathy is usually more widespread, and retrocrural adenopathy is less common in sarcoidosis than in lymphoma (18% versus 70%). The lymph nodes are usually larger than those of sarcoidosis, which have a mean diameter of 1.6 cm. Moreover, the elevated ACE level in sarcoidosis may help in the differential diagnosis of multifocal splenic lesions (Warshauwer et al. 1995).

6.4.2 Other

Warhauwer et al. (1998) reported a case of a spotted spleen (due to delayed reaction to the drug phenytoin) on CT. Splenic manifestations of porphyria, hypersensitivity state and other complications of drug therapy or use are not discussed in detail because of the extremely low prevalence.

References

Albala MM, Anamur M, Bernardo JR (1989) Delayed spontaneous splenic rupture in sarcoidosis. R I Med J 72:175–177
Armbruster C, Vetter N (1991) Wegenersche Granulomatose mit Milzbeteiligung und Thyreoiditis lymphomatosa Hashimoto. Pneumologie 45:28–31
Aspestrand F, Charania B, Scheel B, et al. (1989) Focal changes of the spleen in one case of Gaucher's disease-assessed by ultrasonography, CT, MRI and angiography. Radiologe 29:569–571
Bell MD, Wright RK (1992) Fatal virus-associated hemophagocytic syndrome in a young adult producing non-traumatic splenic rupture. J Forensic Sci 37:1407–1417
Buskila D, Gladman DD, Hannah W, et al. (1989) Primary

malignant lymphoma of the spleen in systemic lupus erythematosus. J Rheumatol 16:993–996
Cohen BA, Mitty HA, Mendelson DS (1984) Computed tomography of splenic infarction. J Comput Assist Tomogr 8:167–168
Crystal RG (1994) Sarcoidosis. In: Isselbacher KJ, Braunwald E, Wilson JD, et al. (eds) Harrison's principles of internal medicine, 13th edn. McGraw-Hill, New York, pp 1679–1684
Cubo T, Ramia JM, Pardo R, et al. (1997) Spontaneous rupture of the spleen in amyloidosis. Am J Emerg Med 15:443–444
Dachman AH, Fishman EK, Friedman AC (1993) Miscellaneous disorders. In: Dachman AH, Friedman AC (eds) Radiology of the spleen. Mosby Year Book, St. Louis, pp 207–212
Du Cret RP, Adkins MC, Halvorsen RA Jr, et al. (1991) Ectopic splenomegaly in Felty's syndrome. Clin Nucl Med 16:160–161
Edelstein RA, Filling-Katz MR, Pentchev P, et al. (1988) Cholesteryl ester storage disease: a patient with massive splenomegaly and splenic abscess. Am J Gastroenterol 83:687–692
Fishman D, Isenberg DA (1997) Splenic involvement in rheumatic diseases. Semin Arthritis Rheum 27:141–155
Fonner BT, Nemcek AA, Bochman C (1995) CT appearance of splenic infarction in Wegener's granulomatosis. AJR Am J Roentgenol 164:353–354
Ford GA, Bradley JR, Appleton DS, et al. (1986) Spontaneous splenic rupture in polyarteritis nodosa. Postgrad Med J 62:965–966
Franssen CFM, Ter Maaten JC, Hoorntje SJ (1993) Spontaneous splenic rupture in Wegener's vasculitis. Ann Rheum Dis 52:314
Gregorini G, Campanini M, Tira P, et al. (1990) Spleen involvement in Wegener's granulomatosis: two case reports. APMIS Suppl 19:23
Guyader D, Gandon Y, Robert J-Y, et al. (1992) Magnetic resonance imaging and assessment of liver iron content in genetic hemochromatosis. J Hepatol 15:304–308
Hahn BH (1994) Systemic lupus erythematosus In: Isselbacher KJ, Braunwald E, Wilson JD, et al. (eds) Harrison's principles of internal medicine, 13th edn. McGraw-Hill, New York, pp 1643–1648
Haskard DO, Higgens CS, Temple LN, et al. (1983) Spontaneous rupture of the spleen in rheumatoid arthritis. Ann Rheum Dis 42:411–414
Hawkins PN, Aprile C, Capri G, et al. (1998) Scintigraphic imaging and turnover studies with iodine-131-labelled serum amyloid P component in systemic amyloidosis. Eur J Nucl Med 25:701–708
Hill SC, Reinig JW, Barranger JA, et al. (1986) Gaucher's disease: sonographic appearance of the spleen. Radiology 160:631–634
Hill SC, Damaska BM, Ling A, et al. (1992) Gaucher's disease: abdominal MR imaging findings in 46 patients. Radiology 184:561–566
Hofbauer LC, Diebold J, Heufelder AE (1995) Rheumatoide Arthritis, neutropenie und splenomegalie: Felty-syndrom. Dtsch Med Wochenschr 120:1689–1694
Isselbacher KJ, Braunwald E, Wilson JD, et al. (eds) Harrison's principles of internal medicine, 13th edn. McGraw-Hill, New York
Jacobs JE, Birnbaum BA, Furth EE (1997) Abdominal visceral calcification in primary amyloidosis: CT findings. Abdomin Imaging 22:519–521
Kalaitzoglou I, Drevelengas A, Palladas P, et al. (1998) MRI appearance of pulmonary Wegener's granulomatosis with concomitant splenic infarction. Eur Radiol 8:367–370
Kessler A, Mitchell DG, Israel HL, et al. (1993) Hepatic and splenic sarcoidosis: ultrasound and MR imaging. Abdom Imaging 18:159–163
Kozicky OJ, Brandt LJ, Lederman M, et al. (1987) Splenic amyloidosis: a case report of spontaneous splenic rupture with a review of the pertinent literature. Am J Gastroenterol 82:582–587
Lam KY, Chan ACL, Wat MS (1996) Langerhans' cell histiocytosis forming an asymptomatic solitary nodule in the spleen. J Clin Pathol 49:262–264
Leavitt RY, Fauci AS, Block DA, et al. (1990) The American College of Rheumatology criteria for the classification of Wegener's granulomatosis. Arthritis Rheum 33:1101–1107
Lipsky PE (1994) Rheumatoid arthritis. In: Isselbacher KJ, Braunwald E, Wilson JD, et al. (eds) Harrison's principles of internal medicine, 13th edn. McGraw-Hill, New York, pp 1648–1653
Lorberboym M, Pastores GM, Kim CK, et al. (1997) Scintigraphic monitoring of reticuloendothelial system in patients with type-1 Gaucher's disease on enzyme replacement therapy. J Nucl Med 38:890–895
Malleson P, PettyRE, Nadel H, et al. (1988) Functional asplenia in childhood onset systemic lupus erythematosus. J Rheumatol 15:1648–1652
Mampaey S, Warson F, Van Hedent E, et al. (1999) Langerhans' cell histiocytosis of the liver and the spleen in an adult: imaging findings and evolution Eur Radiol 9:96–98
McHugh K, Manson D, Eberhard BA, et al. (1991) Splenic necrosis in Wegener's granulomatosis. Pediatr Radiol 21:588–589
McLelland J, Chu AC (1990) Multi-system Langerhans' cell histiocytosis in adults. Clin Exp Dermatol 15:79–82
Morayati SJ, Fink-Benett D (1986) Indium-111 leukocyte scintigraphy in Wegener's granulomatosis involving the spleen. J Nucl Med 27:864–1966
Muwakkit S, Gharagozloo A, Souid AK, et al. (1994) The sonographic appearance of lesions of the spleen and pancreas in an infant with Langerhans' cell histiocytosis. Pediatr Radiol 24:222–223
Nakamura H, Ohishi A, Asano K, et al. (1994) Partial splenic embolization for Felty's syndrome: a 10-year follow-up. J Rheumatol 21:1964–1966
Omarini LP, Frank-Burkhardt SE, Seemayer TA, et al. (1995) Niemann-Pick disease type C: nodular splenomegaly. Abdom Imaging 20:157–160
Pastor Santovena S, Fernandez-Ramos J, Gonzalez-Reimers, et al. (1993) Ultrasonographic features of type-B Niemann-Pick disease. Eur J Radiol 16:215–216
Powell LW, Isselbacher KJ (1994) Hemochromatosis. In: Isselbacher KJ, Braunwald E, Wilson JD, et al. (eds) Harrison's principles of internal medicine, 13th edn. McGraw-Hill, New York, pp 2069–2073
Rosenthal DI, Barton NW, McKusick KA, et al. (1992) Quantitative imaging of Gaucher's disease. Radiology 185:841–845
Ruel M, Bobrie G, Jarrousse B, et al. (1989) Iconographie splénique au cours de la granulomatose de Wegener. Presse Med 18:725
Russell TJ, Ferrera PC (1998) Spontaneous rupture of an amyloid spleen in a patient on continuous ambulatory peritoneal dialysis. Am J Emerg Med 16:279–280
Rust S, Walter M, Funke H, et al. (1998) Assignment of Tangier disease to chromosome 9q31 by a graphical linkage exclusion strategy. Nat Genet 20:96–98
Schubert F (1994) Echogenic splenic tumours in type-B Niemann-Pick disease. Australas Radiol 38:127–129

Scott GC, Berman JM, Higgins JL (1997) CT patterns of nodular hepatic and splenic sarcoidosis: a review of the literature. J Comput Assist Tomogr 21:369–372

Siegelman ES, Mitchell DG, Rubin R, et al. (1991) Parenchymal versus reticuloendothelial iron overload in the liver: distinction with MR imaging. Radiology 179:361–366

Taybi H, Lachman RS (1996) In: Taybi H, Lachman RS (eds) Radiology of syndromes, metabolic disorders, and skeletal dysplasias. Mosby Year Book, St. Louis, pp 588–592

Terk MR, Esplin J, Lee K, et al. (1995) MR imaging of patients with type-1 Gaucher's disease: relationship between bone and visceral changes. AJR Am J Roentgenol 165:599–604

Tolaymat A, Al-Mousily F, Haafiz AB, et al. (1995) Spontaneous rupture of the spleen in a patient with systemic lupus erythematosus. J Rheumatol 22:2344–2345

Van Krieken JHJM, Breedveld FC, Te Velde J (1988) The spleen in Felty's syndrome: a histological, morphometrical, and immunohistochemical study. Eur J Haematol 40:58–64

Van Linthoudt D, Greder B, Ott H (1990) Overlap syndrome with multiple calcifications of the spleen. Clin Rheumatol 9:88–91

Venbrux AC, Dachman AH, Fishman EK (1993) Vascular disease. In: Dachman AH, Friedman AC (eds) Radiology of the spleen. Mosby Year Book, St. Louis, pp 171–205

Warshauwer DM, Dumbleton SA, Molina PL, et al. (1994a) Abdominal CT findings in sarcoidosis: radiologic and clinical correlation. Radiology 192:93–98

Warshauwer DM, Semelka RC, Ascher SM (1994b) Nodular sarcoidosis of the liver and spleen: appearance on MR images. J Magn Reson Imaging 4:553–557

Warshauwer DM, Molina PL, Hamman SM, et al. (1995) Nodular sarcoidosis of the liver and spleen: analysis of 32 cases. Radiology 195:757–762

Warshauwer DM, Molina PL, Worawanttanakul S (1998) The spotted spleen: CT and clinical correlation in a tertiary care center. J Comput Assist Tomogr 22:694–702

Williams PH, Fairhurst JJ (1995) Sonographic and radiographic appearance of lesions in an infant with Langerhans'cell histiocytosis. Pediatr Radiol 25:401–402

Wilson H, Yawn DH (1979) Rupture of the spleen in amyloidosis. JAMA 241:790–791

Yoon DY, Choi BI, Han JK, et al. (1994) MR findings of secondary hemochromatosis: transfusional vs erythropoietic. J Comput Assist Tomogr 18:416–419

7 The Spleen in Infectious Disorders

A. DREVELENGAS

CONTENTS

7.1 Introduction

The spleen is an infrequent target of infection. However, an increasing number of immunocompromised patients, including those with acquired immunodeficiency syndrome (AIDS), organ transplants, chemotherapy for malignant disease and congenital immunodeficiency syndrome, exhibit a marked increased incidence of splenic infections.

Despite this, the diagnosis of splenic infections is often not considered due to its rarity and the presence of predisposing conditions that obscure its clinical presentation. The purpose of this chapter is to describe the various appearances of splenic infections on ultrasound (US), computed tomography (CT) and magnetic resonance imaging (MRI) and to assist radiologists evaluating patients with suspected splenic infection.

7.2 Abscesses

7.2.1 Bacterial Abscesses

Splenic abscess is defined as any infectious suppurative process involving identifiable macroscopic filling defects either in the parenchyma of the spleen or the subcapsular space (NELKEN et al. 1987). Splenic abscesses are uncommon and arise from: (a) systemic bacteraemia, e.g. endocarditis or sepsis that originates in another site and is now causing infection in a previously normal spleen; (b) extension from a contiguous infection (infected pancreatitis, perinephric abscess); and (c) superinfection (presumably of haematogenous origin) in a spleen damaged by trauma or by infarction (such as occurs in haemoglobinopathies) (RABUSHKA et al. 1994; URRUTIA et al. 1996). The most common bacteria are streptococci, staphylococci and salmonella (Fig. 7.1), but every pyogenic organism has been incriminated.

The frequency of splenic abscess has recently increased because of a rising number of immunocompromised patients due to aggressive chemotherapy, intravenous drug abuse and AIDS

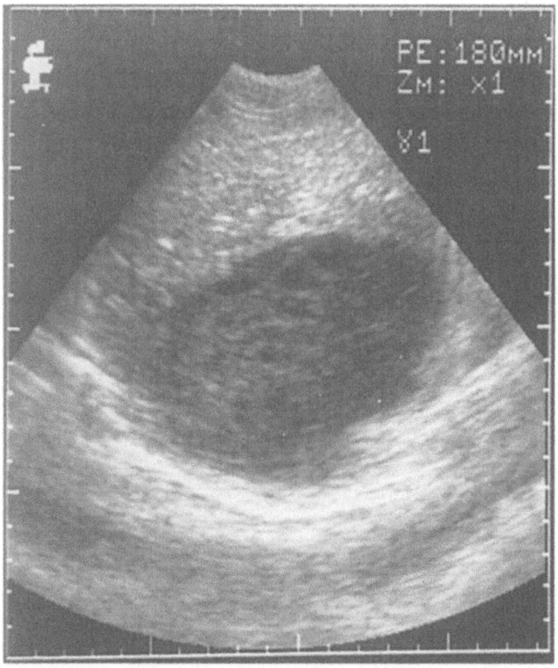

Fig. 7.1. Bacterial abscess. Ultrasound of the spleen shows a large hypoechoic lesion with internal echoes and irregular posterior borders

A. DREVELENGAS; Department of Radiology, Papanicolaou Hospital, Thessaloniki, Greece

(Rabushka et al. 1994). In all these groups, the abscess may reach a very large size with minimal symptoms and signs. The major symptoms are subacute onset of fever, chills and left upper-quadrant pain and tenderness.

At microscopic examination, an abscess consists of dead leucocytes (pus) surrounded by a highly vascularised fibrous capsule, which limits further spread and forms the wall of the abscess. The US and CT appearance of a pyogenic abscess varies with the stage at which it is seen. Similar to abscesses elsewhere in the body, the US appearances vary greatly. Typically, they appear as focal echo-free defects or as lesions with solid and cystic components (Gupta et al. 1987). They may also appear similar to cysts, but the abscess wall is often thick and irregular, and they may contain echoes due to debris, septations or gas bubbles (Gupta et al. 1987; Cox et al. 1989) (Fig. 7.2). Gas is an uncommon feature of pyogenic abscesses but, when seen, it is diagnostic; it is seen as a collection of very bright echoes.

CT is the imaging modality of choice, because it is the most reliable method of identifying small amounts of gas (Dachman et al. 1986; Downer and Peterson 1993; Rabushka et al.1994). Bacterial abscesses present as a hypodense collection of fluid or necrotic tissue (Franquet et al. 1990) (Fig. 7.3). CT attenuation measurements range from 20 HU to 40 HU (Fig. 7.4). Layers of different attenuation values secondary to layering of the proteinaceous material within the abscess are frequently noted (Urrutia et al. 1996). Minimal peripheral contrast enhancement may be present when a capsule has developed, although it is less often seen in splenic than in hepatic abscesses. The presence of gas is diagnostic, although the majority of splenic abscesses do

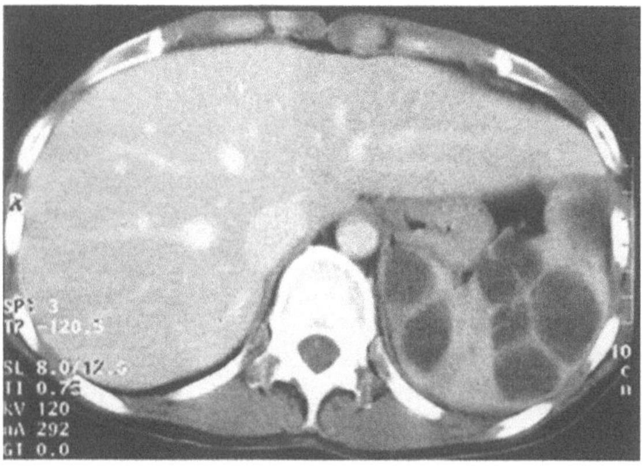

Fig. 7.2. Splenic abscesses. Post-contrast computed tomography shows multiple, well-demarcated, hypodense lesions

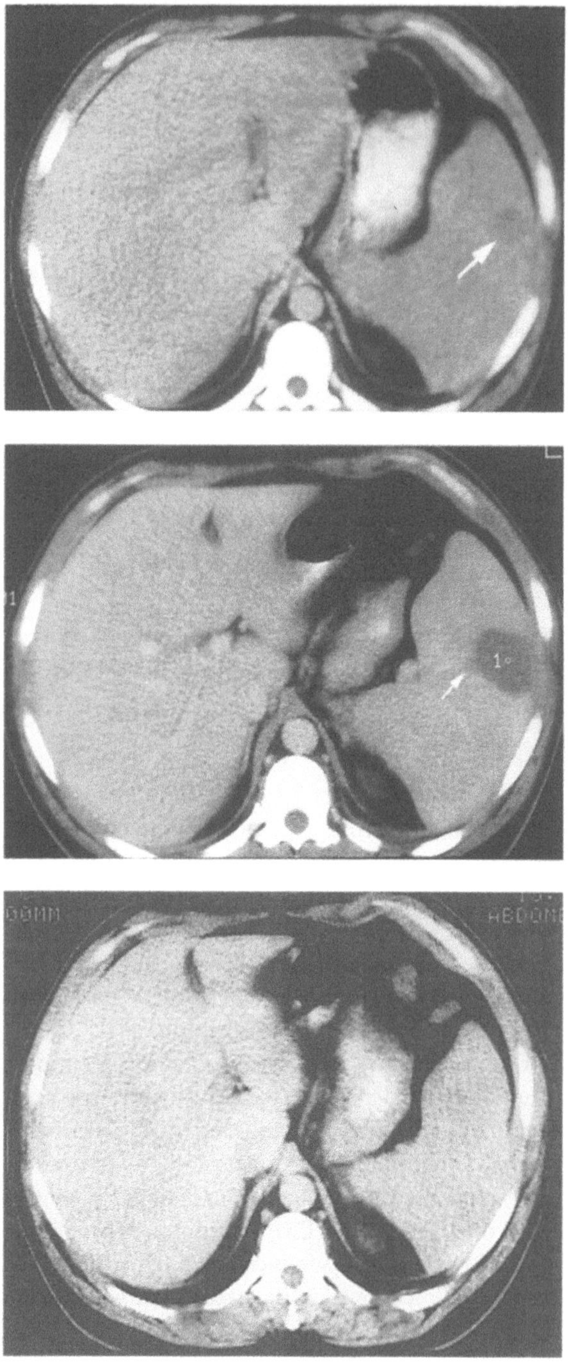

a

b

c

Fig. 7.3. Splenic abscess of *Staphylococcus*. **a** Enhanced computed tomography (CT) shows a subtle hypoattenuating mass within the spleen of a 40-year-old man with a 2-week history of fever and general fatigue (*arrow*). **b** A second contrast CT 1 week later shows an increase of the low-attenuation mass, with the development of a small satellite lesion (*arrow*). Note that the attenuation of the hypodense mass is 36 HU. **c** Post-treatment enhanced CT shows the complete resolution of the lesion

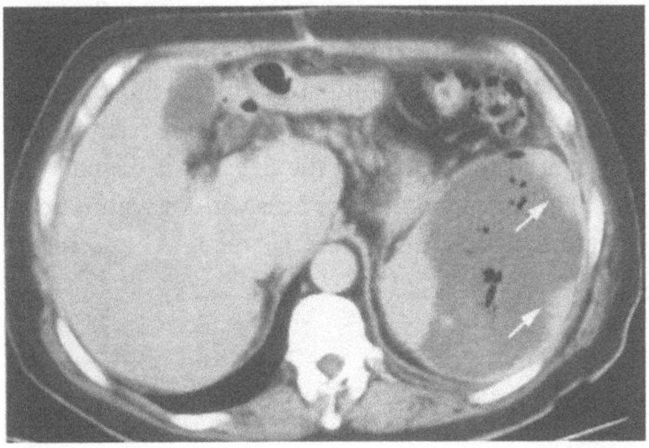

Fig. 7.4. Pyogenic abscess of the spleen. Enhanced computed tomography demonstrates a large, low-attenuation mass containing gas bubbles. Note also the irregular borders of the lesion (*arrows*)

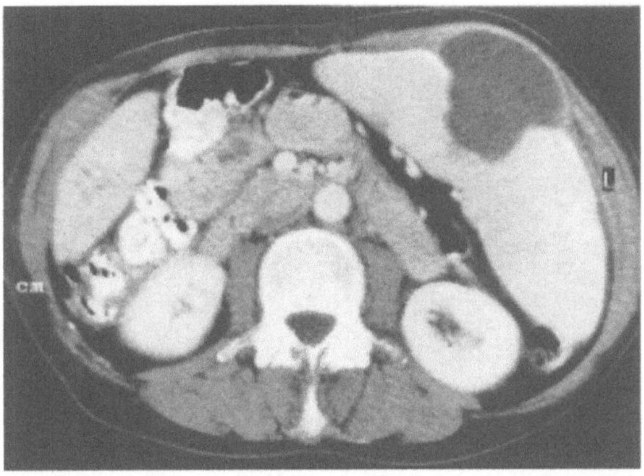

Fig. 7.5. Salmonella abscess. Enhanced computed tomography shows a large, hypodense lesion ventrally within the spleen, with bulging of the overlying abdominal wall (courtesy of K. Mortelé)

not contain air (Rabushka et al. 1994) (Fig. 7.5). MRI is rarely performed in patients with suspected splenic abscesses, since CT is highly sensitive and many patients are clinically not stable.

A multicentre study and review of the literature showed that CT had a sensitivity of 96%, which was significantly superior to the sensitivity of ultrasonography (76%, $P < 0.01$), liver and spleen scanning (75%, $P < 0.01$), gallium scanning (71%, $P < 0.001$) and indium scanning (50%, $P < 0.05$; Nelken et al. 1987). The authors also postulated that the chest radiograph was surprisingly sensitive, showing abnormalities in 82% of the patients, independent of the type of abscess or predisposing clinical condition. Abnormalities included mass effects in the left upper quadrant, left pleural effusion, elevation of the hemidiaphragm, left lower-lobe infiltrate and, rarely, extragastric gas bubbles in the left upper quadrant. Plain abdominal films showed similar changes in 69% of the patients. No specificity, however, was provided by either of these studies (Nelken et al. 1987).

Traditional treatment for splenic abscess has been splenectomy and antibiotic therapy. Recently, diagnostic fine-needle aspiration and drainage has shown promising results. With this method, an immediate gram stain should be used to identify the most likely causative organism in order to start the appropriate systemic antibiotics without any delay.

7.2.2 Fungal Abscesses

Fungal microabscesses have been found to constitute up to 26% of splenic abscesses and occur almost exclusively in immunocompromised patients (Nelken et al. 1987). Candida fungus is the most frequently encountered, followed by Aspergillus and Cryptococcus fungi.

Splenomegaly is common, and the liver and kidneys are often involved. Persistent fever, malaise and weight loss are some of the clinical findings.

At microscopic examination, concentric rings with central necrotic hyphae can be seen; these rings are surrounded by variable hyphae and a rim of peripheral inflammation (Henry and Symmer 1992). At gross examination, the entire spleen may be seen to have innumerable small (less than 5 mm in diameter) fungal deposits.

On US, the fungal abscesses are demonstrated as multiple, small, rounded, hypoechoic areas throughout the spleen (Goerg et al. 1990) (Fig. 7.6). On CT, multiple small lesions of relatively low attenuation, which typically range from a few millimetres to 2 cm in size, are seen (Fig. 7.7). Occasionally, a central focus of higher attenuation or a "wheel-within-a-wheel" pattern may be demonstrated (Chew et al. 1991; Urrutia et al. 1996).

Use of MRI in fungal infection is limited, and optimal contrast-enhanced resolution of small lesions may be difficult to obtain. MRI may demonstrate multiple small lesions of intermediate signal intensity on T1-weighted images and high signal intensity on T2-weighted images (Fig. 7.8). Ring-like enhancement may be seen with contrast-enhanced CT or MRI.

In hepatosplenic candidiasis, four patterns are discerned on US (Pastakia et al. 1988). The type-1 pattern, a "wheel within a wheel", is seen early in the

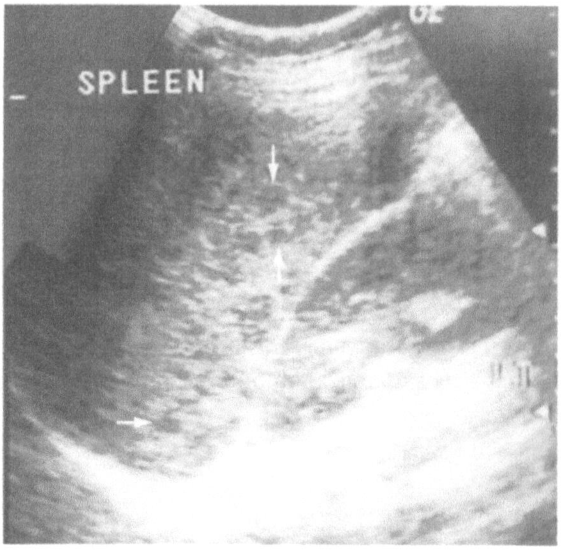

Fig. 7.6. Fungal microabscesses in a patient with non-Hodgkin's lymphoma. A sonogram shows multiple, small, rounded, hypoechoic lesions throughout the splenic parenchyma (*arrows*)

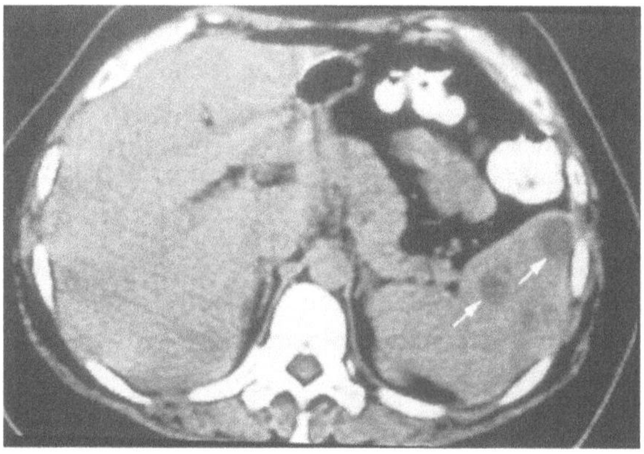

Fig. 7.7. Fungal abscesses in a 35-year-old patient with known leukaemia. Enhanced computed tomography demonstrates multiple small, focal areas of decreased attenuation throughout the spleen (*arrows*)

course of the disease. It consists of a peripheral hypoechoic zone that matches a ring of fibrosis found on pathologic examination and that forms the first wheel. Within this, there is a second wheel, which appears echogenic on US and has proved to be a zone of inflammatory cells. When necrosis occurs in the centre of the dense nidus of inflammatory cells, a hypoechoic centre appears and the type-1 pattern is seen (Fig. 7.9). The type-2 pattern is that of the typical bull's-eye lesion. It is the evolution of the type-1 lesion (Fig. 7.10). Type-1 and -2 lesions are seen only when the neutrophil counts of previously neutropenic patients have returned to normal. With healing and disappearance of the central inflammatory mass, the lesion progresses to the type-3 appearance, that of the uniformly hypoechoic lesion consisting of fibrosis. Finally, the type-4 lesion, seen only late in the course of the disease, is a small (2–5 mm) echogenic nodule or scar with or without calcification, which causes variable degrees of posterior acoustic shadowing (Fig. 7.11).

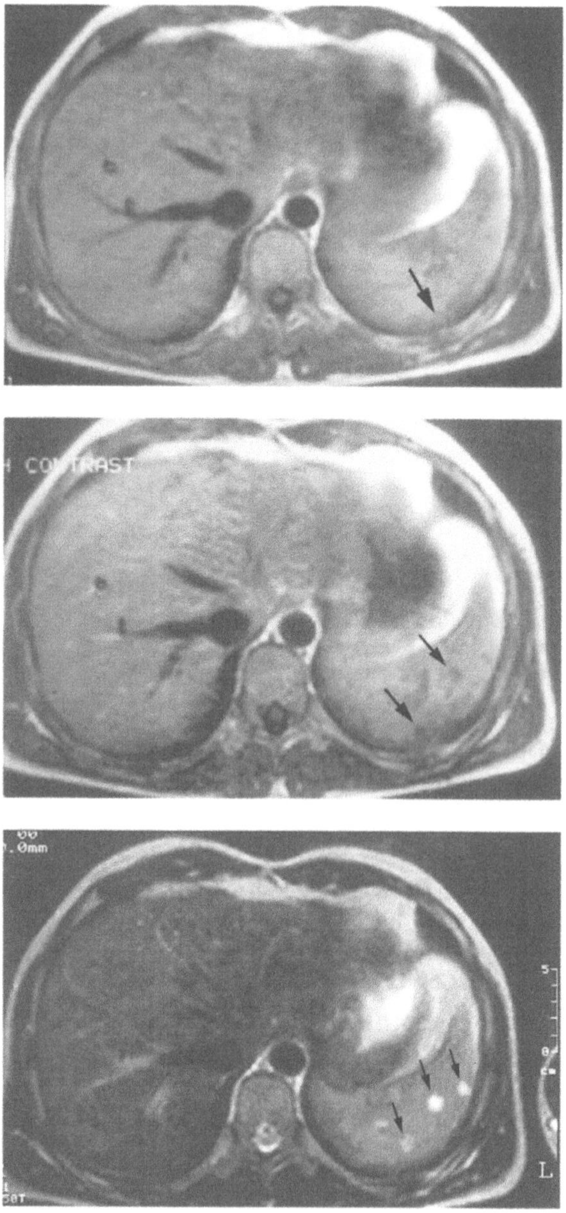

a

b

c

Fig. 7.8. Multiple microabscesses of the spleen. **a** A T1-weighted MR image shows a slightly enlarged spleen with faintly small low signal intensity lesions at the periphery of the spleen (*arrow*). **b** A post-gadolinium T1-weighted MR image reveals multiple, small, low-intensity lesions within the splenic parenchyma (*arrows*). **c** A T2-weighted image shows multiple small, high-intensity nodules (*arrows*)

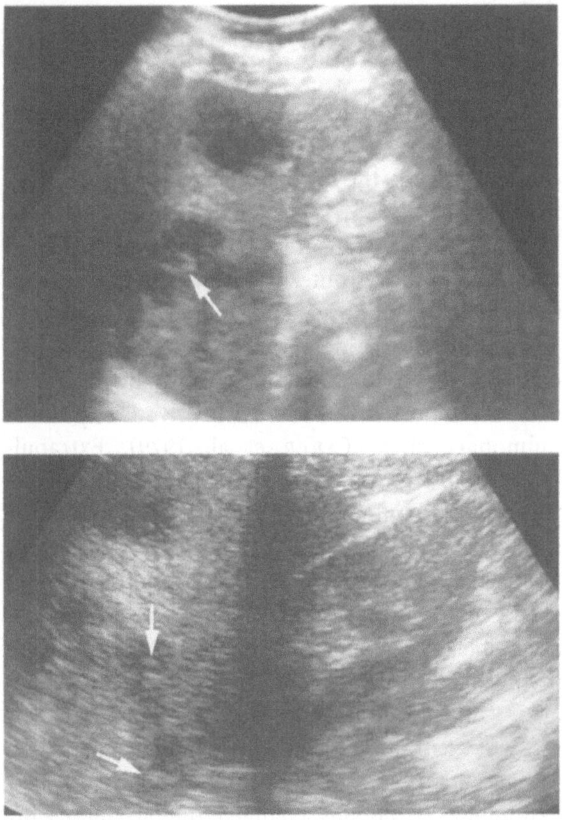
a
b

Fig. 7.9. a. Sonogram of the spleen in a patient with candida abscesses shows the typical wheel-within-a-wheel pattern, which is characterised by a central hypoechoic nidus (*arrow*) **b.** Ultrasound examination of the spleen of a previous patient 1 week later shows the typical bull's-eye lesions (*arrows*)

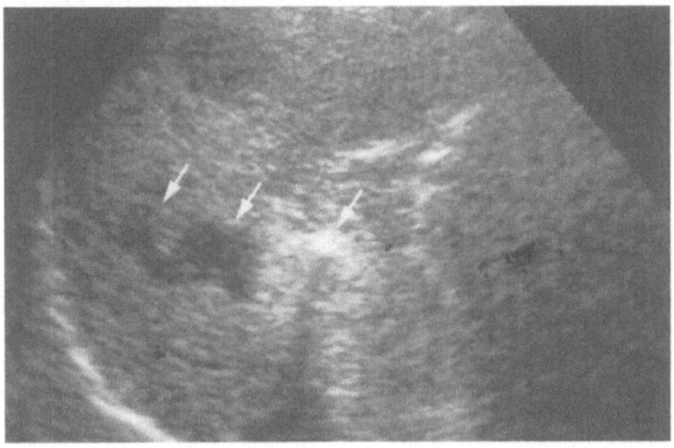

Fig. 7.10. Ultrasound examination of the patient with splenic candidiasis shows multiple uniformly hypoechoic lesions representing the type-3 pattern (*arrows*). The small hyperechoic nidus with the posterior acoustic shadowing represents the type-4 pattern (*arrows*)

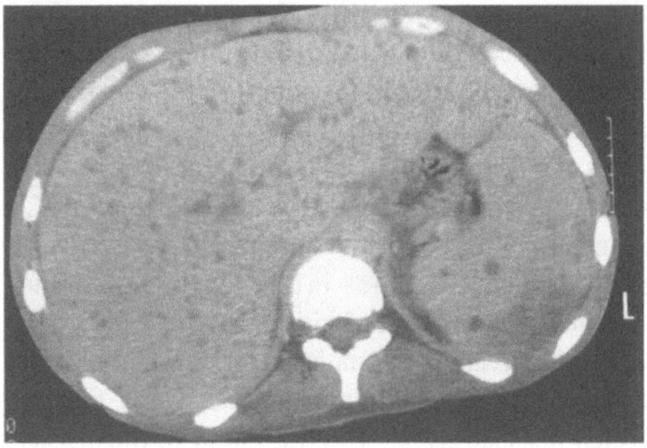

Fig. 7.11. Post-contrast computed-tomography scan of candidiasis microabscesses shows multiple, low-attenuation lesions within the liver and spleen

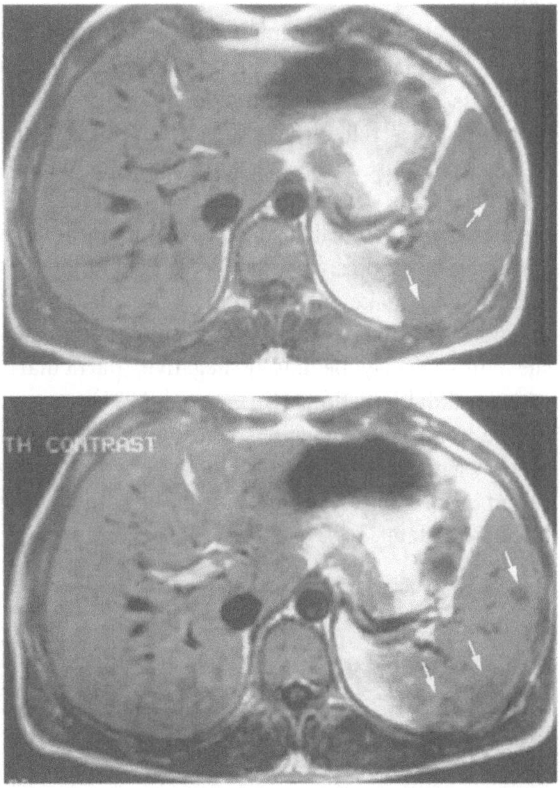

a
b

Fig. 7.12. Magnetic resonance examination in a patient with splenic candidiasis. **a** A T1-weighted image shows some low-signal lesions within the spleen (*arrows*). **b** A T1-weighted image after the administration of paramagnetic agent clearly shows multiple, confluent, low-signal lesions throughout the splenic parenchyma (*arrows*)

On CT, three patterns of hepatosplenic candidiasis have been described in recent literature (Pastakia et al. 1988; Freeman et al. 1993). The most common pattern consists of multiple, scattered, rounded areas of decreased attenuation (Fig. 7.12). For maximum imaging sensitivity, patients should be studied using US and enhanced and non-enhanced CT, because some lesions are better depicted using US while others are better using CT. The second type is the bull's-eye pattern and is only demonstrated occasionally. Numerous areas of increased attenuation, each measuring 2–5 mm in diameter, are seen late in the course of the disease and are identified at histopathological examination as areas of calcification. In addition to these three types of focal lesions in liver and spleen (as seen on CT scans), another pattern of abnormality was seen on non-enhanced CT scans in the livers of immunocompromised patients. This consisted of periportal areas of increased attenuation. The histopathological correlate of this finding was focal linear fibrosis, which was also seen late in the course of the disease.

The MR images in splenic candidiasis show multiple, small lesions of intermediate signal intensity on T1-weighted images and high signal intensity on T2-weighted images. After the administration of paramagnetic agents, the lesions become more apparent (Fig. 7.13).

Fungal abscesses in neutropenic patients are not always detectable with imaging techniques, even with disseminated infection. Percutaneous needle biopsy is not a reliable method of establishing the diagnosis because of the substantial number of false-negative results (Pastakia et al. 1988). Therefore, if there is strong clinical suspicion of fungal infection and imaging studies are negative, surgical biopsy is indicated to make the diagnosis. The histological diagnosis is often necessary, because blood and tissue cultures may be falsely negative, particularly with candidal infections (Chew et al. 1991).

The treatment is usually splenectomy; antifungal therapy with close radiological follow-up may be sufficient in some cases. Without prompt treatment, the infection is fatal.

7.3 Tuberculosis

Tuberculosis (TB) is a chronic bacterial infection (caused by *Mycobacterium tuberculosis*) that is characterised by the formation of granulomas in infected tissues and by cell-mediated hypersensitivity. *M. tuberculosis* is transmitted from person to person via the respiratory route. The usual site of disease is the lung, but other organs may be involved.

Prior to the epidemic of human immunodeficiency virus (HIV) infection, approximately 15% of newly reported cases of TB involved only extrapulmonary sites (Farer et al. 1979). Extrapulmonary TB is more of a diagnostic and therapeutic problem than pulmonary TB. In part, this is because it is less common and less familiar to most clinicians (Alvarez and McCabe 1984; Weir and Thorton 1985). In addition, extrapulmonary TB involves less accessible sites and, because of the nature of the sites involved, fewer bacilli can cause much greater damage. With the onset of the HIV epidemic, the rate of extrapulmonary involvement increased (Hopewell 1995). It is very interesting that the epidemiology of TB has changed due to increasing numbers of HIV-positive people. Numerous reports in the past several years have shown an increased rate of TB in persons who are infected with HIV. Patients with AIDS are susceptible to a wide range of usual, unusual and opportunistic infections (Mildvan et al. 1982; Lerner and Tapper 1984). Recently, an increasing number of patients with AIDS with disseminated infection from atypical mycobacteria, particularly *Mycobacterium avium*

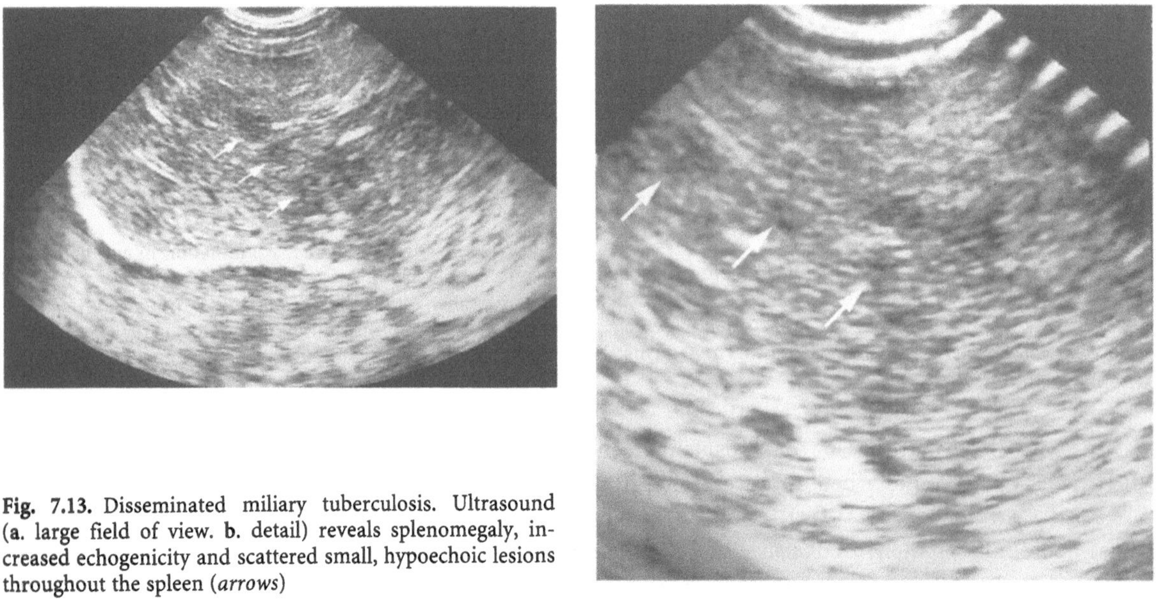

a b

Fig. 7.13. Disseminated miliary tuberculosis. Ultrasound (**a**. large field of view. **b**. detail) reveals splenomegaly, increased echogenicity and scattered small, hypoechoic lesions throughout the spleen (*arrows*) *intracellulare* (MAI), have been reported (GREENE et al. 1982; ZAKOWSKI et al. 1982). Since *M. avium* and *M. intracellulare* are difficult to distinguish by the usual laboratory methods, they are referred to as a single group (GREENE et al. 1982). MAI is ubiquitous in the environment, and person-to-person transmission does not occur.

HIV infection predisposes patients with latent TB to develop clinical TB. In patients with HIV infection, up to 70% with TB will show extrapulmonary manifestations (BUCKNER et al. 1991). However, disseminated extrapulmonary involvement by TB or MAI infection is indicative of a diagnosis of AIDS in HIV-positive patients (RABUSHKA et al. 1994). Disseminated infection from MAI has been recognised recently as a common life-threatening complication of AIDS.

A TB granuloma pathologically consists of giant cells and epithelioid cells and is characterised by a tendency for fibrosis and caseation, a unique form of non-liquefying necrosis. The clinical presentation of splenic TB is usually a febrile illness of undetermined origin; however, abdominal pain or discomfort, anorexia and weight loss may also occur (LEDER and LOW 1995).

TB of the spleen is extremely common in patients with disseminated disease; however, it is not usually identified at initial presentation (THOENI and MARGULIS 1979). When present, there usually is *miliary hepatosplenic* dissemination in association with miliary pulmonary TB (LEDER and LOW 1995). In miliary involvement of the spleen, the lesions usually are below the resolution capability of imaging modalities and are much more frequently found on autopsy (in 80–100% of cases).

Miliary TB manifests only as moderate splenomegaly (RABUSHKA et al. 1994). Ultrasonography may reveal increased echogenicity, the "bright-spleen" pattern or small hypoechoic lesions (Fig. 7.14).

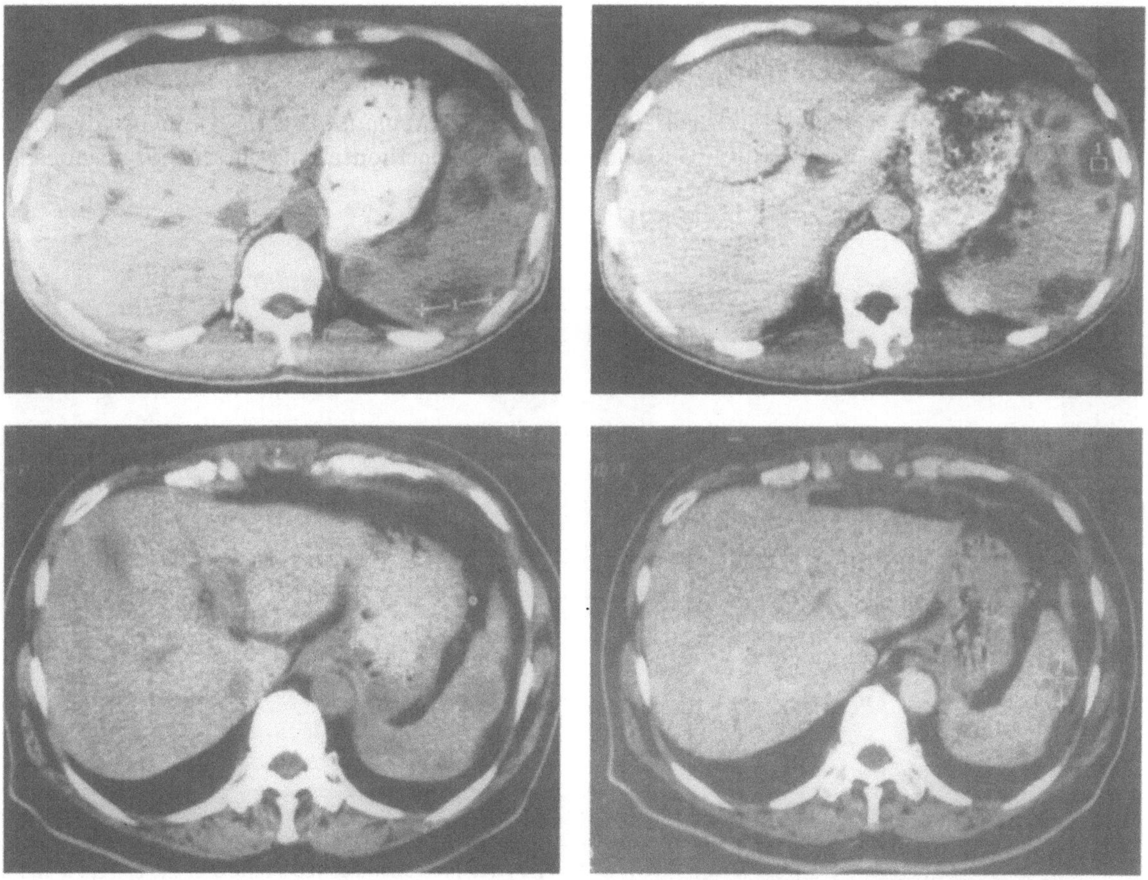

a b c d

Fig. 7.14. Pathologically proven macronodular splenic tuberculosis in two different patients (a, b: case 1; c, d: case 2). **a** Unenhanced computed tomography (CT) of the upper abdomen shows splenomegaly with multiple round and ovoid, low-density lesions within the splenic parenchyma. **b** Contrast-enhanced CT shows slight rim enhancement. No enhancement is seen in the centres of the lesions. **c** Unenhanced CT of another patient with splenic tuberculosis demonstrates multiple round and ovoid, lower-density lesions in the spleen. **d** Contrast enhanced CT shows no enhancement of the lesions (WANG et al. 1998)

On CT, the individual lesions may appear as tiny, low-density foci widely scattered throughout the spleen. When the lesions increase in size, they may appear as small, focal splenic nodules of low attenuation. Occasionally, small peripheral wedge-shaped areas of low attenuation may be present; these represent infarcts from septic emboli, although differentiation from bland infarcts is often impossible.

The *macronodular form* (tuberculoma or pseudotumour) is a rare manifestation of splenic TB and occurs without overt pulmonary involvement (Hulnick et al. 1985; Choi et al. 1989; Kapoor et al. 1991). On US, the lesions are similarly nonspecific, and are seen as round, hypoechoic areas. On CT, the disease appears as a diffuse spleen enlargement containing multiple, low-density, 1- to 3-cm, round lesions or as a single mass. Early in the evolution of the lesion, its appearance is more typically like an abscess with single or multiple low-density, septated, or "honeycomb-like" lesions with irregular, ill-defined margins. After intravenous contrast administration, the lesions show minimal or slight central uptake. With evolution of the disease, the lesion typically appears as an abscess with single or multiple low densities with ring-like enhancements (Fig. 7.15; Denath 1990; Kapoor et al. 1991; Buxi et al. 1992). On MRI, a tuberculoma appears as a hypointense lesion with a hypointense rim on T1-weighted images and appears hyperintense with a less intense rim on T2-weighted images. Pathologically, the centre of the lesion corresponds to caseation necrosis, and the peripheral rim corresponds to granulation tissue (Kawamori et al. 1992). Following treatment with an anti-TB agent, CT scans may show punctate or extensive calcifications representing healed granulomas (Hulnick et al. 1985; Fig. 7.16). In fact, those calcifications are a very common finding and, in endemic areas, are presumed to be due to past tuberculosis. As the appearance of splenic TB is nonspecific, other associated imaging findings, such as hepatic involvement, renal abnormalities, intestinal disease or enlarged lymph nodes with low-density centres, may be helpful in the differential diagnosis.

Abdominal imaging findings of non-TB mycobacteria in AIDS patients have been described in several studies. Focal splenic lesions have been reported in 30% of patients with TB and in 7% of patients with MAI infection. CT demonstration of focal lesions is the exception rather than the rule. Marked splenomegaly was noted in 20% of patients with MAI infection but was uncommon in those with TB infection (Rabushka et al. 1994). In a study, large, bulky retroperitoneal and mesenteric adenopathy

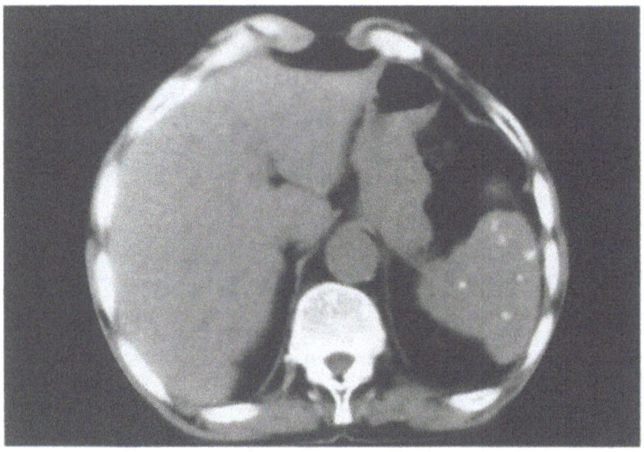
a

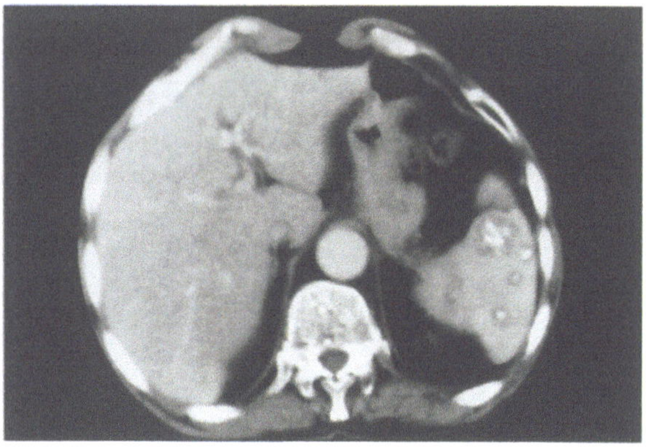
b

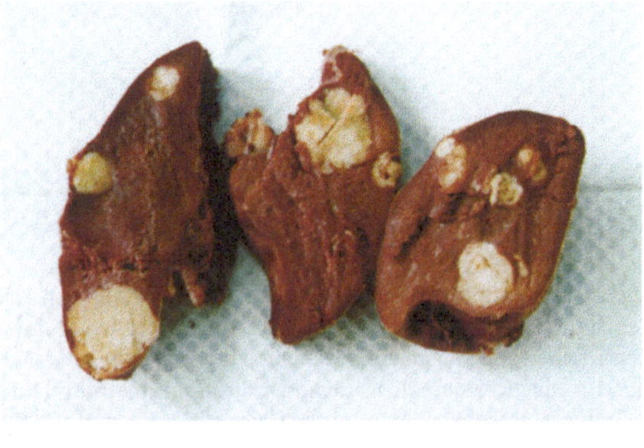
c

Fig. 7.15. Macronodular tuberculosis of the spleen. **a** and **b** unenhanced and contrast-enhanced CT-scan of the upper abdomen in another patient with macronodular tuberculosis of the spleen. Multiple calcifications, which are centrally located in rounded nonenhancing lesions within the spleen. **c** pathological specimen of the spleen in the same patient with macronodular tuberculosis.

is demonstrated in 82% of patients with MAI and AIDS (NYBERG et al. 1985).

Abdominal CT findings suggestive of disseminated TB infection include: multiple necrotic lymph nodes; multiple focal lesions in the spleen, liver, kidneys and pancreas; segmental ileocaecal wall thickening; and extraluminal gas due to duodenal fistula. Findings suggestive of disseminated MAI infection include multiple nodes 10 mm or more in diameter with soft-tissue density, marked hepatomegaly, marked splenomegaly and diffuse jejunal-wall thickening (RADIN 1991).

Distinction between TB and MAI infection is important because of the therapeutic implications (Table 1). Standard anti-mycobacterial therapy is far more effective in AIDS patients with TB infection than in those with MAI. MAI is usually resistant to standard anti-tuberculous therapy, and treatment often requires new and investigational drugs (GREENE et al. 1982). It is also interesting that peliosis of the spleen, a rare condition characterised by dilated, cystic, blood-filled spaces in the spleen, can be seen in patients with AIDS and may appear indistinguishable from mycobacterial infection (RABUSHKA et al. 1994).

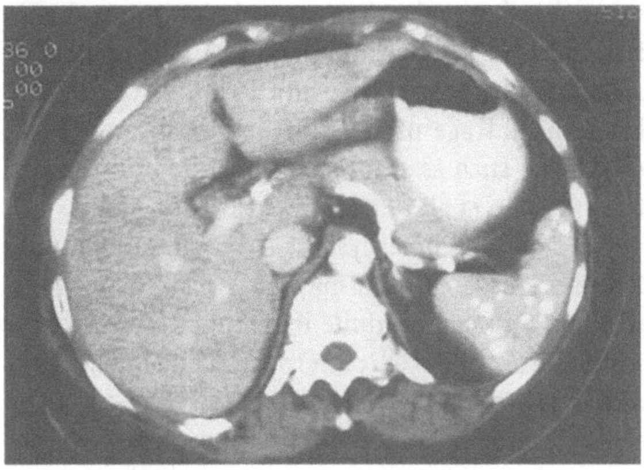

Fig. 7.16. Splenic tuberculosis. Post-contrast computed tomography reveals extensive calcification of the spleen

7.4 Echinococciasis

Echinococciasis is a tissue infection of humans caused by the larva stage of *Echinoccocus granulosus* or *E. multilocularis*. This infection is endemic to the Mediterranean region. The eggs of the worm (*E. granulosus*) may be excreted in the faeces of infected dogs. Cattle, sheep, goats and humans serve as the intermediate hosts. When ingested by an appropriate intermediate host, the embryos from the eggs penetrate the intestinal mucosa and enter the portal circulation. Most are filtered out by the liver or lung, but some escape into the general circulation, to involve other tissues. The life cycle of *E. multilocularis* is similar, except that small rodents serve as the natural intermediate hosts.

Table 1. Abdominal computed tomography (CT) findings in patients with acquired immune deficiency syndrome and disseminated mycobacterial infection

CT findings	*Mycobacterium tuberculosis*	*Mycobacterium avium intracellulare*
Splenomegaly	Rarely	More common
Focal lesions (liver, spleen, kidney, pancreas)	Often	Rarely
Lymph nodes enlargement	Common	Common
Necrotic lymph nodes	Often	Rarely
Small-bowel wall thickening	Segmental ileocaecal	Diffuse jejunal

The organs of involvement, in order of frequency, are the liver, lung, brain, spleen and other parenchymatous organs. Splenic echinococciasis has been found in about 2% of all patients with echinococciasis (BONAKDARPOUR 1967). In most cases of splenic hydatid cystic disease, concurrent liver cysts are also present (RABUSHKA et al. 1994). Systemic dissemination and intraperitoneal spread from a ruptured liver cyst constitute the two most important sources of splenic infestation (FRANQUET et al. 1990).

Clinical findings are nonspecific and frequently include abdominal pain, fever and splenomegaly. However, if a hydatid cyst ruptures or leaks fluid, an anaphylactoid reaction associated with eosinophilia may develop (FRANQUET et al. 1990).

On microscopic examination, an echinococcus cyst is a three-layered structure consisting of the inner germinal layer, the endocyst of hyalin and the pericyst, which is a thin band of vascularised, fibrotic, compressed spleen. Daughter cysts develop from germinal layers and are responsible for the multilocular form on gross pathologic examination. Scolices and fragments of the germinal layer constitute the so-called hydatid sand within the cyst.

Imaging findings have been based on sporadic case reports. In general, those findings are similar to those previously described for liver echinococcosis (DE DIEGO et al. 1982; KALOVIDOURIS et al. 1986; LEWALL et al. 1987). Those findings are well documented and, in endemic areas, radiologists are familiar with them. The radiographic appearance of splenic hydatidosis varies and is influenced by the location and age of the cyst and associated complications, such as secondary infection and rupture (Caballero et al. 1986).

A single anechoic cyst is a typical sonographic finding. This single cyst may vary in size from 1 cm to 20 cm and may be quite indistinguishable from a simple cyst. A mixed pattern of echogenicity produced by the presence of infolded membranes, scolices and hydatid sand may produce a highly echogenic (solid) pattern on sonography because of the large acoustic impedance differences between the intra-cystic components (Franquet at al 1990; Fig 7.17). Separation of the membrane produces a pathognomonic appearance for hydatid disease: the "water-lily sign". This sign results from the detachment and collapse of the inner germinal layer from the exocyst. The collapsed germinal layer is seen as an undulating, linear collection of echoes either floating in the cyst or lying in the most dependent portion (Niron and Ozer 1981). The development of daughter cysts from the lining germinal membrane produces a characteristic appearance of cysts enclosed within a cyst. This appearance is extremely characteristic and is known as a honeycomb cyst (Babcock et al. 1978).

CT findings of splenic hydatid disease are nonspecific, although the usefulness of CT in the diagnosis is well established. The CT attenuation in hydatidosis depends on intracystic content. Hydatid cysts usually have homogeneous fluid content showing water attenuation values on CT. The presence of debris, sand and inflammatory cells is presumed to

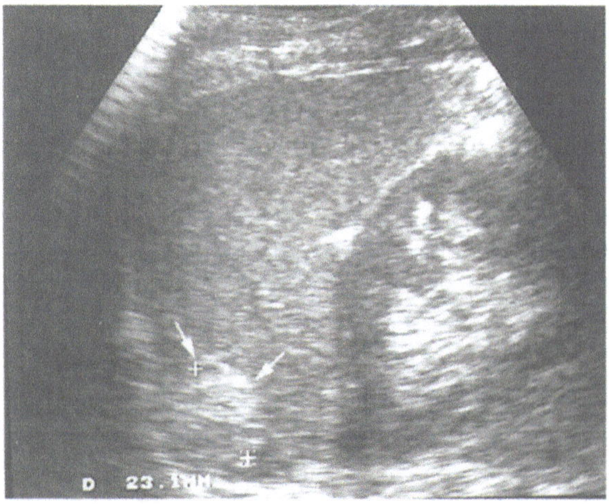

Fig. 7.17. Ultrasound of the spleen shows the echogenic pattern of a hydatid cyst (*arrows*)

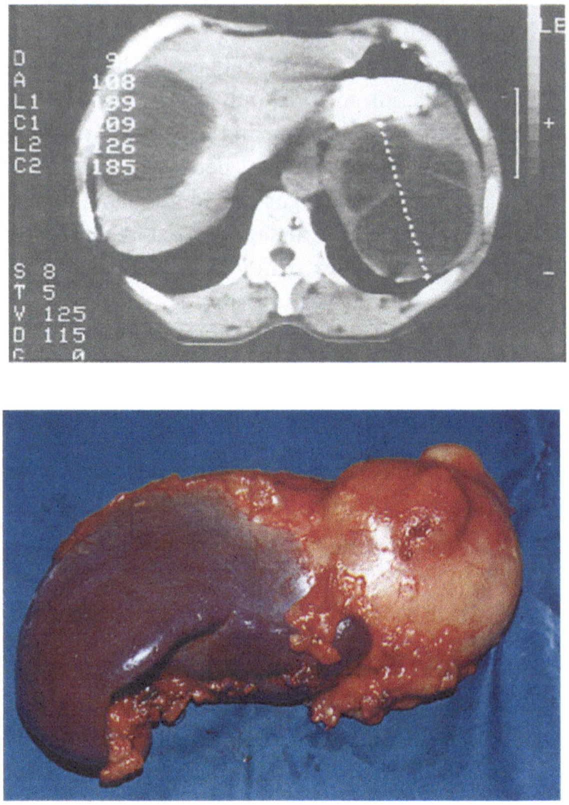

a

b

Fig. 7.18. Echinococcal disease. **a** A non-enhanced computed tomography scan demonstrates a cystic lesion occupying nearly the entire spleen. Internal septa can be seen. A second hydatid cyst is depicted within the liver. **b** A macroscopic specimen of the spleen shows a hydatid cyst

cause the high CT values (Lewall et al. 1987). No enhancement is seen after the administration of contrast material, except for the possible ring-like enhancement of the external cyst wall and the enhancement of the internal trabeculae (Fig 7.18). Wall calcification may occur after the death of a parasite, sometimes many years after the initial infection. The presence of a complete ring of calcification suggests an inactive lesion (Itzchuk et al. 1983). CT is the modality of choice in depicting subtle cyst-wall calcification (Fig. 7.19).

The MRI appearance of hydatid cysts is nonspecific and overlaps with that of other cystic lesions. Typically, a well-defined, rounded mass with signal intensity equal to that of water is seen on both T1- and T2-weighted sequences. However, depending on the protein or haemorrhage content of the cystic fluid, signal intensity on T1-weighted images may vary, whereas signal intensity on T2 images remains quite high due to fluid content (Rabushka et al. 1994). The presence of a hypointense rim on T1-weighted and T2-weighted images, corresponding to

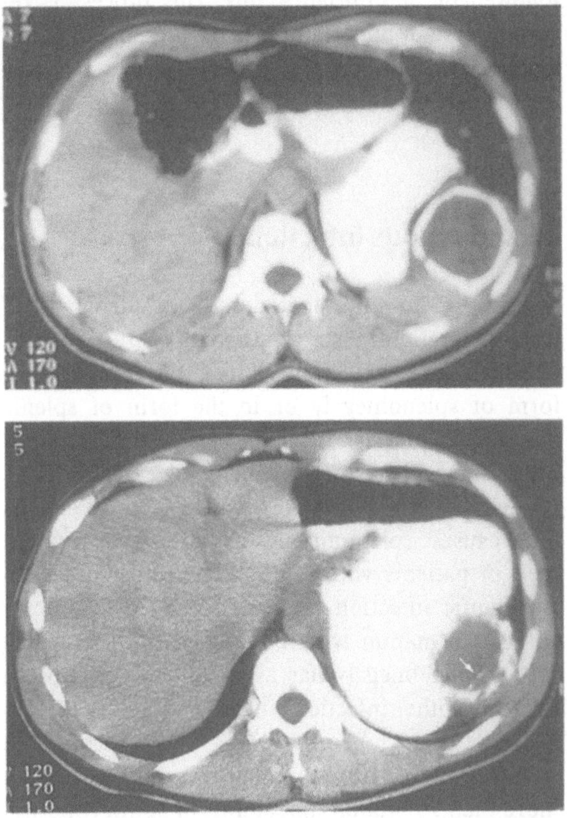

a

b

Fig. 7.19. Hydatid cyst. **a** A contrast-enhanced computed tomography scan shows a round splenic cyst with rim-like calcification. **b** A slightly superior image shows a small daughter cyst, which is also calcified (*arrow*)

wall calcification, and a multiloculated appearance are considered to be distinctive features of this lesion (Hoff et al. 1987).

The problem in the diagnosis of splenic hydatidosis is in differentiating it from other cystic lesions that have similar appearances. The differential diagnosis includes epidermoid cyst, pseudocyst, large solitary abscess or haematoma, intrasplenic pancreatic pseudocyst and cystic neoplasm of the spleen (Dachman et al. 1986). As the appearance of splenic echinococcosis is nonspecific, the presence of daughter cyst, hepatic involvement and positive specific serologic tests may be helpful in the differential diagnosis.

7.5 *Pneumocystis carinii* Infection of the Spleen

Pneumocystis carinii (PC) is an opportunistic pathogen whose natural habitat is the lung. PC is more closely related to fungi than to protozoa. The organism is an important cause of pneumonia in the immunocompromised host. PC pneumonia is the most common opportunistic infection in patients with AIDS.

Extrapulmonary involvement in patients with AIDS (even with prophylactic administration of pentamidine) and in other immunocompromised patients is rare but has been described with increasing frequency in the literature (Lubat et al. 1990; Radin et al. 1990). It seems likely that dissemination of PC infection in AIDS patients will be seen with increasing frequency in the future. The lymph nodes and spleen are the most common sites of involvement, suggesting a primarily lymphatic mode of dissemination. However, many patients have involvement outside the reticuloendothelial system, indicating a haematogenous route of spread; organs involved include the kidneys, pancreas, pericardium, heart, thymic capsule, thymus and gastrointestinal tract. Most patients with extrapulmonary involvement have a history of PC pneumonia (Brooke 1992).

Splenic involvement, as part of disseminated, intra-abdominal PC infection, is usually asymptomatic but sometimes produces fever and abdominal pain. Intrasplenic PC infection is often discovered incidentally in the patient with AIDS who is undergoing CT examination for a fever of unknown origin.

CT shows an enlarged spleen with focal low-attenuation lesions. This appearance is nonspecific. The focal lesions may progressively calcify either in rim-like or punctate fashion (Brooke 1992; Rabushka et al. 1994; Fig. 7.20). In some cases, calcifications that are obvious on unenhanced CT are barely perceptible after enhancement with intravenous contrast material. The appearance ranges from several scattered punctate foci to innumerable calcifications throughout the organ. Occasionally, the spleen may be almost completely calcified (Radin et al. 1990). It has been suggested that a granulomatus response to PC infection and consequent gross calcifications is an indication of improved host defence, perhaps due to treatment with 3'-azido-3'-deoxythymidine in HIV-positive patients (Klein et al. 1989). Grossly detectable calcifications have been described only once before in an extrapulmonary PC infection in AIDS (Carter et al. 1988). There is some evidence that low-density lesions and calcifications represent different manifestations of extrapulmonary PC infection rather than active and healed phases (Radin et al. 1990).

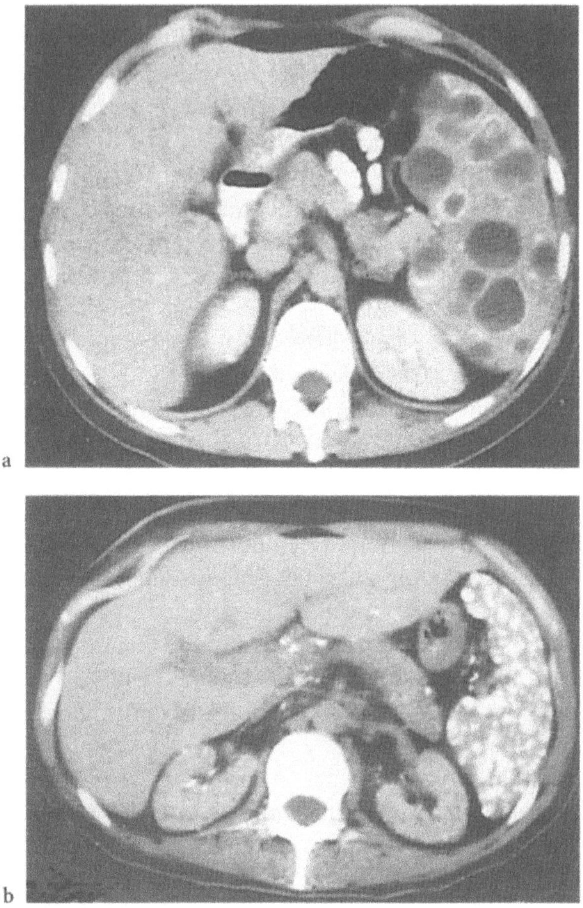

Fig. 7.20. Disseminated *Pneumocystis carinii* infection. **a** Rim calcification around splenic microabscesses. **b** In another patient with disseminated *P. carinii* infection, multiple splenic microcalcifications are apparent (Jeffrey 1992).

Associated findings are punctate calcifications in the liver, kidneys, lymph nodes, thyroid and adrenal glands (Rabushka et al. 1994). Diffuse punctate calcifications in the liver, spleen and kidneys may even be visible on plain films.

Sonography shows diffuse, tiny, echogenic foci without shadowing in the spleen. In patients with the most dense splenic calcifications, the ultrasonic beam is completely reflected at the surface of the spleen.

The differential diagnosis in patients with AIDS includes other infections, especially mycobacterial and fungal abscess, lymphoma and Kaposi's sarcoma (Radin et al. 1990). Splenic PC infection should be considered when calcifications or focal lesions are detected in the spleen in an immunodeficient patient, even if there is no history or evidence of PC pneumonia. The diagnosis of PC infection is confirmed by percutaneous fine-needle aspiration followed by appropriate stains. This process is recommended by most authors in the presence of radiological evidence for PC in order to start the appropriate treatment.

7.6 Miscellaneous Infections

In addition to the above-described splenic infections, there are also a number of rare microorganisms causing splenic infections either in the form of splenomegaly or in the form of splenic abscesses. Table 2 shows some of the atypical microorganisms which cause splenic involvement.

Melioidosis is likely to be one of the infections that causes splenomegaly or abscess formation seen in patients with AIDS. Cat-scratch disease is a zoonotic infection also characterised by microabscess formation within the spleen (Dunn et al. 1997). Splenomegaly has also been reported to be related to other infectious disorders, such as brucellosis and campylobacter.

Infection with *Schistosoma mansoni* occurs in more than 70 million inhabitants of South America, the Caribbean, the Arabic peninsula and Africa. The spleen is usually enlarged and, in some patients, small hyperechoic foci scattered throughout the spleen are seen (Richter et al. 1992).

Malaria, a protozoan infection characterised by chills, fever, sweating and anaemia, also causes liver and splenic enlargement. In chronic, untreated or partially treated malaria, splenic enlargement takes place more gradually. The spleen is stronger because of the presence of fibrosis and decreased vascularity of the organ. In these cases, a splenic rupture usually occurs in two stages: first, the formation of a subcapsular haematoma occurs, most often caused by trauma; second, the rupture of this haematoma into the peritoneal cavity occurs spontaneously or due to minimal trauma (Fig. 7.21). Defective haemostasis due to thrombocytopenia or treatment of fever with aspirin may contribute to intrasplenic haemorrhage.

Table 2. Miscellaneous splenic infections

Infections	Imaging findings
Melioidosis	Splenomegaly/abscess
Cat scratch	Splenic microabscesses
Brucellosis	Splenomegaly
Campylobacter	Splenomegaly
Schistosomiasis	Splenomegaly/hyperechoic foci
Malaria	Splenomegaly/splenic rupture

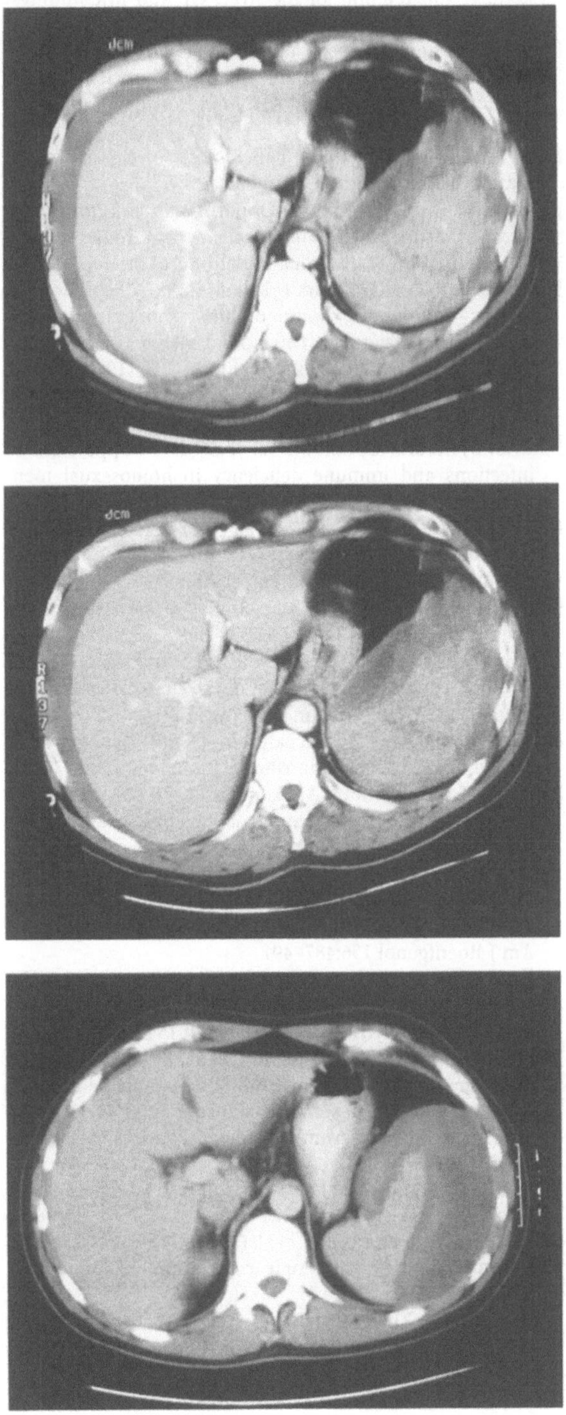

a b c

Fig. 7.21. Spontaneous rupture of the spleen due to malaria in two patients. a, b A contrast-enhanced computed-tomography (CT) scan shows splenic fracture and free peritoneal fluid (haemoperitoneum). c Case 2. A contrast-enhanced CT scan shows large subscapular haematoma (De Aguirre et al. 1998)

The actual treatment of splenic rupture is focused on splenic preservation, especially for patients living in or travelling to malaria-endemic areas. Splenectomy should be reserved for patients with severe rupture or with recurrent splenic bleeding.

7.7 Conclusion

Recently, an increasing number of patients with specific infections have been reported. This is due to the widespread use of improved imaging techniques and to the increase in the number of immunocompromised patients.

Cross-sectional imaging with US and CT is required for the depiction of inflammatory disease of the spleen. MRI may be used as a complementary diagnostic tool in patients who are allergic to iodinated contrast material. Furthermore, MRI may be increasingly used as newer pulse sequences and organ-specific contrast agents are developed.

References

Alvarez S, McCabe WR (1984) Extrapulmonary tuberculosis revisited: a review of experience at Boston City and other hospitals. Medicine (Baltimore) 63:25

Babcock DS, Kaufman L, Cosnow I (1978) Ultrasound diagnosis of hydatid disease (echinococcosis) in two cases. AJR Am J Roentgenol 131:895

Bonakdarpour A (1967) Echinococcus disease: report of 112 cases from Iran and a review of 611 cases from the United States. AJR Am J Roentgenol 99:660–667

Brooke J (1992) Abdominal imaging in the immunocompromised patient. Radiol Clin North Am 30:579–596

Buckner CB, Leithiser RE, Walker WW, et al. (1991) The changing epidemiology of tuberculosis and other mycobacterial infection in the United States: implications for the radiologist. AJR Am J Roentgenol 156:255–264

Buxi TBS, Vohra RB, Sujatha Y, et al. (1992) CT appearances in macronodular hepatosplenic tuberculosis: a review with five additional new cases. Comput Med Imaging Graph 16:381–387

Caballero P, Ocon E, Robledo AG, et al. (1986) Splenic hydatid cyst opening to the colon. AJR Am J Roentgenol 147:859–860

Carter TR, Cooper PH, Petri WA Jr, et al. (1988) *Pneumocystis carinii* infection of the small intestine in a patient with acquired immune deficiency syndrome. Am J Clin Pathol 89:679–683

Chew FS, Smith PL, Barboriak D (1991) Candidal splenic abscesses. AJR Am J Roentgenol 156:474

Choi BI, Im JG, Han MC, et al. (1989) Hepatosplenic tuberculosis with hypersplenism: CT evaluation. Gastrointest Radiol 14:265–267

Cox F, Perlman S, Sathyanarayana (1989) Splenic abscesses in cat scratch disease: sonographic diagnosis and follow up. J Clin Ultrasound 17:511

Dachman AH, Ros PR, Murary P J (1986) Nonparasitic splenic cysts: a report of 52 cases with radiologic-pathologic correlation. AJR Am J Roentgenol 149:537–542

De Aguirre Z, De Droogh E, Van Den Ende J, et al. (1998) Splenic rupture as a complication of *P. falciparum* malaria after residence in the tropics. Acta Clin Belg 53:374–377

De Diego JC, Lecumberri FJO, Franquet TC (1982) Computed tomography in hepatic echinococcosis. AJR Am J Roentgenol 138:699–702

Denath FM (1990) Abdominal tuberculosis in children: CT findings. Gastrointest Radiol 15:303–306

Downer WR, Peterson MS (1993) Case report: massive splenic infarction and liquefactive necrosis complicating polycythemia vera. AJR Am J Roentgenol 161:79–80

Dunn MW, Berkowitz FE, Miller JJ, et al. (1997) Hepatosplenic cat-scratch disease and abdominal pain. Pediatr Infect Dis J 16:269–272

Farer LS, Lowell AM, Meador MP (1979) Extrapulmonary tuberculosis in the United States. Am J Epidemiol 109: 205–217

Franquet T, Montes M, Lecumberri FJ (1990) Hydatid disease of the spleen: imaging findings in nine patients. AJR Am J Roentgenol 154:525–528

Freeman JL, Jafri SZH, Roberts JL, et al. (1993) CT of congenital and acquired abnormalities of the spleen. Radiographics 13:597–610

Goerg C, Schwerk WB, Goerg K (1991) Pictorial essay: sonography of focal lesions of the spleen. AJR Am J Roentgenol 156:949–953

Greene JB, Sidhu GS, Lewin S, et al. (1982) *Mycobacterium avium intracellulare*: a cause of disseminated life-threatening infection in homosexuals and drug abusers. Ann Intern Med 97:539–546

Gupta RK, Pant CS, Ganguly SK (1987) Ultrasound demonstration of amebic splenic abscess. J Clin Ultrasound 15:555–557

Henry K, Symmer W (1992) Systemic pathology, 3rd edn. Churchill Livingstone, New York, pp 574–603

Hoff FL, Aisen AM, Walden ME, et al. (1987) MR imaging in hydatid desease of the liver. Gastrointest Radiol 12:39–42

Hopewell PC (1995) A clinical view of tuberculosis. Radiol Clin North Am 33:641–653

Hulnick DH, Megibow AJ, Naidich DP, et al. (1985) Abdominal tuberculosis: CT evaluation. Radiology 157:199–204

Itzchuk Y, Rubinstein Z, Shilo R (1983) Ultrasound in tropical diseases. In: Sanders RC, Hill MC (eds) Ultrasound annual. Raven, New York, pp ••

Jeffrey RB, Jr (1992) Abdominal imaging in the immunocompromised patient. Radiol Clin North Am 30:579–596

Kalovidouris A, Pissiotis C, Pontifex G, et al. (1986) CT characterization of multivesicular hydatid cyst. J Comput Assist Tomogr 10:428–431

Kapoor R, Jain AK, Chaturvedi U, et al. (1991) Case report: ultrasound detection of tuberculomas of the spleen. Clin Radiol 43:128

Kawamori Y, Matsui O, Kitigawa K, et al. (1992) Macronodular tuberculoma of the liver: CT and MR findings. AJR Am J Roentgenol 158:311

Klein JS, Warnock M, Webb WR, et al. (1989) Cavitating and noncavitating granulomas in AIDS patients with *Pneumocystis pneumonitis*. AJR Am J Roentgenol 152:753–754

Leder AR, Low VHS (1995) Tuberculosis of the abdomen. Radiol Clin North Am 33:691–705

Lerner CW, Tapper ML (1984) Opportunistic infection complicating acquired immunodeficiency syndrome: clinical features of 25 cases. Medicine (Baltimore) 63:155–164

Lewall DB, Bailey TM, McCorkell SJ (1987) Echinococcal matrix: computed tomographic, sonographic and pathologic correlation. J Ultrasound Med 5:33–35

Lubat E, Megibow AJ, Baltazar EJ, et al. (1990) Extrapulmonary *Pneumocystis carinii* infection in AIDS: CT findings. Radiology 174:157–160

Mildvan D, Mathur U, Enlow RW, et al. (1982) Opportunistic infections and immune deficiency in homosexual men. Ann Intern Med 96:700–704

Nelken N, Ignatius, Skinner M, et al. (1987) Changing clinical spectrum of splenic abscess: a multicenter study and review of the literature. Am J Surg 154:27–33

Niron EA, Ozer H (1981) Ultrasound appearances of liver hydatid disease. Br J Radiol 54:335–338

Nyberg DA, Federle MD, Jeffrey RB (1985) Abdominal CT findings of disseminated *Mycobacterium avium intracellulare* in AIDS. AJR Am J Roentgenol 145:297–299

Pastakia B, Shawker TH, Thaler M (1988) Hepatosplenic candidiasis: wheels within wheels. Radiology 166:417–421

Rabushka LS, Kawashima A, Fishman EK (1994) Imaging of the spleen. CT with supplemental MR examination. Radiographics 14:307–332

Radin DR (1991) Intraabdominal *Mycobacterium tuberculosis* vs *Mycobacterium avium intracellulare* infections in patients with AIDS: distinction based on CT findings. AJR Am J Roentgenol 156:487–491

Radin DR, Baecer LE, Katt EC, et al. (1990)Visceral and nodal calcification in patients with AIDS-related *Pneumocystis carinii* infection AJR Am J Roentgenol 154:27–31

Richter J, Monteiro E da S, Braz RM, et al.(1992) Sonographic organometry in Brazilian and Sudanese patients with hepatosplenic schistosomiasis mansoni and its relation to the risk of bleeding from oesophageal varices. Acta Trop 51:281–291

Thoeni RF, Margulis AR (1979) Gastrointestinal tuberculosis. Semin Roentgenol 14:283–294

Urrutia M, Mergo PJ, Ros LH, et al. (1996) Cystic masses of the spleen: radiologic-pathologic correlation. Radiographics 16:107–129

Wang Y, He G, Zhan W, Jiang H, Wu D, Wang D, Tang A (1998) CT findings in splenic tuberculosis. J Belge Radiol 81:90-91

Weir MR, Thornton GF (1985) Extrapulmonary tuberculosis: experience of a community hospital and review of the literature. Am J Med 79:467

Zakowski P, Fligiel S, Berlin GW, et al. (1982) Disseminated *Mycobacterium avium intracellulare* infection in homosexual men dying of acquired immunodeficiency. JAMA 248:2980–2982

8 Trauma of the Spleen

B. CORTHOUTS and H. DEGRYSE

CONTENTS

8.1 Introduction

Potentially serious abdominal injury is encountered on an almost daily basis in major emergency departments. Approximately 10% of the thousands of yearly fatalities are considered the direct result of abdominal injury, and survivor morbidity is significantly influenced by abdominal trauma (BUDNICK and CHAIKEN 1985). Among the involved organs, the spleen is very commonly injured in both blunt and penetrating abdominal trauma. As it is the role of the emergency physician, together with other members of the trauma team (including the radiologist) to accurately detect all significant traumatic injuries, assessment of splenic injury represents one of the most common and challenging problems in diagnostic imaging of the spleen.

8.2 Splenic Injury in Abdominal Trauma

Classically, abdominal trauma is divided into blunt and penetrating categories. This subdivision is relevant, as both the mechanism of injury and the incidence of particular organ injuries (and, consequently, diagnostic approaches) are substantially different in each category (NEWTON and PARISKY 1992).

In penetrating trauma, the incidence of organ involvement is approximately proportional to the cross-sectional area of the organ in question. Hence, splenic injury is relatively infrequent in penetrating abdominal trauma and accounts for approximately 7% of cases (ANDERSON and BALLINGER 1985).

Blunt abdominal trauma has become increasingly common with the advent of high-speed transportation during recent decades. In adults, the spleen is by far the most commonly injured organ in blunt abdominal trauma; it is involved in 25% of the cases with abdominal organ injuries (ANDERSON and BALLINGER 1985). In children who sustain blunt abdominal trauma, incidence of splenic injury is preceded by hepatic involvement (SIVIT and BULAS 1993).

As for other solid viscera, injury to the spleen may result from direct compression, avulsion of vascular attachments by sudden deceleration forces or laceration by fractured adjacent skeletal structures. In addition to the manifestations related to associated injury of other abdominal organs, signs of splenic trauma usually result from hypovolemia, blood loss or local or referred symptoms of hemoperitoneum (ROBERTS et al. 1996). Tachycardia, hypotension and even profound shock (occurring in up to 16% of patients with abdominal trauma) are due to blood loss. Generalized abdominal pain is common, whereas localized left upper quadrant pain is seen in 30% of cases. Rebound tenderness, diffuse abdominal rigidity, progressive abdominal distention and decreased bowel sounds are all results of irritation because of hemoperitoneum.

Management of these patients (including the need to perform imaging studies, the choice of the most appropriate imaging modality and, most important, the choice between conservative versus surgical treatment) must be dictated by the patient's clinical condition (NEWTON and PARISKY 1992; KOHN et al. 1994; MCLOUGHLIN and MATHIESON 1995; BENYA

B. CORTHOUTS and H. DEGRYSE; Department of Radiology, University Hospital Antwerp, Wilrijkstraat 10, B-2650 Edegem, Belgium and Bulas 1996; Bond et al. 1996; Emery 1997). Hemodynamically unstable patients who fail to respond to initial fluid resuscitation should not undergo diagnostic studies but should proceed immediately to surgery to identify and correct the source of bleeding. In other patients, detailed assessment of potential splenic damage by imaging is indicated.

Overwhelming sepsis following splenectomy is now a well-recognized entity, with reported prevalence of 4.25% and mortality of 2.25% (Pimpl et al. 1989; Umlas and Cronan 1991; Gay and Sistrom 1992). This observation has encouraged clinicians to use types of treatment that preserve the spleen (Pickhardt et al. 1989; Lawson et al. 1995; Bond et al. 1996; Hagiwara et al. 1996; Clancy et al. 1997; Emery 1997).

Delayed splenic rupture is defined as bleeding occurring more than 48 h after trauma in previously hemodynamically stable patients, with no injury or minor injury seen at initial imaging (Scatamacchia et al. 1989; Lawson et al. 1995; Emery 1997). The reported frequency of this entity varies between 1% and 14%. Its major significance lies in markedly higher mortality rates than with acute splenic injury (5–15% versus 1%; Emery 1997).

8.3 Diagnostic Imaging in the Initial Diagnosis

First of all, it should be remembered that, before making any decision concerning diagnostic imaging of patients with abdominal trauma, one must be sure that the patient is reasonably stable. Hemodynamic instability bypasses radiologic evaluation and requires emergent surgery. In view of the actual tendency toward non-operative management of stable patients after blunt abdominal trauma, diagnostic imaging plays a central role in the assessment of potential abdominal injury.

8.3.1 Conventional Radiography in Splenic Injury

In the setting of penetrating trauma, plain radiographs may be indicated for detection, localization and determination of the trajectory of projectiles, bullets or other devices (Newton and Parisky 1992). Further evaluation of organ damage is done by ultrasonography or computed-tomography (CT) scan.

Due to lack of both sensitivity and specificity for detecting organ injury or hemoperitoneum, controversy exists regarding whether plain radiographs should be obtained as part of the initial investigation in patients with blunt abdominal trauma. Occasionally, medial displacement of the stomach, elevation of the left hemidiaphragm, downward displacement of the splenic flexure of the colon or overlying rib fractures may suggest potential splenic injury.

Hemoperitoneum resulting from splenic damage may obscure the normally sharply outlined inferior border of the spleen, but this sign does not allow further assessment of splenic injury. As a consequence, ultrasonography and CT scan have largely replaced conventional radiographies in the evaluation of patients with blunt or penetrating abdominal trauma (McLoughlin and Mathieson 1995).

8.3.2 Ultrasonography of Splenic Injury

On ultrasonography of the injured spleen with either laceration or hematoma, areas of both increased and decreased echogenicity are seen. This variable presentation depends on multiple factors, of which the age of the lesion plays a major role. Initial hematomas are hyperechoic but gradually progress to low echogenicity and finally sonolucency within 96 h after the trauma (Newton and Parisky 1992). Subcapsular hematomas or perisplenic fluid collections present as anechoic to hypoechoic areas surrounding the spleen. Subcapsular hematomas or splenic lacerations that are adjacent to the diaphragm may escape ultrasonographic detection. Furthermore, when ultrasonography is performed too early, small subcapsular hematomas may be missed (Benya and Bulas 1996).

Ultrasonography is less costly than CT scans and can be performed in the emergency department when using a portable unit, thereby minimizing movement of a critically ill patient. Despite its relatively high sensitivity for hemoperitoneum and solid-organ injury, the limitations of ultrasonography outweigh its apparent immediate advantages. Accuracy of the examination depends on the skill of the performing radiologist and the sophistication of the equipment; cooperation of the patient is required, and ultrasonography is less accurate in detailed visualization of the retroperitoneal organs, especially in association with concomitant fractures or air in overlying bowel loops. Therefore, the actual role of ultrasonography is restrained to determination of resolution or progression in patients with established diagnoses (NEWTON and PARISKY 1992).

8.3.3
CT of Splenic Injury

Among the various imaging techniques, CT scan offers in a single, relatively non-invasive examination a simultaneous view of both the entire abdomen and the retroperitoneum, with detailed resolution. In addition, unsuspected findings, such as spinal or pelvic fractures or other concomitant pathologies, may be disclosed by a CT scan. CT has a decreased interoperator variability and allows better assessment of bowel, pancreas and bone than other imaging techniques do. By shortening examination times and improving bolus contrast enhancement, helical CT has become a major advancement in the evaluation of trauma patients. New helical CT scanners enable a complete abdominal examination in 1 min, while a complete body examination, including scanning of head, thorax and abdomen, can be accomplished within 15 min. As a consequence, CT scan is actually considered the gold standard for non-invasive imaging of blunt abdominal trauma (BENYA and BULAS 1996; EMERY 1997; BECKER et al. 1998). The reported sensitivity of CT scans in the detection of splenic injury varies from 96% to nearly 100% (GAY and SISTROM 1992; NEWTON and PARISKY 1992; LAWSON et al. 1995; MCLOUGHLIN and MATHIESON 1995; EMERY 1997; SHUMAN 1997).

8.3.3.1
CT-Scan Technique in Blunt Abdominal Trauma

In centers where peritoneal lavage is used as part of the initial diagnostic work-up, it might be advisable to perform the CT scan before the peritoneal lavage, as residual lavage fluid may mimic hemoperitoneum on subsequent CT scans. In order to maximize capability for lesion detection, CT scans of the abdomen require administration of both intravenous and oral contrast material. Oral contrast material enables improved assessment of injury to the stomach, bowel and pancreas and better evaluation of hemoperitoneum, especially in thin patients. The use of non-ionic intravenous contrast material is advocated in trauma patients to minimize the risk of vomiting (SHUMAN 1997).

Dilute (1%) water-soluble gastrograffin is commonly used as oral contrast material. If the patient is unable to drink, the contrast material may be administered through a nasogastric tube. Administration of up to 500 ml of contrast material 45 min before scanning and an additional 200 ml just before the start of the examination is recommended. Intravenous contrast material is administered via a rapid drip or bolus technique at 2–4 ml/s for a total volume of 150–180 ml (NEWTON and PARISKY 1992; SHUMAN 1997; BECKER et al. 1998). With helical CT, optimum organ enhancement is obtained when the initiation of scanning starts 70–90 s after the beginning of the injection. In the upper abdomen, scans are advised at 1-cm intervals, from the level of the hemidiaphragm to the level of the kidneys, followed by scans at intervals of 1.5 cm or 2.0 cm to the level of the ischia. Review of all images at various window settings (lung, bone, soft tissue) is recommended for optimal detection of pneumoperitoneum, bone and subtle abdominal organ injury.

8.3.3.2
CT Findings and Grading of Splenic Injury

With good technique, including appropriate administration of contrast material, CT is up to 98% sensitive for the detection of splenic injury, and accurately shows the injury's extent. Subcapsular hematomas present as crescentic regions of low attenuation that flatten or indent the splenic margin (Fig. 8.1). They are usually lateral in location, which

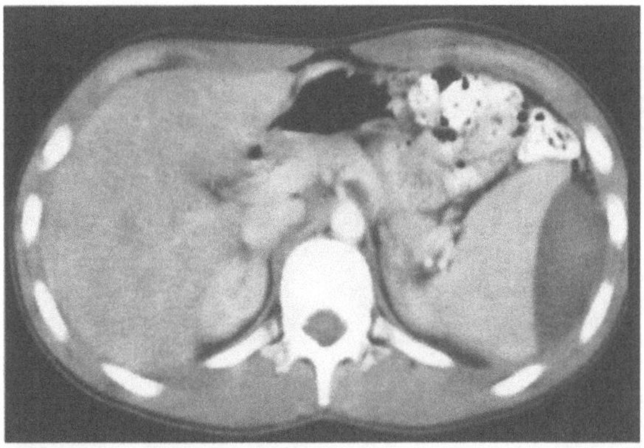

Fig. 8.1. Contrast-enhanced computed-tomography scan of the upper abdomen. Subcapsular hematoma of the spleen. Large, lenticular mass adjacent to and compressing the splenic parenchyma. Inhomogeneous density of the lesion due to clot formation. Absence of perisplenic fluid proves the integrity of the splenic capsule

helps to distinguish them from congenital splenic clefts, which almost always occur medially (Gay and Sistrom 1992) (Fig. 8.2). Intrasplenic hematomas are seen as rounded areas which reveal variable attenuation values depending on the age of the lesion. Early lesions appear as hypodense areas within normally perfused splenic parenchyma; thereafter, they become inhomogeneous and, later, they contain high-attenuation clots (Figs. 8.3, 8.4). The picture of multiple hematomas must be differentiated from the mottled appearance of the spleen that is observed on scans performed too early (20–50 s) after bolus administration of contrast material. In case of doubt, later phase scans (70–100 s) will enable differentiation (Gay and Sistrom 1992; Shuman 1997).

Laceration is considered when linear, low-density areas are seen within the splenic parenchyma (Figs. 8.5–8.10). The term "shattered spleen" or "fragmented spleen" refers to disruption of the entire spleen by multiple lacerations that connect opposed splenic surfaces. Perisplenic fluid is present in all patients with splenic lacerations. Very high-attenuation intrasplenic fluid usually corresponds to extravasated intraparenchymal contrast material and, therefore, indicates active bleeding (Fig. 10).

Non-enhancing portions of the spleen are suggestive of injury or thrombosis of the artery in contact with the affected segment. Multiple scoring systems for CT grading of the extent of splenic injury have been proposed in the literature (Buntain et al.

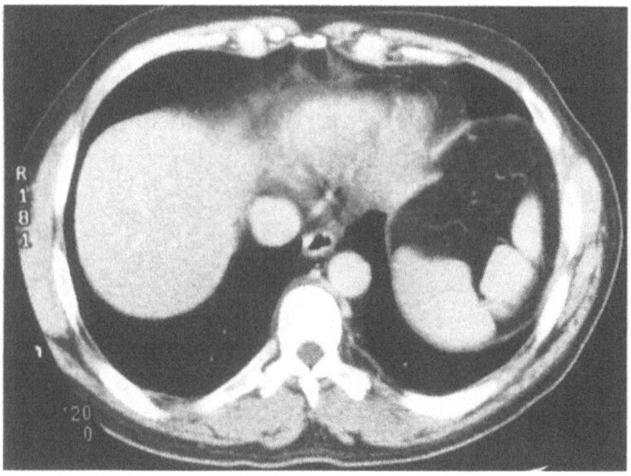

Fig. 8.2. Contrast-enhanced computed-tomography scan of the upper abdomen. Congenital splenic clefts or pseudo-fragmentation of the spleen. The smooth and well-defined borders of the fragments aid in differentiation from splenic rupture

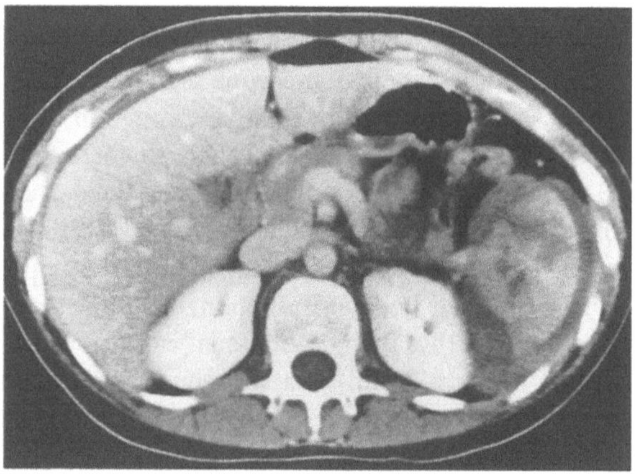

Fig. 8.4. Contrast-enhanced computed-tomography scan of the upper abdomen. Intrasplenic hematomas (*arrowheads*), splenic rupture (*arrows*) and perisplenic hematoma in a victim of a car accident

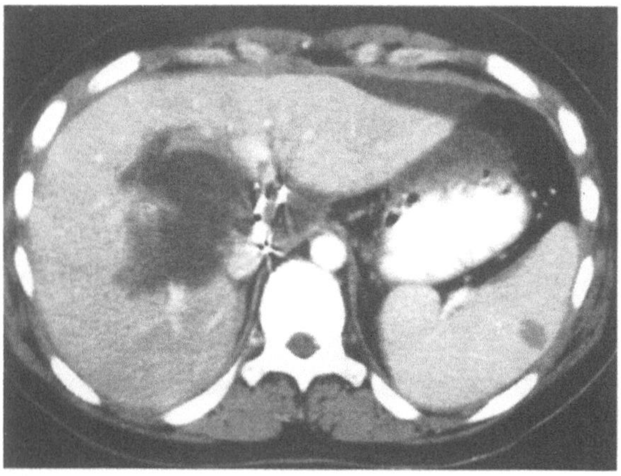

Fig. 8.3. Contrast-enhanced computed-tomography scan of the spleen. Blunt abdominal trauma with sequelae of large hepatic and small splenic hematomas. Presence of free peritoneal fluid (blood)

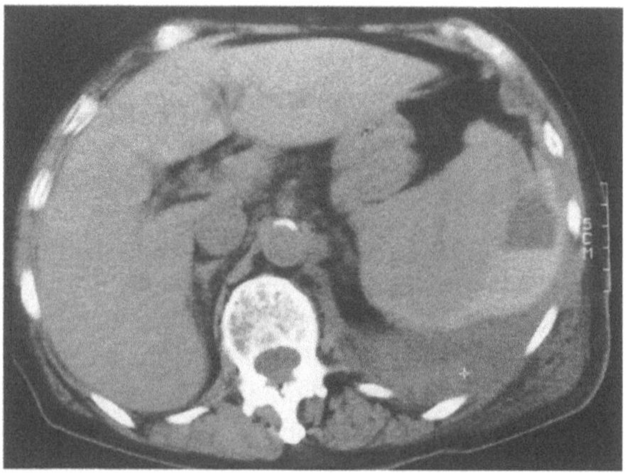

Fig. 8.5. Non-enhanced computed-tomography scan of the upper abdomen. Fluid level (*hematocrit sign*) in a recent perisplenic hematoma after puncture of a pleural effusion (courtesy of F. Vanhoenacker)

1988; Resciniti et al. 1988; Mirvis et al. 1989; Scatamacchia et al. 1989; Moore et al. 1995). The most commonly used grading systems are those proposed by Mirvis et al. (1989) and, more recently, by Moore et al. (1995). These are summarized in Tables 8.1 and 8.2, respectively.

8.3.3.3
Do CT Grading Systems Enable Prediction?

While it is generally accepted that CT is a reliable method of identifying and quantifying splenic injury and that the information provided by CT at admission may greatly facilitate patient management, the

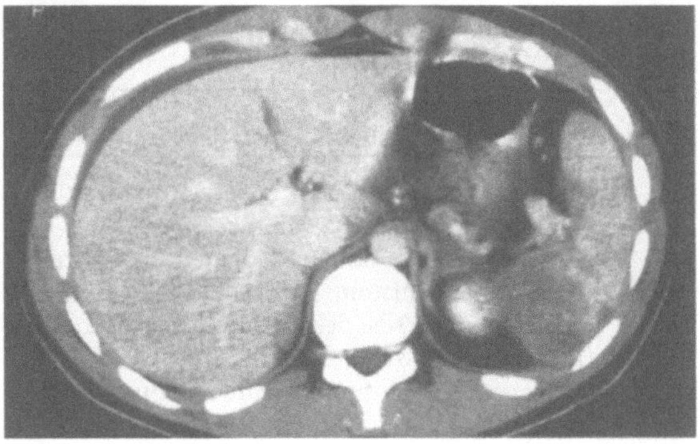

Fig. 8.8. Contrast-enhanced computed-tomography scan of the upper abdomen. Laceration of the spleen. Presence of multiple non-enhancing areas within the posterior part of the spleen. Presence of perihepatic free fluid

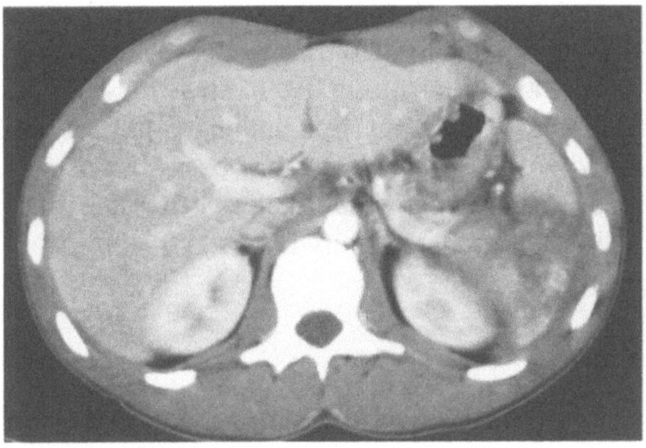

Fig. 8.6. Contrast-enhanced computed-tomography scan of the upper abdomen in a case of laceration of the spleen. Triangular, non-enhancing, parenchymal defect extending into the hilum of the spleen. Minute amount of perisplenic blood

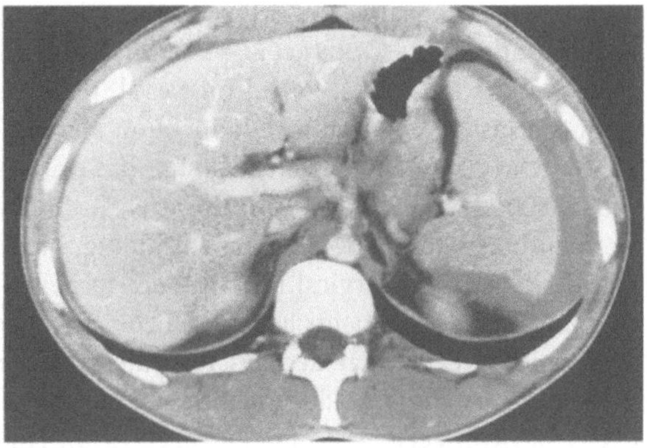

Fig. 8.9. Contrast-enhanced computed-tomography scan of the upper abdomen. Perisplenic hematoma with layers of different attenuation, proving metachronous bleeding. No obvious parenchymal laceration or intrasplenic hematoma. A capsular avulsion was found on surgical exploration (courtesy of M. Mespreuve)

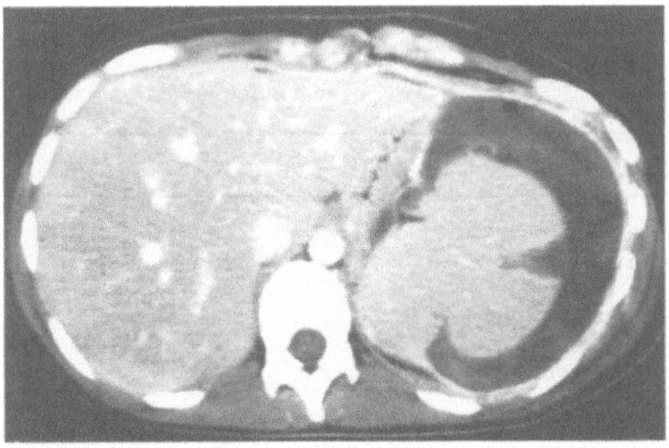

Fig. 8.7. Contrast-enhanced computed-tomography scan in a case of splenic laceration. Presence of two wedge-shaped parenchymal defects on the lateral border of the spleen and a large perisplenic hematoma

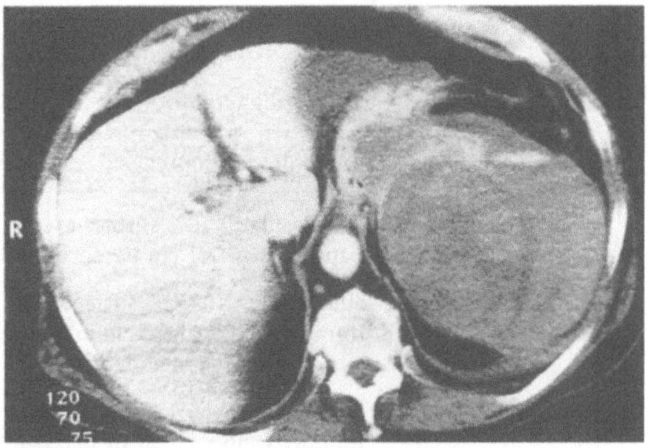

Fig. 8.10. Contrast-enhanced computed-tomography scan of the upper abdomen. Intrasplenic hematoma extending into the region of the hilum. The stomach is displaced medially. The hyperdensity ventral to the hematoma represents extravasation of contrast, indicating active bleeding (*arrow*). The inhomogeneous, rounded densities in the hematoma represent blood clots (*arrowheads*)

Table 1. Computed-tomography grading of splenic injury, according to MIRVIS et al. (1989)

Grade	Criteria
1	Capsular avulsion; superficial laceration(s) or subcapsular hematoma <1 cm
2	Parenchymal laceration(s) 1–3 cm deep; central/ subscapular hematoma(s) <3 cm
3	Laceration(s) >3 cm deep; central/subcapsular hematoma(s) >3 cm
4	Fragmentation of three or more sections; devascularized (non-enhanced) spleen

role of CT grading systems for splenic injury remains controversial. Despite promising initial observations, general agreement exists that, to date (at least in adults), the CT grade of splenic injury cannot be used to select those patients who can be managed non-operatively (RESCINITI et al. 1988; MIRVIS et al. 1989; BECKER et al. 1994, 1998; KOHN et al. 1994).

In contrast, in children sustaining blunt abdominal trauma, CT grading of splenic injury has proven useful (BENYA and BULAS 1996). However, it should be mentioned that, in children sustaining blunt splenic injury, non-surgical management in hemodynamically stable patients has gained considerable acceptance over several decades regardless of the grade of injury and has a documented success rate of over 95% (KOHN et al. 1994; BECKER et al. 1998). This may be partially explained by the fact that delayed rupture is exceedingly rare in children and that the spleen has a tremendous ability to heal. In view of the increasing popularity of non-surgical management of splenic injury (including in adults), however, the issue has become less important. In recent reports, it has been stated that dynamic helical CT scans of the spleen might be valuable in selecting patients who would benefit from angiographic embolization. The following criteria were used: active contrast extravasation, vascular abnormalities of the spleen and increase in the CT grade of splenic injury on follow-up CT (SHANMUGANATHAN et al. 1998).

Commonly used CT grading systems for splenic injury that are based on the estimated size of hematomas and lacerations are incapable of predicting the clinical outcome of non-surgical treatment of splenic injuries (UMLAS and CRONAN 1991; GAVANT et al. 1997). CT findings cannot be used to predict delayed splenic rupture, as initial CT scans in these patients are either normal or disclose only minimal abnormalities (LAWSON et al. 1995). Although the CT grading does not influence initial treatment of splenic injury, which is guided by clinical parameters, it has a role in long-term management, because CT enables one to follow healing of the injury over time (BENYA and BULAS 1996). Since most trauma surgeons will permit resumption of full physical activity only when healing has been documented, this establishes an important role for CT in the follow-up of splenic injury (FEDERLE 1995).

8.3.4 Angiography

The role of celiac angiography is to provide a complete anatomical cartography and to prove active extravasation if endovascular embolization is considered as treatment in splenic trauma patients (Chap. 13.3). The so-called patchy starry-night appearance of the spleen (Fig. 8.11) is a sign of extravasation and should not be treated by embolization.

Table 2. Spleen-injury scale, according to MOORE et al. (1995)

Grade	Injury type	Injury description
I	Hematoma	Subcapsular; <10% surface area
	Laceration	Capsular tear; <1 cm parenchymal depth
II	Hematoma	Subcapsular; 10–50% surface area
		Intraparenchymal; <5 cm in diameter
	Laceration	1-3-cm parenchymal depth, which does not involve a trabecular vessel
III	Hematoma	Subcapsular; >50% surface area or expanding
		Ruptured subcapsular or parenchymal
		Intraparenchymal; >5 cm or expanding
	Laceration	>3 cm parenchymal depth or involving the trabecular vessels
IV	Laceration	Laceration involving segmental or hilar vessels, producing major devascularization in >25% of the spleen
V	Laceration	Completely shattered spleen
	Vascular	Hilar vascular injury that devascularizes the spleen

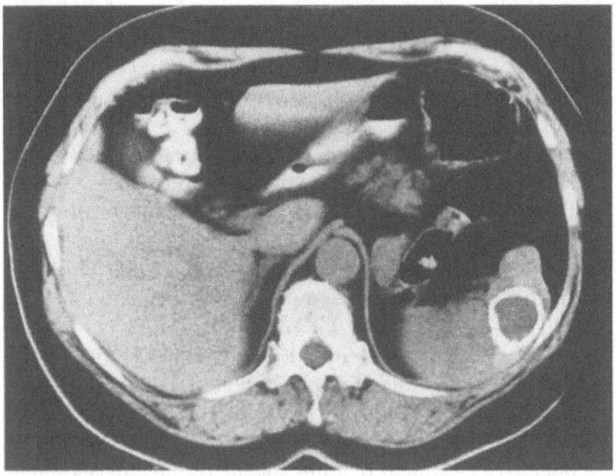

Fig. 8.11. Non-enhanced computed-tomography scan of the upper abdomen. Old hematoma in a patient with previous splenic trauma (courtesy of M. MESPREUVE)

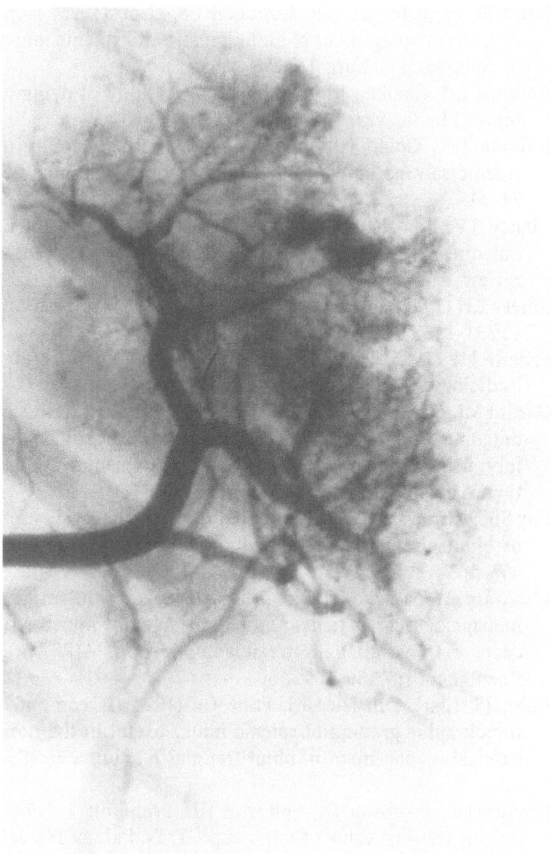

Fig. 8.12. Arterial-phase angiography of the splenic artery after blunt abdominal trauma. Multiple rounded and stellar vascular lakes within the spleen; this symptom is known as the "starry-night spleen", as it resembles the painting of Vincent Van Gogh

8.4 Imaging of Healing Splenic Injury

Ultrasonography and CT scans can be used to follow the resolution of splenic injuries. As may be expected, the course and duration of healing depend on the nature and the extent of the initial injury. With time, splenic hematomas and lacerations become hypodense relative to adjacent splenic tissue. Hematomas may become sharply delineated as their size decreases. Areas of devascularized splenic tissue generally show reperfusion on follow-up CT examination 6 weeks after the initial injury. Following injury, the shape of the spleen may return to normal, or residual contour deformity may persist. Rarely, cyst formation or calcification may occur at the site of splenic injury (Fig. 8.12; Chap. 10). Perisplenic fluid collections commonly resolve within 2–4 weeks after the injury. In splenic hematomas, a period of weeks to months is needed for complete healing. Grade-1 and -2 lesions usually heal within 4 months. More severe grade-3 injuries generally heal within 6 months, whereas grade-4 injuries can take up to 11 months to heal (BENYA and BULAS 1996; ROBERTS et al. 1996).

8.5 Conclusion

Over the past 20 years, development of new diagnostic imaging methods and refinement of existing methods have contributed to our ability to distinguish patients with serious injury from those without injuries following abdominal trauma. Accurate assessment of splenic injury is particularly relevant in this era, in which non-operative management of certain injuries is promoted in order to salvage splenic function whenever possible.

References

Anderson CB, Ballinger WF (1985) Abdominal injuries. In: Zuidema GD, Rutherford RB, Ballinger WF (eds) The management of trauma. Saunders, Philadelphia, pp 101–131

Becker CD, Mentha G, Terrier F (1998) Blunt abdominal trauma in adults: role of CT in the diagnosis and management of visceral injuries. Eur Radiol 8:553–562

Becker CD, Spring P, Glättli A, Schweizer W (1994) Blunt splenic trauma in adults: can CT findings be used to determine the need for surgery? AJR Am J Roentgenol 162:343–347

Benya EC, Bulas DI (1996) Splenic injuries in children after blunt abdominal trauma. Semin Ultrasound CT MR 17:170–176

Bond SJ, Eichelberger MR, Gotschall CS, et al. (1996) Non-operative management of blunt hepatic and splenic injury in children. Ann Surg 223:286–289
Budnick LD, Chaiken BP (1985) The probability of dying of injuries by the year 2000. JAMA 254:3350
Buntain WL, Gould HR, Maull KI (1998) Predictability of splenic salvage by computed tomography. J Trauma 28: 24–34
Clancy TV, Ramshaw DG, Maxwell JG (1997) Management outcomes in splenic injury: a statewide trauma center review. Ann Surg 226:17–24
Emery KH (1997) Splenic emergencies. Radiol Clin North Am 35:831–843
Federle MP (1995) Splenic trauma: is follow-up CT of value? Radiology 194:23–24
Gavant ML, Schurr M, Flick PA, et al. (1997) Predicting clinical outcome of non-surgical management of blunt splenic injury: using CT to reveal abnormalities of splenic vasculature. AJR Am J Roentgenol 168:207–212
Gay SB, Sistrom CL (1992) Computed tomographic evaluation of blunt abdominal trauma. Radiol Clin North Am 30: 367–388
Hagiwara A, Yukioka T, Ohta S, et al. (1996) Non-surgical management of patients with blunt splenic injury: efficacy of transcatheter arterial embolization. AJR Am J Roentgenol 167:159–166
Kohn JS, Clark DE, Isler RJ, Pope CF (1994) Is computed tomographic grading of splenic injury useful in the non-surgical management of blunt trauma? J Trauma 36:385–390
Lawson DE, Jacobson JA, Spizarny DL, Pranikoff T (1995) Splenic trauma: value of follow-up CT. Radiology 194:94–100
McLoughlin RF, Mathieson JR (1995) Imaging and intervention in abdominal emergencies. Baillieres Clin Gastroenterol 9:1–19
Mirvis SE, Whitley NO, Gens DR (1989) Blunt splenic trauma in adults: CT-based classification and correlation with prognosis and treatment. Radiology 171:33–39
Moore EE, Cogbill TH, Jurkovich GJ, et al. (1995) Organ injury scaling: spleen and liver (1994 revision). J Trauma 38:323–324
Newton EJ, Parisky YR (1992) Abdominal trauma. In: Rosen P, Doris PE, Barkin RM, Barkin SZ, Markovchick VJ (eds) Diagnostic radiology in emergency medicine. Mosby Year Book, St. Louis, pp 101–141
Pickhardt B, Moore EE, Moore FA, et al. (1989) Operative splenic salvage in adults: a decade perspective. J Trauma 29:1386–1391
Pimpl W, Dapunt O, Kaindl H, Thalhamer J (1989) Incidence of septic and thromboembolic-related deaths after splenectomy in adults. Br J Surg 76:517–521
Resciniti A, Fink MP, Raptopoulos V, et al. (1988) Non-operative treatment of adult splenic trauma: development of a computed tomographic scoring system that detects appropriate candidates for expectant management. J Trauma 128:828–831
Roberts JL (1996) CT of abdominal and pelvic trauma. Semin Ultrasound CT MR 17:142–169
Scatamacchia SA, Raptopoulos V, Fink MP, Silva WE (1989) Splenic trauma in adults: impact of CT grading on management. Radiology 171:725–729
Shanmuganathan K, Mirvis SE, Tatsuyoshi T, et al. (1998) Non-operative management of blunt splenic injury: CT criteria to select patients for angiographic embolization of the spleen. Radiology 209:409
Shuman WP (1997) CT of blunt abdominal trauma in adults. Radiology 205:297–306
Sivit CJ, Bulas DI (1993) Diagnostic imaging. In: Eichelberger MR (ed) Pediatric trauma: prevention, acute care and rehabilitation. Mosby, St. Louis, pp 226–288
Umlas SL, Cronan JJ (1991) Splenic trauma: can CT grading systems enable prediction of successful non-surgical treatment? Radiology 178:481–487

9 Vascular Pathology of the Spleen

C.C. HOEFFEL

CONTENTS

9.1 Introduction and Anatomy

This chapter refers to lesions involving the splenic vessels and to the consequent splenic parenchymal pathology of such lesions. Splenic vessels include the splenic vein and the splenic artery. The splenic vein is a thin-walled vein coursing in a groove along the upper dorsal surface of the pancreas and is formed by the union of four or five branches leaving the splenic hilum. Occasionally, a vein from the upper pole of the spleen joins the splenic vein more proximally (the superior polar vein). Proximally, the splenic vein receives the short gastric veins and the gastroepiploic vein from the stomach. It receives multiple pancreatic branches and the inferior mesenteric vein as it passes posterior to the tail and body of the pancreas. The splenic vein then unites with the superior mesenteric vein to form the portal vein behind the neck of the pancreas. The splenic vessels pass towards the spleen in the phrenicosplenic and lienorenal ligaments. The splenic artery arises from the coeliac trunk and enters the spleen as four or five branches at the hilum between the gastric and renal impressions. The main splenic artery has always been routinely visible on computed tomography (CT) scans, but its smaller branches may now be seen on images from helical CT scanners. Short gastric branches arise from the distal splenic artery near the splenic hilum. The left gastroepiploic artery also originates from the distal splenic artery and continues within the greater omentum along the great curvature of the stomach to anastomose with branches of the right gastroepiploic artery (STALLARD et al. 1994).

9.2 Splenic-Vein Thrombosis

Splenic-vein thrombosis is most often secondary to pancreatitis, pancreatic carcinoma or hypercoagulable states and is also seen in cirrhosis of the liver, after liver transplantation, after splenectomy (PETIT et al. 1994) or idiopathically (BALTHAZAR et al. 1984, 1985). The splenic vein becomes thrombosed in as many as 45% of patients with pancreatitis (VUJIC 1989). Splenic-vein thrombosis causes development of gastric varices. Three different collateral pathways may be encountered: venous drainage via short gastric veins into the right and left gastric veins and then into the portal vein; collateral circulation through the left and right gastroepiploic veins and superior mesenteric veins; and retroperitoneal venous collateral drainage via the left renal vein and inferior vena cava. As many as 50% of patients with splenic vein thrombosis have oesophageal varices due to inadequate decompression through the short gastric veins (VUJIC 1989).

C.C. HOEFFEL; Department of Radiology A, Hôpital COCHIN, 27 Rue du Faubourg Saint Jacques, F-75014 Paris, France

Early management can prevent the occurrence of bowel infarction and gastrointestinal (GI) bleeding. There are few acute symptoms (left upper quadrant pain, diffuse acute abdominal pain), but gastric varices may result in dramatic GI bleeding (haematemesis or melena).

Enhanced CT and colour Doppler sonography are reliable for the diagnosis of thrombosis of the splenic vein (Rahmouni et al. 1992). Doppler ultrasound (US) is a good technique for assessment of the patency of the splenic vein.

Sonographically, splenic-vein thrombosis is often echogenic. A relatively hypoechoic clot is difficult to identify without the use of colour flow sonography. In fresh thrombosis, the vein is dilated, non-compressible and exhibits no respiratory modulation of its calibre. Doppler sonography of obstruction of the splenic vein shows no flow, while an incompletely occluded splenic vein still retains detectable residual flow, which may present with an elevated and stenotic flow velocity.

Angiography is unnecessary when thrombosis of the splenic vein is confidently diagnosed by bolus CT or Doppler sonography. CT scan is also particularly useful in demonstrating gastric varices that accompany splenic vein occlusion. CT findings of gastric varices, splenomegaly and absence of visualisation of the splenic vein are diagnostic of splenic vein occlusion (Fig. 9.1). Acute thrombosis of the splenic vein on CT is evident as an intraluminal, low-density filling defect seen adjacent to enhancing vasa vasorum of the venous wall. On endoscopy, patients with splenic-vein occlusion have minimal oesophageal varices and prominent gastric varices owing to short gastric and gastroepiploic collaterals.

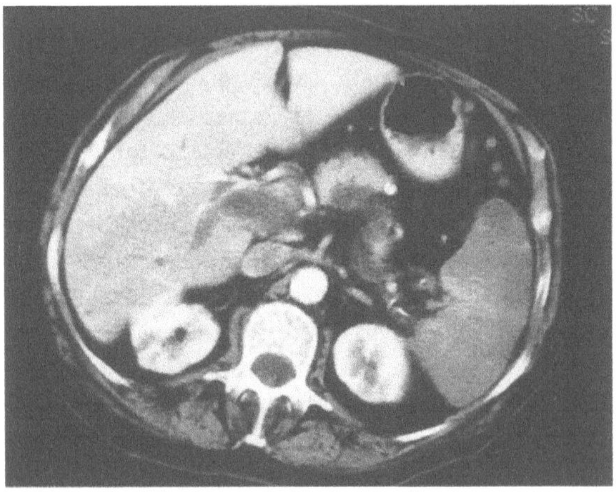

Fig. 9.1. A 60-year-old woman. Helical computed tomography demonstrates thrombosis of the splenic vein and an enlarged, non-enhancing splenic vein associated with collateral circulation via short gastric veins and spleen infarction (a globally low-attenuation spleen). Note the portal-vein thrombosis

The differential diagnosis of left upper-quadrant varices includes portal hypertension and portal-vein thrombosis. The identification of an enlarged left gastroepiploic vein without a recanalised umbilical vein strongly suggests venous thrombosis and not portal hypertension (Marn et al. 1990). In addition, the presence of normally enhanced portal and superior mesenteric veins, with non-visualisation of the splenic vein, supports the diagnosis of splenic-vein thrombosis (Petit et al. 1994).

On magnetic resonance imaging (MRI), gastric varices are seen as multiple, tortuous structures with a signal void on T2-weighted images, whereas the thrombosed splenic vein exhibits hyperintensity on T2-weighted images. Preoperative embolization of the splenic artery reduces the left upper-quadrant varices, facilitating subsequent surgery.

9.3 Splenic-Artery Aneurysm

9.3.1 Aetiology and Frequency

Splenic-artery aneurysm is the most common abdominal visceral artery aneurysm, representing approximately 60% of visceral arterial aneurysms. Because of their association with pregnancy, splenic-artery aneurysms are significantly more common in women, with fewer than 15% being seen in men (Trastek et al. 1982). A rough estimation of the incidence in large autopsy series is about 0.01–0.02%, though the real incidence approximates 10% (Bedford and Lodge 1960). However, their incidence may vary depending on predisposing conditions.

9.3.1.1 Portal Hypertension

The reported incidence of splenic-artery aneurysms in patients with portal hypertension varies from 7.1% to 14.7% (Puttini et al. 1982; Mattar and Lumsden 1995). They appear to be more frequent in cases of splenorenal shunts and of chronic portal hypertension. The precise mechanism of the formation of these aneurysms is still debated, though the theory of a hyperkinetic state seems to be confirmed by Doppler-US studies (Nishida et al. 1986; Ohta et al. 1992).

9.3.1.2
Pregnancy and Multiparity

A history of multiparity is frequent in women with splenic-artery aneurysm, and the risk of rupture of the aneurysm is higher in cases of pregnancy. This strong association is possibly due to hormonal and haemodynamic effects on the arterial wall during pregnancy (Angelakis et al. 1993).

9.3.1.3
Pancreatitis

One of the most life-threatening complications of pancreatitis is the formation of arterial pseudoaneurysms. They may result from erosion of the vessel wall and can be overlooked if dynamic injection of contrast medium and fast data acquisition are not used. A pseudocyst may directly erode into an adjacent artery, immediately transforming the pseudocyst into a large pseudoaneurysm (Fig. 9.2). Pseudoaneurysms may be present in as many as 10% of patients with pancreatitis (Burke et al. 1986).

9.3.1.4
Other Causes

Other causes include arteriosclerotic disease, penetrating gastric ulcer, trauma and vasculitis (Fig. 9.3). Mycotic aneurysms involving the intrasplenic branches of the splenic artery have also been reported (Avery et al. 1991). They are often multiple and associated with other aneurysms involving other abdominal arteries.

9.3.2
Anatomical Characteristics of the Aneurysms and Clinical Presentation

There is no relationship between the morphology and the aetiology of splenic aneurysms. The aneurysms are most often saccular, and over 75% occur at the distal third of the splenic arteries. They are multiple in 20% of cases. However, in portal hypertension, they are more frequently located either at the splenic hilum or distally on splenic-artery branches. Their sizes range from less than 1 cm to 3 cm.

Although most patients are asymptomatic, a pulsatile mass, left upper-quadrant pain and rupture, either in the peritoneal cavity or in the GI tract, have been reported (Bishop et al. 1984; Walker et al. 1988). They may also experience rupture in the Wirsung tract or in a pseudocyst. Risk of rupture of these aneurysms is difficult to evaluate. It is generally admitted that this risk increases with the size of the aneurysm.

9.3.3
Imaging of Splenic-Artery Aneurysms

Splenic-artery aneurysms are often incidentally diagnosed when signet-ring calcifications are seen on abdominal plain films or during US or CT examination of the abdomen (Fig. 9.4b). The usefulness of

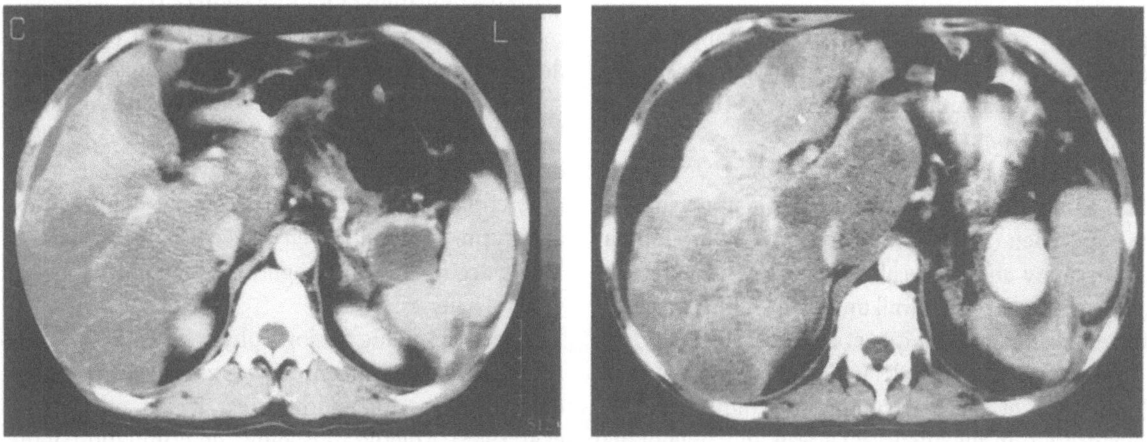

a b

Fig. 9.2. a A helical computed tomography (CT) scan initially shows a pancreatic pseudocyst in the region of the pancreatic tail, adjacent to the splenic artery. **b** Transformation into a big pseudoaneurysm detected on a subsequent helical CT-scan study performed 1 year later in the same patient

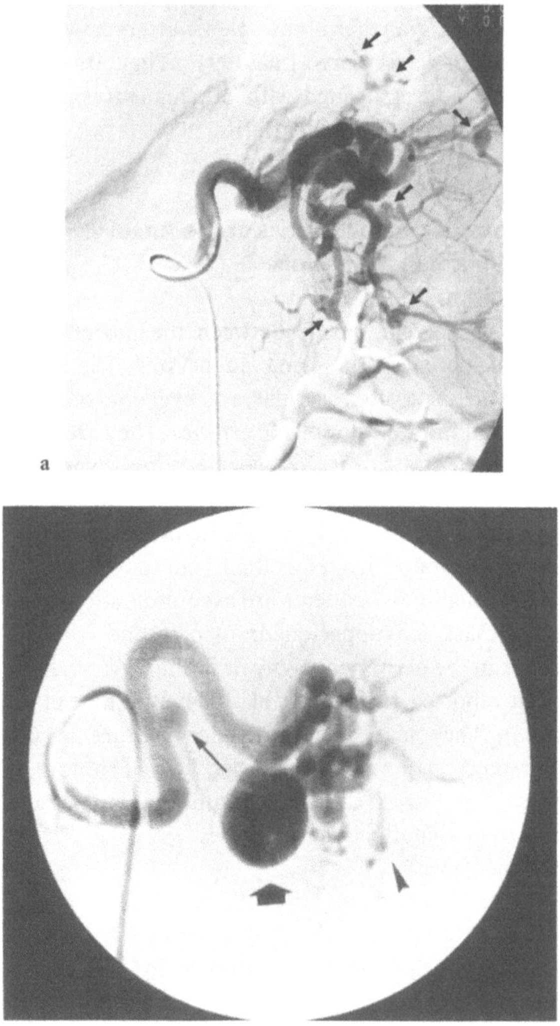

Fig. 9.3. a,b. Angiography, demonstrating multiple aneurysms on the splenic artery or its branches in two different patients (arrows)

grey-scale and colour Doppler sonography in the diagnosis of splenic-artery aneurysm has been emphasised in a number of case reports (Golzarian et al. 1994; Goletti et al. 1996).

Splenic-artery aneurysms appear on US examination as hypoechoic masses in the left upper part of the abdomen (Fig. 9.4a). Pulsed and colour Doppler sonography show a weak, turbulent, pulsatile flow along the aneurysmal wall unless thrombus has filled the entire lumen (Derchi et al. 1984) (Fig. 9.4c).

However, Ishida et al. (1998) have described some limitations of these techniques, including marked calcification in the aneurysmal wall and splenorenal shunts. In cases of splenorenal shunts, small aneurysms may be misinterpreted as a part of the shunt if only grey-scale sonography is used. Demonstration of pulsatile arterial flow helps in differentiating an arterial aneurysm from portal collaterals.

On CT scan, they appear as well-defined, low-density masses with or without calcifications. Differential diagnosis on non-enhanced scans includes pancreatic pseudocyst, cystic pancreatic tumours and splenosis (Murayama and Shimoda 1990). Moreover, the enhancement pattern of splenosis and a splenic aneurysm may be similar. Marked and early arterial enhancement within the residual patent lumen after intravenous contrast-medium administration is the rule unless the lesion is thrombosed (Fig. 9.4d), and it supports the diagnosis of an aneurysm. On a portal phase scan, attenuation values in the lesion decrease in case of an aneurysm. If spiral acquisition is used, multiplanar, mainly two-dimensional (2D) or 3D maximum-intensity projection (Fishmann et al. 1992, 1995) reconstructions optimally demonstrate the relationship and location of the aneurysm (Fig. 9.5).

On MRI, aneurysms show a well-defined ring of low signal intensity at the periphery, corresponding to the aneurysmal wall, while the signal intensity within the aneurysm depends on the presence and velocity of flowing blood and the presence and age of the thrombus. High signal intensity in the mural thrombus on T1-weighted images is consistent with methaemoglobin formation in subacute thrombus and allows the lesion to be differentiated from a pancreatic pseudocyst. Fast-flowing blood within the patent lumen produces a signal void, which persists on all spin-echo sequences. In cases of turbulent or slow flow, gradient-recalled echo sequences or MR angiography (MRA) may be performed. On these sequences, flowing blood is shown as areas of high signal intensity, while signal from background structures is saturated. 3D-MR acquisition of multiple thin (<1cm) slices and reconstruction of the images in selected planes will demonstrate the relation of the aneurysmal sac to the splenic artery and may show the neck of the aneurysm. Either 3D time-of-flight (Kehagias et al. 1998) or phase-contrast acquisition may be used to allow differentiation of the artery causing the pseudoaneurysm. Gadolinium-en hanced 3D MRA is also highly accurate in the diagnosis of the aneurysms of visceral arteries.

Selective splenic angiography is necessary to confirm the diagnosis in equivocal cases or as road map before surgical or endovascular treatment (Short et al. 1985). Angiography allows determination of the precise location, size, presence and diameter of the neck of the aneurysm. In the absence of portal hypertension, selective catheterisation of the other visceral

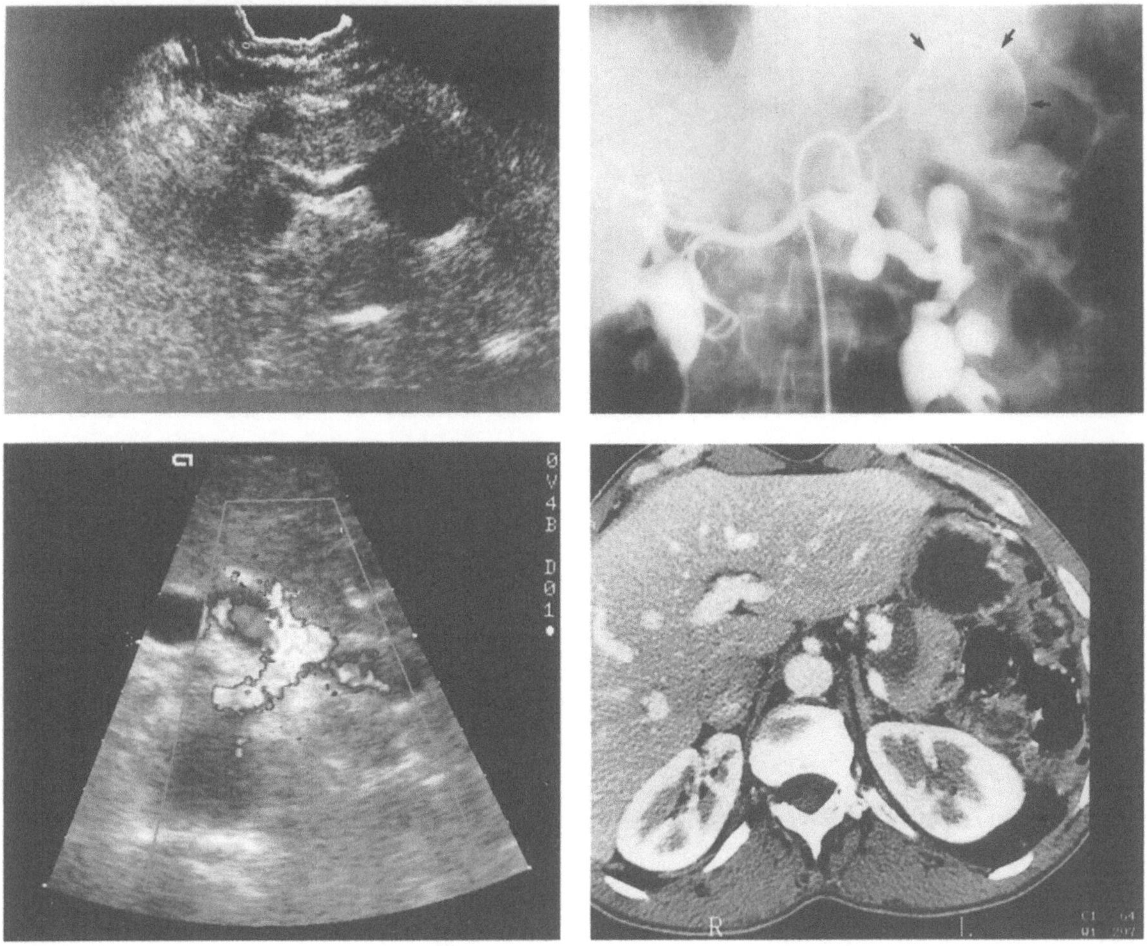

a b c d

Fig. 9.4. Splenic artery aneurysm in three different patients, seen on different imaging modalities. a Ultrasound of a large splenic artery aneurysm seen as a hypoechoic mass on the course of the splenic artery. **b** Angiography of the celiac trunk shows huge calcified splenic artery aneurysm (*arrows*). **c,d** Doppler ultrasound shows hypoechoic mass near the splenic hilium with absence of internal flow, suggesting intraluminal thrombus (**c**). CT scan confirms the diagnosis of a thrombosed aneurysm of the splenic artery (**d**).

arteries should be performed in order to exclude multiplicity (Fig. 9.3).

9.3.4 Treatment

Most authors generally recommend observation by serial CT scans or MRI when the aneurysm diameter is less than 2 cm (Busuttil and Brin 1980). Treatment is recommended in cases of pregnancy or in women of childbearing age, in symptomatic lesions or in large or increasing aneurysms exceeding a diameter of 2 cm. Laparoscopic ligation of the splenic artery is preferred in young pregnant women (Baker et al. 1987; Mandel et al. 1987; Reidy et al. 1990; McDermott et al. 1994; Mattar and Lumsden 1995; Carr et al. 1996).

Surgical treatment consists of aneurysm resection, sometimes in addition to splenectomy or proximal and distal splenic-artery ligation (Trastek et al. 1982; Hashizume et al. 1993). However, the mortality rate in these patients is high due to bad results of emergency treatment of ruptured aneurysms.

Endovascular treatment using coils seems to be the treatment of choice (Baker et al. 1987; Mandel et al. 1987; Reidy et al. 1990). Occlusion must involve the aneurysm, the proximal part of the splenic artery or both. Careful follow-up is required, as splenic infarction and abscess formation are well-known complications of this procedure.

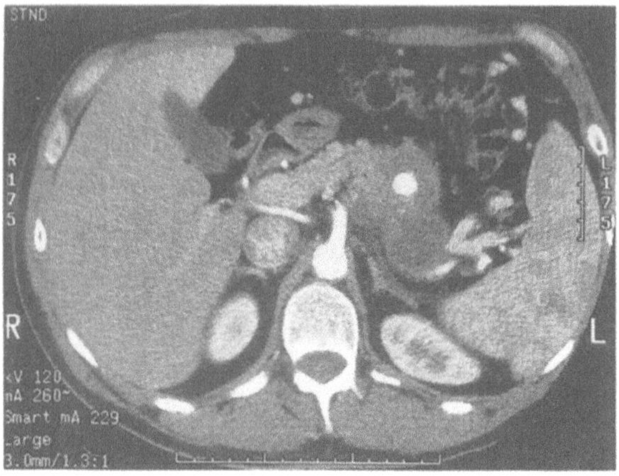

a

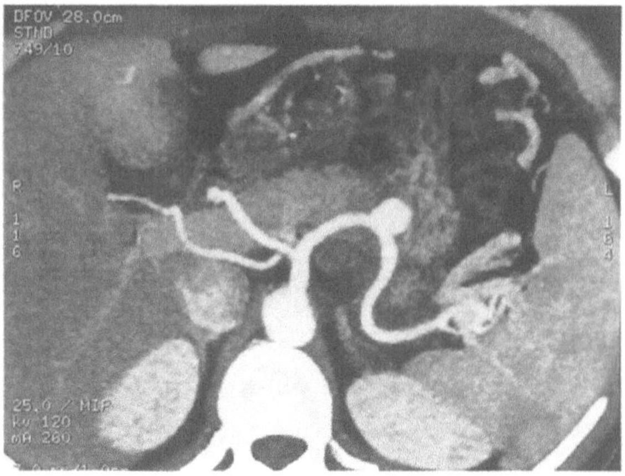

b

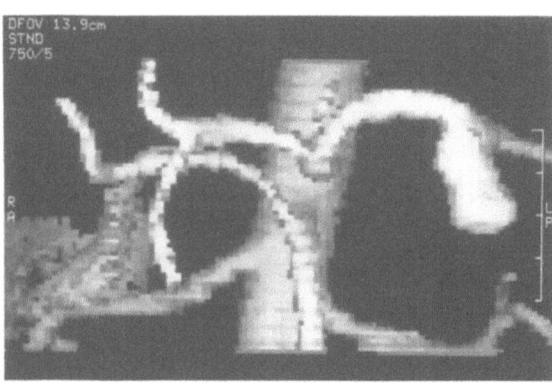

c

Fig. 9.5. Pseudoaneurysm of the splenic artery in a 43-year-old man with chronic pancreatitis. **a** Splenic vessels are encased by pancreatic inflammation. **b** A helical computed tomography scan shows pseudoaneurysm of the splenic artery, caused by pancreatitis. **c** Maximum-intensity projection reformatting and multiplanar reconstructions precisely assess the position and location of the pseudoaneurysm (courtesy of P. Bouillet)

9.4 Splenic Arteriovenous Fistula

9.4.1 Introduction and Clinical Presentation

Arteriovenous fistula between the splenic artery and the splenic vein is a rare finding which is accompanied by a dilated vein or aneurysmal splenic vein that can cause portal hypertension. This condition appears to be more prevalent in women. Pregnancy and multiparity are predisposing factors.

The aetiology can be congenital or acquired. Acquired causes of arteriovenous fistula include fistulisation of a splenic aneurysm into the adjacent splenic vein, local trauma, chronic pancreatitis and splenectomy (Gudmundsen et al. 1988; Sarioglu et al. 1995). Early diagnosis is mandatory, because life-threatening complications may occur if the disease is not treated.

Clinical presentation is usually non-specific, which may prevent early diagnosis. Some non-specific symptoms and signs, such as diarrhoea and abdominal pain, are difficult to explain. GI bleeding and splenomegaly are the most frequent clinical findings at presentation (McClary et al 1986). Ascites and hypersplenism, particularly with thrombocytopenia, are also common. The fistula is usually located at the splenic hilum or on the main splenic artery; rarely, it develops on the distal branches of the splenic artery.

9.4.2 Imaging the Splenic Arteriovenous Fistula

Splenic angiography remains the gold standard in the diagnosis; it can be used to show the exact location and the type of fistula and evaluate the possible associated aneurysms and the extent of the collaterals (Kelekis et al. 1995) (Fig. 9.6a). The invasiveness of arteriography, however, delays its use in some patients, and only 61% of splenic arteriovenous fistulas reported in the literature were correctly diagnosed preoperatively (McClary et al. 1986). Some recent cases have been diagnosed with US or CT (Shleapnik et al. 1990).

Sonography is non invasive and can be rapidly performed in emergency conditions. Typical Doppler findings in splenic arteriovenous fistula

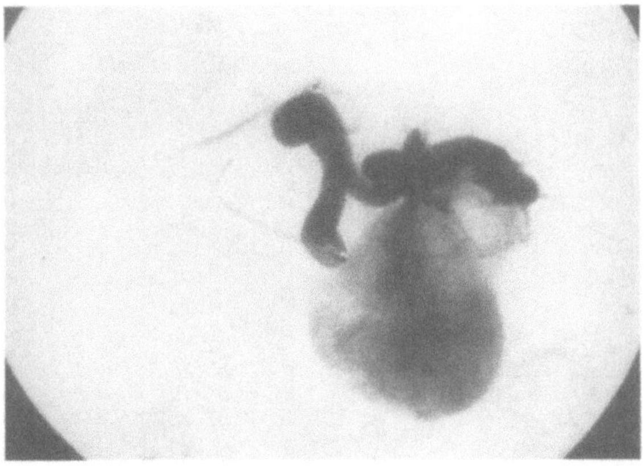

a

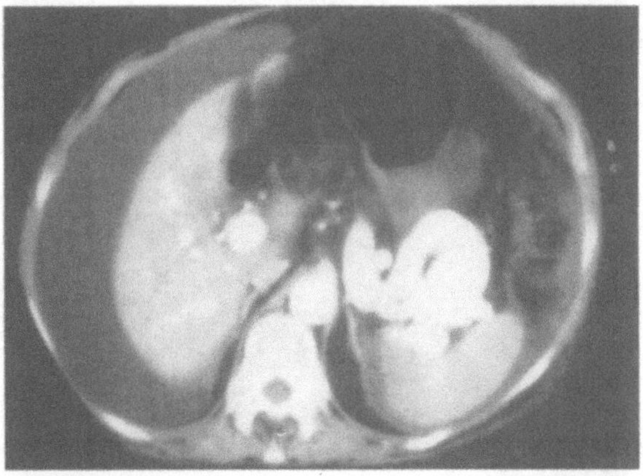

b

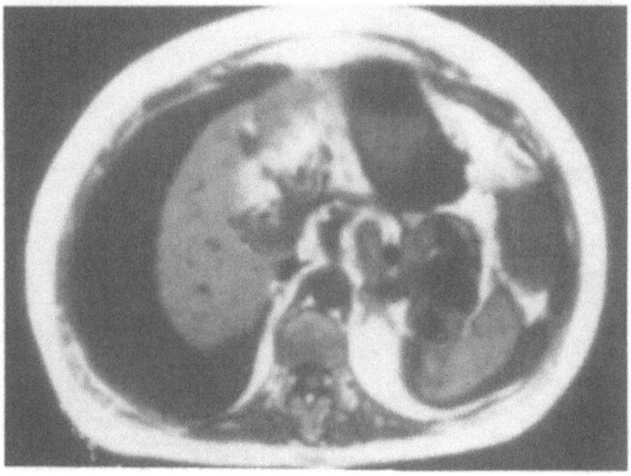

c

Fig. 9.6. Splenic arteriovenous fistula in a 64-year-old woman with a history of multiparity. a Selective angiography of the splenic artery shows the location of the fistula and demonstrates early filling of the splenic vein. **b** A computed-tomography scan at an arterial phase shows two splenic-artery aneurysms and an early enhancement of the dilated splenic vein. c An axial T1-weighted magnetic resonance image reveals a venous dilatation-containing area with a signal void corresponding to the aneurysm (courtesy of D. REGENT)

(CANTARERO et al. 1989; PISCAGLIA et al. 1998) include: a twofold or threefold increase of the flow velocity in the fistula canal with dilatation, elongation or loop formation in the afferent artery, and a fairly pulsatile and high-velocity venous flow immediately distal to the fistula (sometimes extending to the splenic and portal veins, with enlargement of the draining vein). PISCAGLIA et al. (1998) recommend performing Doppler US examination if ectatic vessels in the left upper quadrant and signs of portal hypertension are found in patients without known liver cirrhosis.

CT may show varices and a tortuous, dilated splenic vein. Multiplanar reconstructions are useful in displaying the anatomy of the fistula. AngioCT confirms the diagnosis of fistula, showing early and intense enhancement of the splenic vein (Fig. 9.6b). MR and angioMR also contribute to the diagnosis demonstrating the fistula, the possible associated aneurysms and the venous dilatation (Fig. 9.6c). If the shunt persists for a long period, arterial and venous aneurysms may develop. Treatment consists of either splenectomy and ligation of the fistula or percutaneous embolisation (GARTSIDE and GAMELLI 1987; FAVA et al. 1990).

9.5 Splenic Infarction

9.5.1 Aetiology and General Considerations

Occlusion of the main splenic artery or of one of its branches results in ischemia and infarction. In adults, cardiac emboli are the primary cause of acute splenic infarction (endocarditis, atrial fibrillation or left-ventricular thrombus; JAROCH et al. 1986). Cardiac emboli to the spleen may cause bland or septic infarcts. In these patients, renal infarcts may also be noted in conjunction with splenic infarcts. Other, less frequent causes include local thromboses [especially in haematological diseases (Fig. 9.7) (myelofibrosis, leukaemia and lymphoma)], vasculitis, pancreatitis and splenic torsion (BALCAR et al. 1984; MAGID et al. 1984; RYPENS et al. 1997). In patients younger than 40 years of age, haemo-globinopathies are the most common cause of splenic infarction (BALCAR et al. 1984; JAROCH et al. 1986). Focal or diffuse splenic infarction may occur in cases of pancreatitis with associated vascular compromise due to the inflammation. In these cases, the patient typically

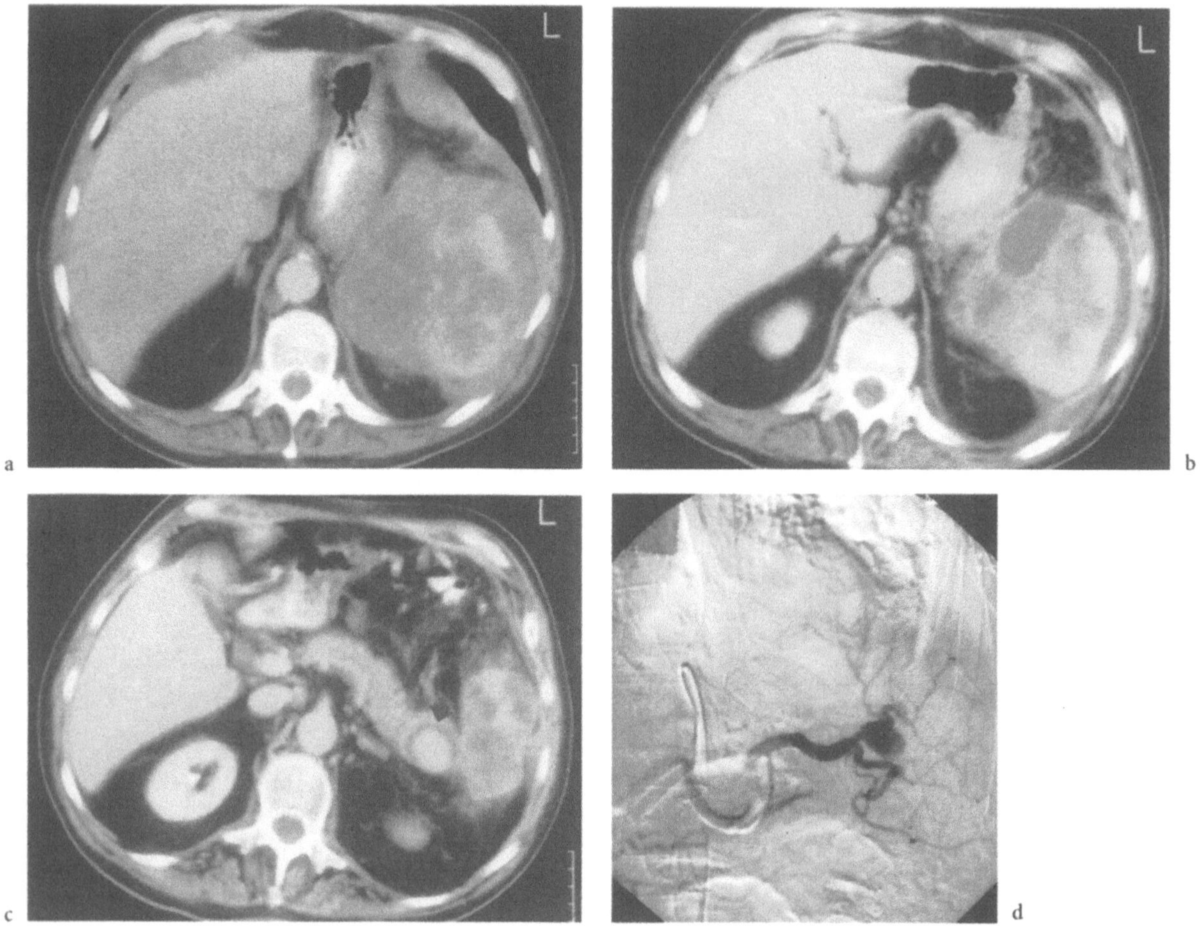

Fig. 9.7a–d. Pseudoaneurysm in a patient with malignant lymphoma damaging the arterial wall of the splenic artery. **a** Initial contrast enhanced CT scan of the upper abdomen. Inhomogeneous enhancement of an enlarged spleen with ill-defined margins, and surrounded by fluid collections. **b,c** Follow-up contrast enhanced CT scan of the upper abdomen. Inhomogeneous enhancement of the spleen, which has slightly decreased in size compared to the previous CT scan. More distinct subcapsular fluid accumulation lateral to the spleen. (**b**) Rounded mass, contiguous to the tail of the pancreas, with homogeneously enhancing central area and surrounded by hypodense rim (arrow). (**c**) **d** Selective angiography of the splenic artery. Aneurysm of the splenic artery in the hilum of the spleen. (Courtesy of M. Olree et al.)

has extensive inflammation around the major splenic vessels, and compression due to inflammation is the presumed cause of infarction (Vujic 1989). Subcapsular haematoma due to splenic infarct may occur. Splenic infarction may also occur as a complication of transcatheter hepatic-arterial embolisation (Weingarten et al. 1984). Splenomegaly alone is a risk factor for infarction. Splenic infarction predisposes a patient to superimposed infection and to splenic rupture. The diagnosis of splenic infarction is of clinical importance in excluding causes of abdominal pain requiring surgical or percutaneous intervention. Clinical presentation usually consists of abrupt onset of left upper-quadrant pain, although infarcts can be silent.

9.5.2 Imaging the Splenic Infarction

The typical appearance of an acute splenic infarction on CT and sonography is a sharply margined peripheral wedge-shaped lesion that demonstrates low attenuation (Fig. 9.8a-d) and decreased echogenicity. Contrast-enhanced CT markedly improves visualisation of a splenic infarct (Balcar et al. 1984). This classical appearance, however, is present in less than half of all acute splenic infarcts (Kazularic and Passega 1986; Goerg and Schwerk 1990). Other reported patterns of splenic infarctions include a multinodular appearance with ill-defined margins and a globally low attenuation (Fig. 9.8) of the spleen (Balcar et al. 1984). Thus, it is more common for splenic infarcts to appear round or irregular, and they frequently have an appearance indistinguishable from that of other splenic lesions,

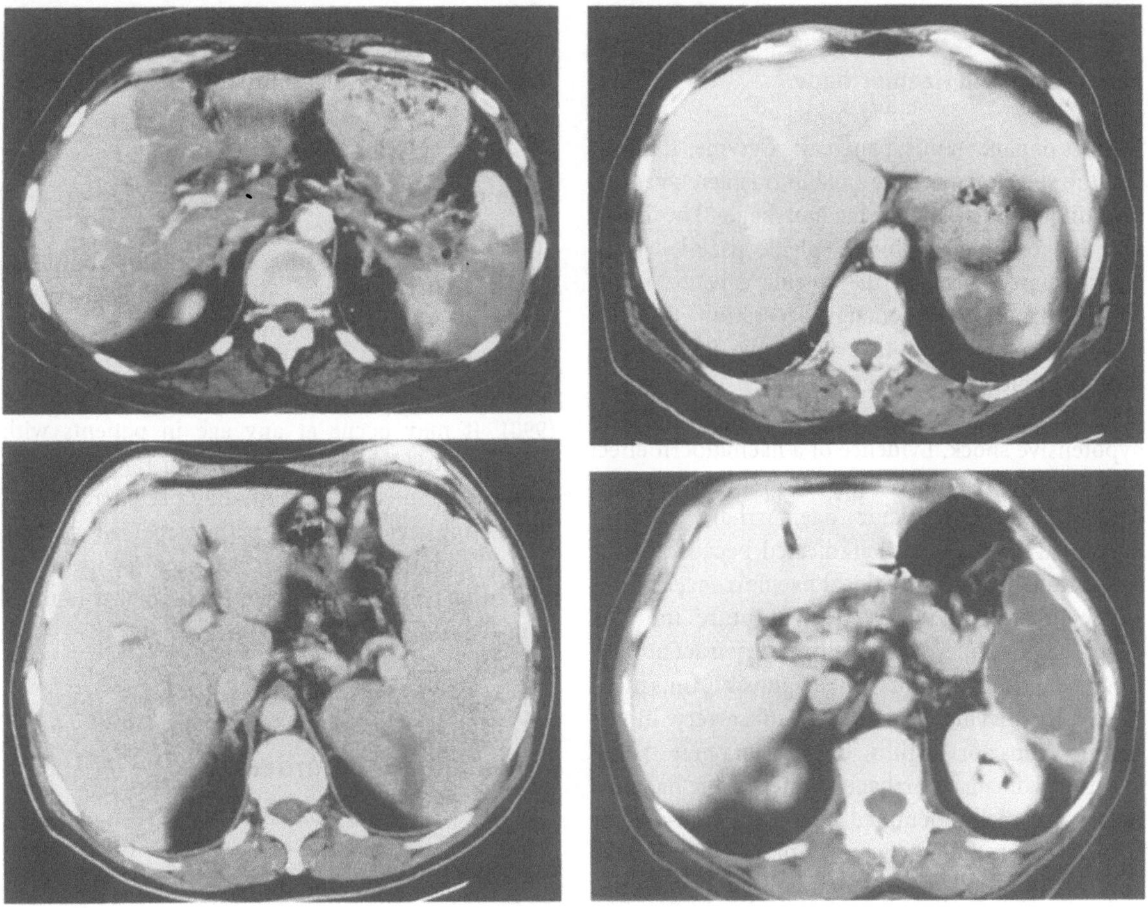

a b c d

Fig. 9.8a–d. Contrast enhanced CT scans showing different imaging patterns of splenic infarction in four different patients. **a** and **b** Peripheral, wedge-shaped pattern, **c** cleftlike appearance of an old infarction and **d** diffuse, low density pattern with capsular rim sign, due to preservation of capsular vascularity.

such as abscesses, haematomas and neoplasms (Balcar et al. 1984). In general, splenic abscesses appear more rounded and exhibit a greater mass effect on the splenic capsule than is caused by infarcts. Guided-needle aspiration may be required for accurate diagnosis in selected cases. There have been a few reports on complications of splenic fine-needle aspiration (Quinn et al. 1986); however, it is a safe and effective method.

The typical MR appearance of an acute splenic infarct is that of a wedge-shaped area of abnormal signal intensity. The variation of signal intensity and its evolution depends on the degree of haemorraghic necrosis and the amount of different blood degradation products within the infarcted area (Rabushka et al. 1994). They are most clearly defined as low-signal-intensity regions on 1-min to 5-min post-gadolinium images.

In the chronic phase, infarcts may disappear completely but, more commonly, splenic infarction significantly changes in size, configuration and echogenicity, density or intensity on subsequent follow-up examinations, depending on the degree of intralesional haemorrhage and fibrosis. Chronic infarcts generally appear as small, wedge-shaped areas of increased echogenicity due to areas of scar formation and fibrosis (Goerg and Schwerk 1990). When serial CT scans demonstrate progressive liquefaction and necrosis with outward expansion, developing subcapsular haemorrhage and free blood in the peritoneal cavity, the possibility of impending rupture or superimposed infections should be considered (Rabushka et al. 1994). In some instances, there may be some calcifications from repeated infarctions related to haemoglobinopathies.

9.6 Splenic Haemorrhage

The leading cause of splenic haemorrhage is trauma, but splenic infarction and pancreatitis may also be complicated by haemorrhage. Other causes of non-traumatic splenic rupture are summarised in Chap. 14.

9.6.1 Pancreatitis and Haemorrhage

In cases of pancreatitis, pancreatic enzymes that dissect the spleen may erode small intrasplenic vessels, resulting in intrasplenic haemorrhage. The blood may be contained within a splenic pseudocyst or it may dissect beneath the splenic capsule. If the haemorrhage is large enough, laceration, capsular disruption or actual rupture of the spleen may occur. If the problem is undiagnosed or if diagnosis is delayed, the patient may rapidly develop signs of hypotensive shock. Evidence of a haematocrit effect (fluid level) within a splenic cyst favours the diagnosis of intrasplenic haemorrhage. Percutaneous drainage is contraindicated because of the risk of causing intraperitoneal haemorrhage.

Pseudoaneurysms may freely rupture into the lesser sac, peritoneal cavity, alimentary tract or pancreatic duct, and their prompt diagnosis is thus mandatory. Involvement of the splenic artery in the splenic hilus or within the spleen may result in intrasplenic haemorrhage. Acute splenic haemorrhages are easily identified on CT as high-density collections. In the management of an acute splenic haemorrhage, splenic-artery embolisation is a valuable adjunct to surgery (Vujic 1989).

9.6.2 Gamna-Gandy Bodies

Portal hypertension causes enlargement of the splenic vein, formation of perisplenic collaterals and, eventually, small areas of intrasplenic haemorrhage. The remnants of these tiny foci of haemorrhage, which are composed of haemosiderin, fibrous tissue and calcium, are referred to as siderotic nodules or Gamna-Gandy bodies. They vary in size but are usually less than 1 cm. They have been described on plain radiographs as multiple small calcifications in an enlarged spleen (Dochez and De Roy 1970; Fig. 9.9a). US may display multiple intrasplenic reflections with accompanying shadowing if the lesions contain sufficient calcium. On CT, non-calcified foci may appear as multiple, punctate, low-attenuation areas (Fig. 9.9b). Calcified foci may appear as multiple high-density lesions. They can be seen on MRI as multiple, punctate, low-intensity lesions on T1-weighted images, T2-weighted images and gradient-echo sequences (Fig. 9.9c). They are more evident on gradient-echo sequences and high-field magnets, and their low signal intensity is due to the superparamagnetic effect of haemosiderin. The blooming artefact on gradient-echo images is pathognomonic for this entity (Minami et al. 1989).

9.6.3 Splenic Sequestration

Acute splenic sequestration is a common complication of sickle cell disease and is a consequence of the trapping of a large amount of blood in the spleen, resulting in sudden splenic enlargement and a rapid decrease in haematocrit (Roshkow and Sanders 1990). It may occur at any age in patients with heterozygous sickle cell disease. On CT scans, the spleen is often enlarged, revealing peripheral hypoattenuating areas that may be interspersed with areas of higher attenuation, representing areas of infarction, pooling of blood or haemorrhage (Adler et al. 1986).

9.7 Miscellaneous Disorders

9.7.1 Atherosclerosis

Atherosclerosis of the splenic artery is a very frequent incidental finding on plain films and computed tomography of the upper abdomen. Although most patients are asymptomatic, complications, such as complete thrombosis and aneurysm formation of the splenic artery, may occur.

9.7.2 Fibromuscular Dysplasia

Fibromuscular dysplasia of the splenic artery is rare. The angiographic appearance is similar to that of the renal arteries with the "*string-of-beads*" configuration (Venbrux et al. 1993).

9.7.3 Splenorenal Shunts

Spontaneous splenorenal shunts may occur in patients with long-standing portal hypertension due to cirrhosis. Dilated perisplenic veins communicating with an enlarged left renal vein may be seen on contrast-enhanced CT, colour Doppler sonography and MRI. Patency of surgically created splenorenal shunts may be evaluated by Doppler US, by selective splenic angiography or left renal vein phlebography.

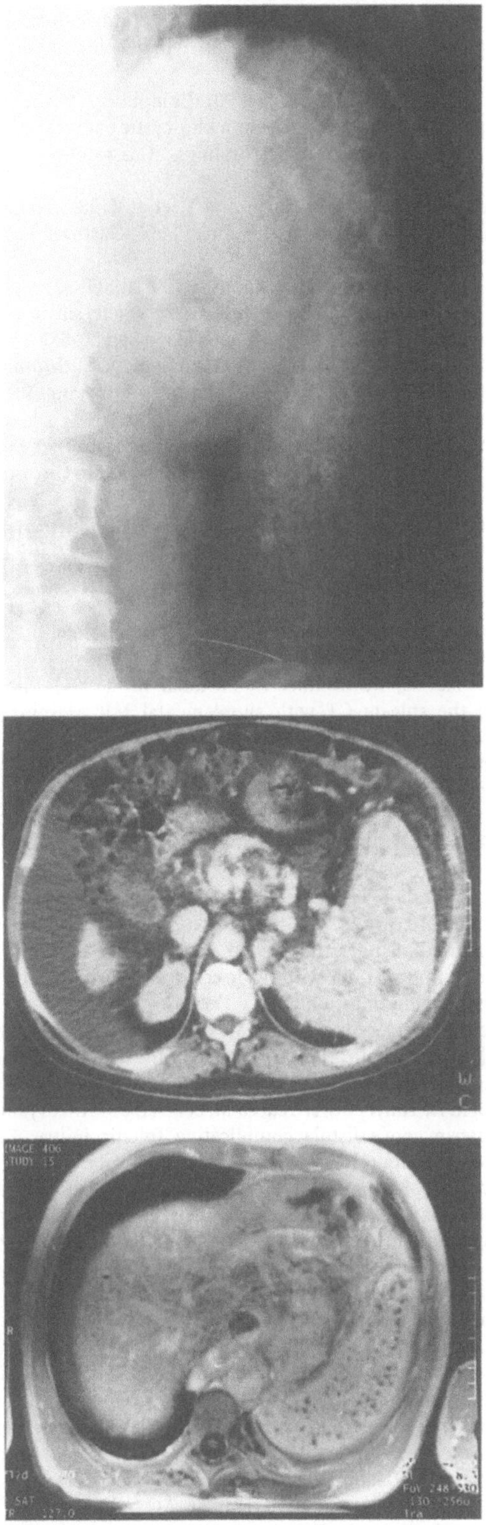

a b c

Fig. 9.9. Gamna-Gandy bodies. **a** Plain film of the abdomen show multiple calcifications in an enlarged spleen (courtesy of C. Dochez). **b** A computed-tomography scan shows multiple, low-density, punctate areas in the spleen. **c** A magnetic resonance T1-weighted image confirms multiple low-intensity splenic lesions (courtesy of K. Mortelé)

9.7.4 Peliosis of the Spleen

Peliosis is a rare condition characterised by multiple, variously sized, blood-filled cysts distributed diffusely throughout the affected organ. The liver is commonly involved, but concomitant splenic involvement has been described in rare cases (Venbrux et al. 1993). Peliosis is associated with the use of drugs, including anabolic steroids, corticosteroids and azathioprine and is also associated with carcinoma and infectious diseases, including tuberculosis, bacillary angiomatosis due to cat-scratch disease, and human immunodeficiency virus.

Imaging findings consist of hepatosplenomegaly and multiple small hepatosplenic lesions. On US, these lesions are hypoechoic, while they are most commonly hypodense on non-contrast-enhanced CT scans. On contrast-enhanced CT, some lesions may not enhance, while others may have a "target" appearance, with central enhancing foci. Non-enhancing lesions seem to represent thrombosed lesions, while the target pattern is probably due to recanalisation of organised thrombi (Venbrux et al. 1993). The signal intensity of peliotic lesions on different MR sequences may vary due to the possibility of intralesional haemorrhage. Portal hypertension and splenic rupture are rare complications.

References

Adler DD, Glazer GM, Aisen AM (1986) MRI of the spleen: normal appearance and findings in sickle-cell anemia. AJR Am J Roentgenol 147:843–845

Angelakis EJ, Bair WE, Barone JE, et al. (1993) Splenic artery aneurysm rupture during pregnancy. Obstet Gynecol Surg 48:145–148

Avery GR, Wilsdon JB, Mitchell L (1991) Case report: CT and angiographic appearances of intrasplenic mycotic aneurysm. Clin Radiol 44:271–272

Baker KS, Tisnado J, Cho SR, et al. (1987) Splanchnic artery aneurysms and pseudoaneurysms: transcatheter embolization. Radiology 163:135–139

Balcar I, Seltzer SE, Davis S, et al. (1984) CT patterns of splenic infarction: a clinical and experimental study. Radiology 151:723–729

Balthazar EJ, Megibow A, Naidich D, et al. (1984) Computed tomographic recognition of gastric varices. AJR Am J Roentgenol 142:1121–1125

Balthazar EJ, Hilton S, Naidich D, et al. (1985) CT of splenic and perisplenic abnormalities in septic patients. AJR Am J Roentgenol 144:53–56

Bedford BT, Lodge B (1960) Aneurysms of the splenic artery. Gut 1:312–320

Bishop NL (1984) Splenic artery aneurysm rupture into the colon diagnosed by angiography. Br J Radiol 57:1149–1150

Burke JW, Erickson SJ, Kellum CD, et al. (1986) Pseudoaneurysms complicating pancreatitis: detection by CT. Radiology 161:447–450

Busuttil RW, Brin BJ (1980) The diagnosis and management of visceral artery aneurysms. Surgery 88:619–624
Cantarero JM, Llorente JG, Hidalgo EG, et al. (1989) Splenic arteriovenous fistula: diagnosis by duplex Doppler sonography. AJR Am J Roentgenol 153:1313–1314
Carr SC, Pearce WH, Vogelzang RL, et al. (1996) Current management of visceral artery aneurysms. Surgery 120:627–634
Derchi LE, Biggi E, Cicio GR, et al. (1984) Aneurysms of the splenic artery: non-invasive diagnosis by pulsed Doppler sonography. J Ultrasound Med 3:41–44
Dochez C, De Roy G (1970) Calcification of the spleen. Fortschr Geb Rontgenstr Nuklearmed 112:274–275
Fava C, Grosso M, Spalluto F, et al. (1990) Percutaneous treatment of splenic arteriovenous fistula. Description of a case. Radiol Med (Torino) 80:559–562
Fishmann EK, Wyatt SH, Ney DR, et al. (1992) Spiral CT of the pancreas with multiplanar display. AJR Am J Roentgenol 159:1209–1215
Fishmann EK, Soyer P, Bliss DF, et al. (1995) Splenic involvement in pancreatitis: spectrum of CT findings. AJR Am J Roentgenol 164:631–635
Gartside R, Gamelli RL (1987) Splenic arteriovenous fistula. J Trauma 27:671–673
Goerg C, Schwerk WB (1990) Splenic infarction: sonographic patterns, diagnosis, follow-up, and complications. Radiology 174:803–807
Goletti O, Ghiselli G, Lippolis PV, et al. (1996) Intrasplenic posttraumatic pseudoaneurysm: echo colour Doppler diagnosis. J Trauma 41:542–545
Golzarian J, Braude P, Bank WO, et al. (1994) Case report: colour Doppler demonstration of pseudoaneurysms complicating pancreatic pseudocysts. Br J Radiol 67:91–93
Gudmundsen TE, Lie M, Ostensen H (1988) Splenic arteriovenous fistula. Case report. Eur J Surg 154:603–604
Hashizume M, Ohta M, Ueno K, et al. (1993) Laparoscopic ligation of splenic artery aneurysm. Surgery 113:352–354
Ishida H, Konno K, Hamashima Y,et al. (1998) Splenic artery aneurysm: value of colour doppler and the limitation of gray-scale ultrasonography. Abdom Imaging 23:627–632
Jaroch MT, Broughan TA, Hermann RE (1986) The natural history of splenic infarction. Surgery 100:743–750
Kauzlaric D, Passega E (1986) Atypical sonographic findings in splenic infarction. J Clin Ultrasound 14:461–462
Kehagias DT, Tzalonikos MT, Moulopoulos LA, et al. (1998) MRI of a giant splenic artery aneurysm. Br J Radiol 71:444–446
Kelekis D, Brountzos EN, Kelekis N, et al. (1995) Splenic aneurysm with arteriovenous fistula. A case report. Hepatogastroenterology 42:352–355
Magid D, Fishman EK, Siegelman SS (1984) Computed tomography of the spleen and liver in sickle cell disease. AJR Am J Roentgenol 143:245–249
Mandel SR, Jacques PF, Sanofsky S, et al. (1987) Non-operative management of peripancreatic arterial aneurysms. A 10-year experience. Ann Surg 205:126–128
Marn CS, Glazer GM, Williams DM, et al. (1990) CT-angiographic correlation of collateral venous pathways in isolated splenic vein occlusion: new observations. Radiology 175:375–380
Mattar SG, Lumsden AB (1995) The management of splenic artery aneurysms: experience with 23 cases. Am J Surg 169:580–584
McClary D, Finelli DS, Croker B, et al. (1986) Portal hypertension secondary to a spontaneous splenic arteriovenous fistula: case report and review of the literature. Am J Gastroenterol 81:572–575
McDermott VG, Shlansky-Goldberg R, Cope C (1994) Endovascular management of splenic artery aneurysms and pseudoaneurysms. Cardiovasc Intervent Radiol 17:179–184
Minami, Itai J, Ohtomo K, et al. (1989) Siderotic nodules in the spleen. MR imaging of portal hypertension. Radiology 172:681–684
Murayama S, Shimoda Y (1990) Completely thrombosed splenic artery aneurysm mimicking cystic pancreatic mass: computed tomographic findings. Gastrointest Radiol 15:205–206
Nishida O, Moriyasu F, Nakamura T, et al. (1986) Hemodynamics of splenic artery aneurysm. Gastroenterology 90:1042–1046
Ohta M, Hashizume M, Tanoue K, et al. (1992) Splenic hyperkinetic state and splenic artery aneurysm in portal hypertension. Hepatogastroenterology 39:529–532
Petit P, Bret P, Atri M, et al. (1994) Splenic vein thrombosis after splenectomy: frequency and role of imaging. Radiology 190:65–68
Piscaglia F, Valgimigli M, Serra C, et al. (1998) Duplex Doppler findings in splenic arteriovenous fistula. J Clin Ultrasound 26:103–105
Puttini M, Aseni P, Brambilla G, et al. (1982) Splenic artery aneurysms in portal hypertension. J Cardiovasc Surg Torino 23:490–493
Quinn SF, Van Sonnenberg E, Casola G, et al. (1986) Interventional radiology of the spleen. Radiology 161:289–291
Rabushka LS, Kawashima A, Fishman EK (1994) Imaging of the spleen: CT with supplemental MR examination. Radiographics 14:307–332
Rahmouni A, Mathieu D, Golli M, et al. (1992) Value of CT and sonography in the conservative management of acute splenoportal and superior mesenteric venous thrombosis. Gastrointest Radiol 17:135–140
Reidy JF, Rowe PH, Ellis FG (1990) Splenic artery aneurysm embolisation. The preferred technique to surgery. Clin Radiol 41:281–282
Roshkow JE, Sanders LM (1990) Acute splenic sequestration crisis in two adults with sickle cell disease: US, CT, and MR imaging findings. Radiology 177:723–725
Rypens F, Devière J, Zalcman M, et al. (1997) Splenic parenchymal complications of pancreatitis: CT findings and natural history. J Comput Assist Tomogr 21:89–93
Sarioglu A, Tanyel FC, Ariyurek M, et al. (1995) Aneurysmatic arteriovenous fistula complicating splenic injury. Eur J Pediatr Surg 6:183–185
Shleapnik M, Shpitz B, Siegal A, et al. (1990) Bleeding oesophageal varices and portal hypertension caused by arteriovenous fistula of splenic artery. HPB Surg 3:53–57
Short DH, Puyau MK, Sauls JL, et al. (1985) Use of digital subtraction angiography in the diagnosis of splenic artery aneurysms. Am Surg 51:606–608
Stallard DJ, Tu RK, Gould MJ, et al. (1994) Minor vascular anatomy of the abdomen and pelvis: a CT atlas. Radiographics 14:493–513
Trastek VF, Pairolero PC, Joyce JW, et al. (1982) Splenic artery aneurysms. Surgery 91:694–699
Venbrux AC, Dachman AH, Fishman EK (1993) Vascular disease. In: Dachman AH, Friedman AC (eds) Radiology of the spleen. Mosby Year Book, St. Louis, pp 171–205
Vujic I (1989) Vascular complications of pancreatitis. Radiol Clin North Am 27:81–91
Walker TG, Geller SC, Waltman AC (1988) Splenic artery pseudoaneurysms causing lower gastrointestinal hemorrhage. AJR Am J Roentgenol 150:433–434
Weingarten MJ, Fakhry J, MacCarthy J, et al. (1984) Sonography after splenic embolization: the wedge-shaped acute infarct. AJR Am J Roentgenol 142:957–959

10 Tumoral Pathology of the Spleen

K. J. Mortelé, P. J. Mergo, M. Kunnen, and P. R. Ros

CONTENTS

10.1 Introduction

The spleen can be either primarily or secondarily involved with neoplasia. However, compared with other abdominal organs, primary tumoral anomalies of the spleen are relatively uncommon. Both benign and malignant primary neoplastic involvement of the spleen have been described, although the malignant causes are considered to be more frequent, with lymphoma being the most common primary splenic malignant tumor (Taylor et al. 1991). Of nonlymphoid primary neoplastic lesions, those of vascular origin constitute the majority, with hemangiomas and angiosarcomas being the tumors most frequently encountered (Ferrozzi et al. 1996). Other, more uncommon primary lesions encountered in the spleen include benign entities, such as cyst, lymphangioma, hamartoma and, less commonly, lesions with variable biologic behavior, such as hemangiopericytoma, epithelioid vascular tumor and littoral cell angioma. Far more commonly, however, the spleen will be secondarily involved by metastatic disease.

Despite the relative rarity of splenic lesions, their identification and characterization can have important implications, particularly in patients with lymphoma, in whom the presence of splenic involvement can determine the type of treatment administered (Mirowitz et al. 1991). Because of this, and since tumoral pathologies of the spleen tend to be small and infiltrating, detection and characterization of suspected splenic disease with various imaging modalities has always been a challenge for the radiologist (Rabushka et al. 1994). The available literature, however, indicates that imaging modalities, such as ultrasound (US), computed tomography (CT) and conventional magnetic resonance imaging (MRI), are relatively insensitive in the detection of splenic lesions (Mirowitz et al. 1991). On MRI, for example, splenic lesions have been found to have T1 and T2 relaxation times and proton-density values very similar to those of normal splenic parenchyma. Consequently, little inherent tissue contrast exists for detection of most splenic lesions, which often results in underestimation of the extent of involvement. Fortunately, a gamut of primary splenic neoplasms exhibit some specific imaging appearances allowing one to characterize them.

10.2 Benign Lesions

10.2.1 Cyst

10.2.1.1 Clinical Manifestations

Splenic cysts are usually asymptomatic and are incidentally found at radiologic examination,

K.J. Mortelé, M. Kunnen; Department of Radiology, University Hospital Ghent, De Pintelaan 185, B-9000 Ghent, Belgium
P.J. Mergo; Department of Radiology, University of Florida College of Medicine, Health Science Center, P.O. Box 100374, Gainesville, FL 32610-0374, USA
P.R. Ros; Department of Radiology, Harvard Medical School, Brigham and Women's Hospital, 75 Francis Street, Boston, MA 02115, USA

surgery or autopsy (Rabushka et al. 1994). Occasionally, a splenic cyst may present as a left upper-quadrant mass, causing a sense of epigastric fullness or intermittent dull pain (Urrutia et al. 1996).

10.2.1.2 Incidence

Splenic cysts can be divided into two categories (Table 10.1): primary cysts, which possess a cellular lining, and secondary (false) cysts, which have no cellular lining (Taylor et al. 1991). The primary cysts are either non-parasitic (congenital) or parasitic (echinococcal). Congenital (also called epidermoid, mesothelial or true) cysts are characterized pathologically by the presence of an inner endothelial lining (Griscom et al. 1977). They are developmental in origin and are thought to arise from an infolding of the peritoneal mesothelium during development, representing collections of peritoneal mesothelial cells trapped within the splenic sulci (Shirkhoda et al. 1995). They are usually discovered in childhood or adolescence, and they are more common in female than in male patients (Younger and Hall 1990). Although the vast majority of cases are sporadic, familial occurrence has been described (Gilmartin 1978). In most series, congenital cysts make up approximately 20% of non-parasitic cysts. In 80% of cases, congenital splenic cysts are unilocular and solitary (Warshauer and Koehler 1998). Occasionally, trabeculae or septations may be seen (Kelekis et al. 1997).

10.2.1.3 Imaging

US classically shows an anechoic and well-defined mass (Eshaghi and Ros 1989) (Fig. 10.1). Less commonly, low-level internal echoes are demonstrated secondary to the deposition of cholesterol crystals (Urrutia et al. 1996). On CT, a large, unilocular, mass the density of water and with imperceptible walls is seen (Fig. 10.2). Following administration of intravenous contrast material, no enhancement is noticed except in the internal septae (Dachman et al. 1986). MRI T1- and T2-weighted images show a well-defined, rounded mass with signal intensities equal to that of water (Grumbach and McDowell 1994; Fig. 10.3). Cysts complicated by protein or hemorrhage may have regions of high signal intensity on T1-weighted images, regions of mixed signal intensity on T2-weighted images, or both (Kelekis et al. 1997). Cysts do not enhance on post-gadolinium (Gd) images (Kelekis et al. 1997).

Post-traumatic cysts (false cysts, non-pancreatic pseudocysts of the spleen) are presumed to be the end stage of an intrasplenic hematoma, previous infarction or infection of the spleen (Dachman et al. 1986). Post-traumatic cysts account for 80% of all splenic cysts (Garvin and King 1981). In contrast to congenital splenic cysts, post-traumatic cysts do not contain an inner endothelial lining but are delineated by a thick, fibrous wall (Dachman et al. 1986). False cysts are usually smaller than true cysts and may contain internal debris. Calcifications may be seen within the thick fibrous wall (Urrutia et al. 1996). Although it is usually difficult to distinguish post-traumatic cysts from true splenic cysts by

Table 10.1. True and false cysts

	True cyst	False cyst
Synonyms	Congenital cyst; epidermoid cyst; mesothelial cyst	Secondary cyst; post-traumatic cyst
Pathology	Inner endothelial lining; unilocular, solitary; large	Thick, fibrous wall; usually smaller
Incidence	Childhood, adolescence	Adults
Imaging	Anechoic (US) Calcifications (14%)	Internal debris (US) Peripheral egg-shell calcifications (50%)

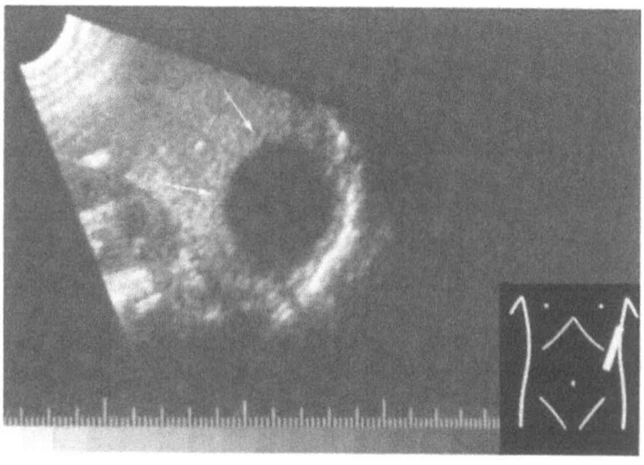

Fig. 10.1. Epidermoid cyst of the spleen. A sagittal sonogram shows a round and sharply circumscribed anechoic lesion (*arrows*) in the inferior portion of the spleen, consistent with an epidermoid cyst

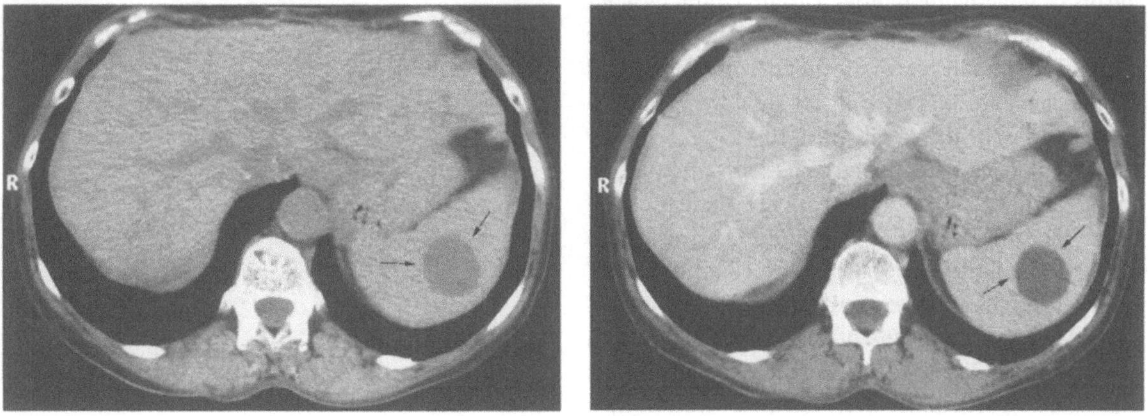

a b

Fig. 10.2. Epidermoid cyst of the spleen. Non-enhanced (**a**) and contrast-material-enhanced (**b**) computed-tomography images of an asymptomatic patient show a well-defined, low-attenuation mass (*arrows*) without enhancement

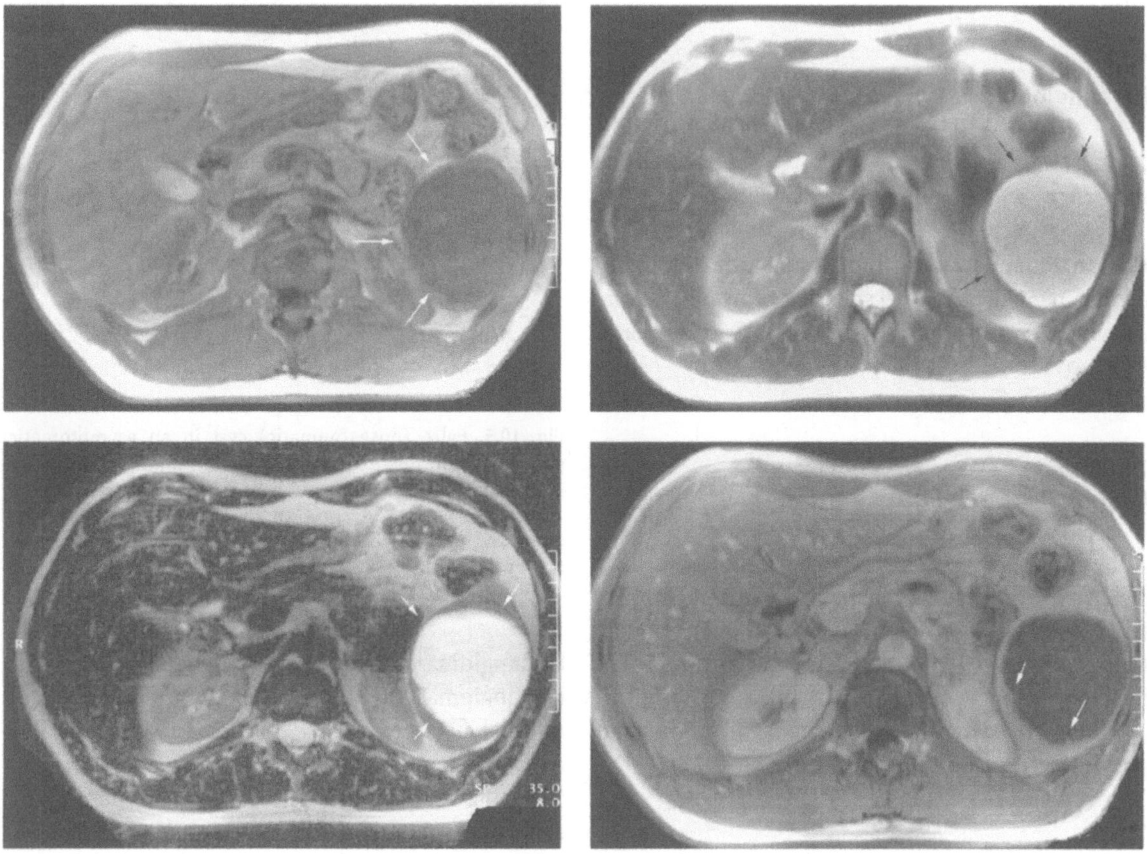

a b c d

Fig. 10.3. Epidermoid cyst of the spleen. (**a**) T1-weighted fast low-angle shot [FLASH; repetition time/echo time (TR/TE) = 130/4, 70°], (**b**) T2-weighted half-Fourier single-shot turbo spin-echo (TSE) and (**c**) heavily T2-weighted TSE (TR/TE = 2200/259) images show a well-defined rounded and septated mass (*arrows*) with very low, high and very high signal intensities, respectively. (**d**) A T1-weighted FLASH image (TR/TE = 130/4, 70°) performed during the portal venous phase of intravenous gadolinium-diethylenetriaminepentaacetic acid administration shows no enhancement, except in the internal septae (*arrows*). After removal, this was shown to be an epithelial cyst means of imaging modalities, certain characteristics may help differentiate these two entities. On US, false cysts may contain internal echoes from debris and show echogenic foci with distal shadowing due to calcifications in their wall (Fig. 10.4). CT typically shows a sharply demarcated mass with attenuation values identical to or slightly higher than those of water (DACHMAN et al. 1986). Peripheral eggshell-like calcifications may be present (Fig. 10.5). CT reportedly demonstrates cyst-wall calcifications in 14% of true cysts and 50% of false cysts (DAWES and MALANGONI 1986; Fig. 10.6). On MRI, false cysts may show (particularly early in their evolution) a variable signal intensity on T1-weighted images, depending on the degree of proteinaceous material or hemorrhage present (KELEKIS et al. 1997). Such high attenuation cysts may occur in up to 33% of false cysts (RABUSHKA et al. 1994).

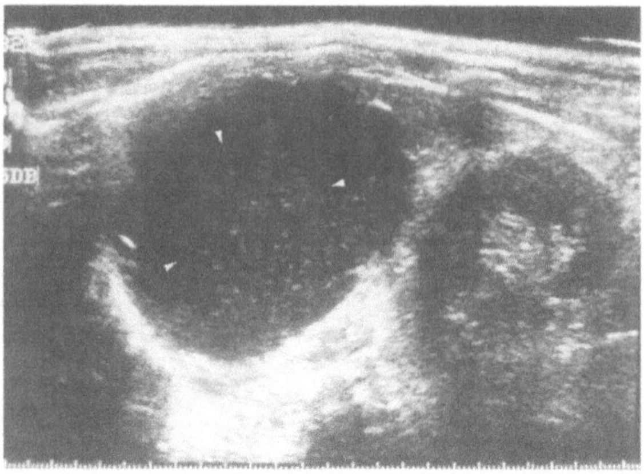

Fig. 10.4. False (post-traumatic) cyst. A sonogram in a patient with a previous history of upper abdominal trauma shows a large, hypoechoic mass with a thick but regular wall and internal echoes (*arrowheads*)

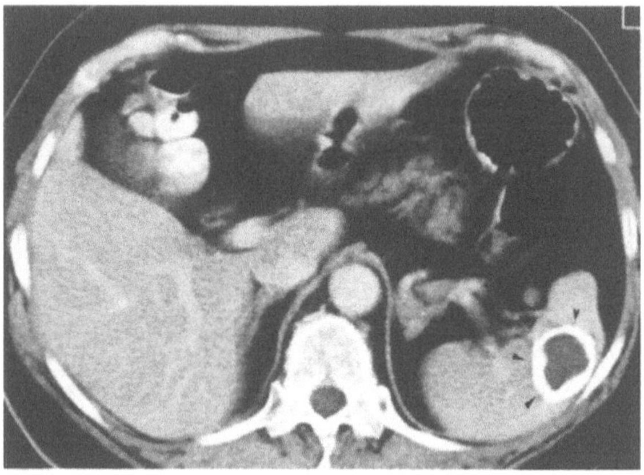

Fig. 10.5. False (post-traumatic) cyst in an asymptomatic patient. A contrast-enhanced computed-tomography image shows uniform low attenuation of the cystic splenic lesion, with extensive calcification (*arrowheads*) within the wall presumed to be secondary to trauma (courtesy of M. MESPREUVE)

10.2.2 Hemangioma

10.2.2.1 Incidence

Hemangioma represents the most common primary benign neoplasm of the spleen, reportedly occurring in 0.01–0.14% of cases at autopsy (PINES and RABINOVITCH 1942).

10.2.2.2 Clinical Manifestations

Although they are usually asymptomatic and discovered incidentally, hemangiomas can produce splenomegaly, pain and, less commonly, splenic rupture (HUSNI 1961). Associated findings reported include anemia, thrombocytopenia, consumptive coagulopathy (Kasabach-Merritt syndrome) and portal hypertension (SHANBERGE et al. 1971).

10.2.2.3 Pathology

Hemangiomas are characterized by an unencapsuled proliferation of vascular channels of variable size that are lined with a single layer of endothelium and filled with red blood cells (DISLER and CHEW 1991). These vascular channels vary in size from capillary to cavernous (ROS et al. 1987). In the spleen, cavernous hemangiomas are more common than capillary-type hemangiomas (ROS et al. 1987). Although areas of internal fibrosis are less frequently found than in hepatic hemangiomas, cystic areas are very common (URRUTIA et al. 1996). The contents of these cystic elements range from serous to hemorrhagic. Splenic hemangiomas may be single or multiple (as part of a generalized angiomatosis, such as Klippel-Trenaunay-Weber syndrome), sometimes replacing the entire spleen (hemangiomatosis), and may range from a few millimeters to many centimeters in size (PAKTER et al. 1987; FREEMAN et al. 1993). Most lesions are under 2 cm in diameter; when larger, they rupture, causing hemorrhage in about 25% of cases (HUSNI 1961).

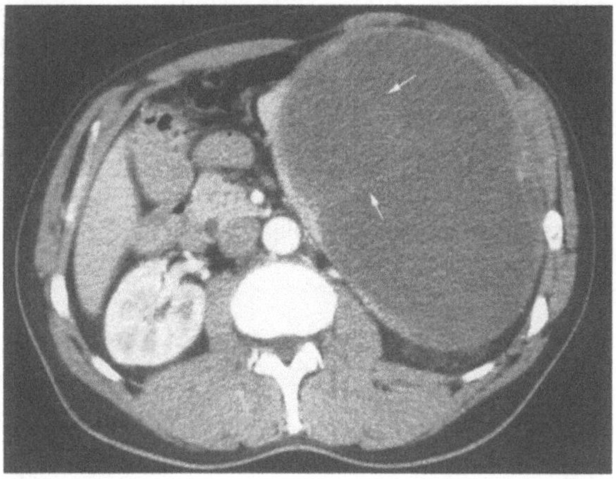

Fig. 10.6. False (post-traumatic) cyst. An enhanced computed tomography scan of the upper abdomen in a 57-year-old man demonstrates a well-delineated, low-attenuation mass with thin septations (*arrows*) and small calcifications occupying nearly the entire spleen. The surgical specimen showed no endothelial lining of the cyst

10.2.2.4 Imaging

The appearance depends on the gross morphology and may range from solid to mixed (cystic and solid components) to purely cystic (Duddy and Calder 1989). *Sonograms* usually show an inconsistent and nonspecific appearance of echogenicity and sharp margination, sometimes with cystic regions (Goerg et al. 1991) (Fig. 10.7). Color Doppler flow US may demonstrate blood flow within the solid portions (Niizawa et al. 1991). *CT* shows low-attenuation lesions resembling cysts with delayed enhancement of the solid portions following contrast-material administration (Ros et al. 1987). Calcifications may be curvilinear or eggshell-like and are most often detected in cystic hemangioma, whereas the mottled central foci of calcium are more typical of plain solid lesions (Ros et al. 1987). *MRI* characteristics resemble those of hepatic hemangiomas, which are known to show low to isointense signal intensity on T1-weighted images and markedly high signal intensity on T2-weighted images (Harris and Simpson 1989). However, due to the moderately high signal intensity of the spleen in T2-weighted images, splenic hemangiomas are minimally hyperintense relative to the spleen on T2-weighted images. Due to the relatively low signal intensity of spleen on these images, splenic hemangiomas are minimally hypointense to isointense to background spleen on T1-weighted images (Kelekis et al. 1997) (Fig. 10.8). T2-weighted images may show heterogeneous

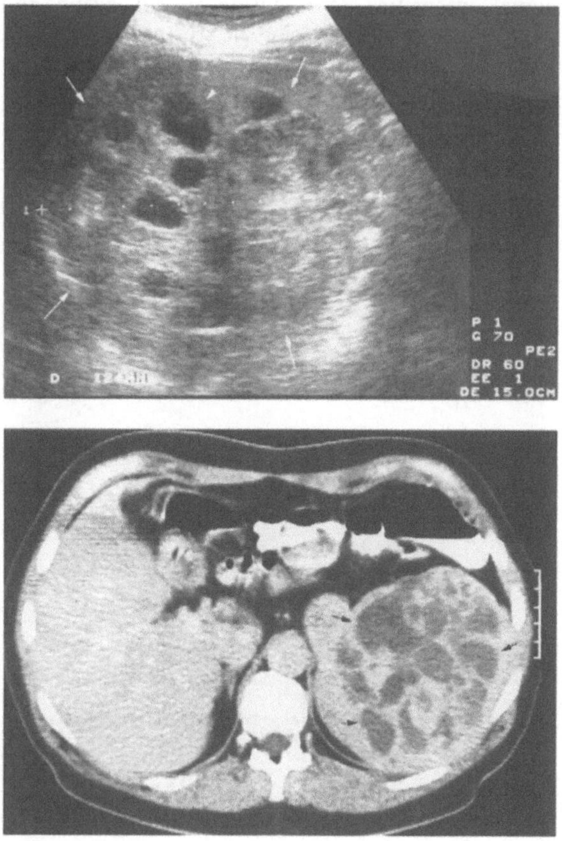

a

b

Fig. 10.7. Mixed hemangioma. **a** A sagittal sonogram shows a large, complex, hyperechoic mass (*arrows*) with scattered internal hypoechoic areas (*arrowheads*). **b** A contrast-enhanced computed tomography scan shows a complex mass with heterogeneous density. The small areas of low-attenuation probably represent cavernous portions of the mass (*arrows*) (courtesy of A. M. De Schepper)

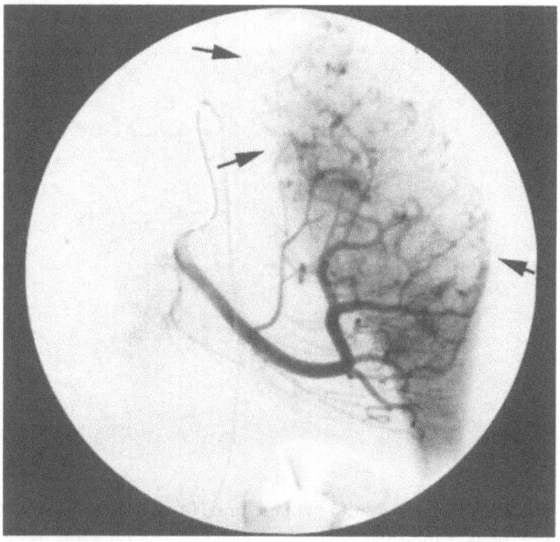

Fig. 10.8. Hemangioma. A digital subtraction angiogram of the splenic artery shows a hypovascular space occupying lesion with a characteristic internal "cotton-wool" vascular blush.

signal intensities representing mixed cystic and solid components (Peene et al. 1991). On dynamic scanning following rapid bolus of Gd-diethylenetriaminepentaacetic acid, three patterns of enhancement are described: (1) immediate, homogeneous, persistent enhancement; (2) early peripheral enhancement with uniform delayed enhancement; and (3) peripheral enhancement with centripetal progression but persistent enhancement of a central fibrous scar (Kelekis et al. 1997). The angiographic findings of splenic hemangioma are considered nonspecific, with hypovascular and hypervascular patterns as previously described (Rosenthal et al. 1973) (Fig. 10.9).

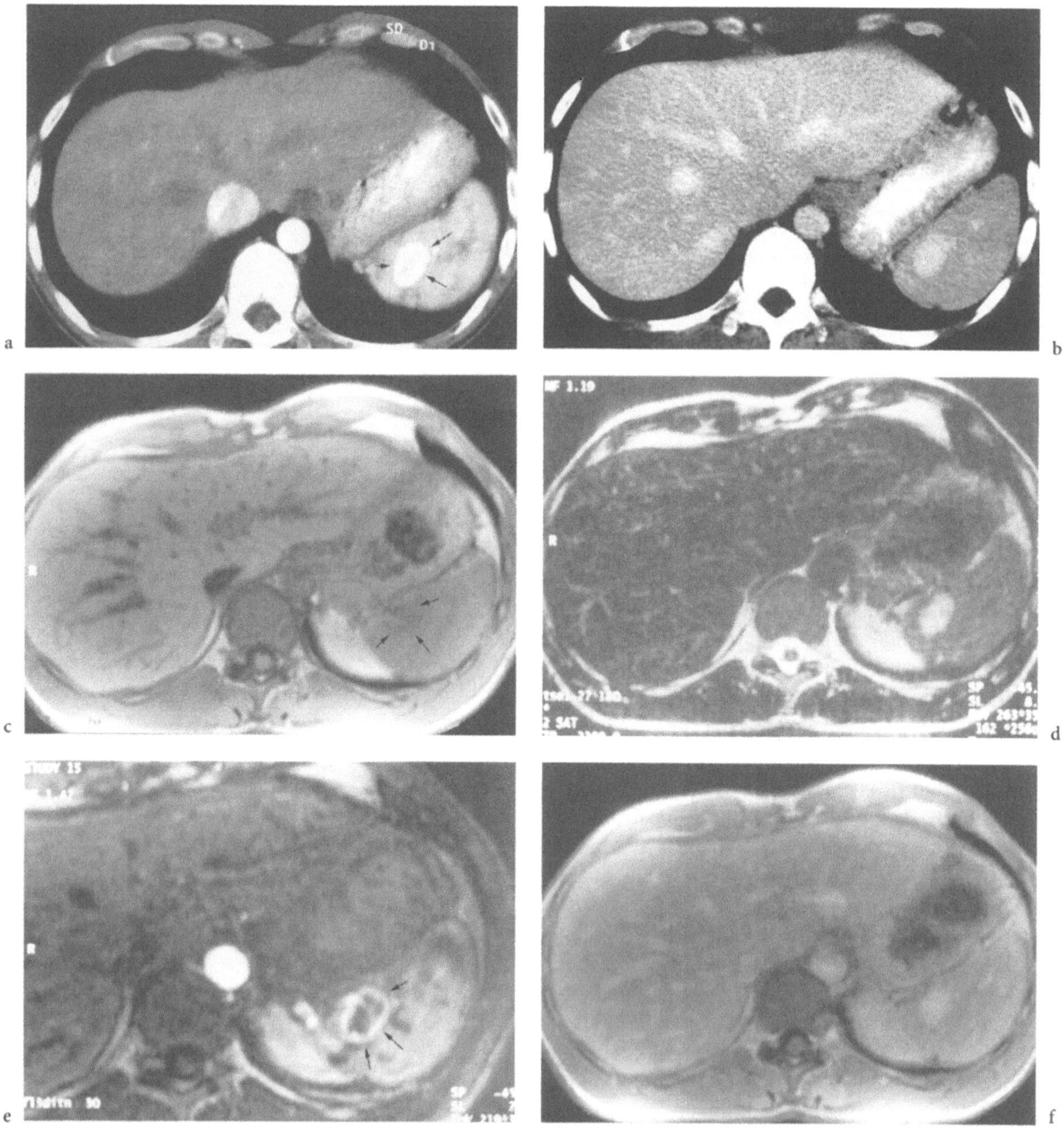

Fig. 10.9. Capillary solid hemangioma. (**a**) Arterial phase, and (**b**) portal venous phase contrast-enhanced computed tomography images both demonstrate a discrete, round, solid nodule (*arrows*) with marked homogeneous enhancement due to the typical hypervascularity of these lesions. (**c**) T1-weighted fast low-angle shot [FLASH; repetition time/echo time (TR/TE) = 130/4, 70°] and (**d**) heavily T2-weighted turbo spin-echo (TR/TE = 2200/259) demonstrate low and high signal intensities, respectively. (**e**) A T1-weighted three-dimensional FLASH image performed during per-fusion phase and (**f**) a T1-weighted FLASH image performed during equilibrium phase of intravenous gadolinium-diethylenetriaminepentaacetic acid administration demonstrate an intense peripheral enhancement (*arrows*) on the initial image but complete and homogeneous enhancement on the equilibrium image

10.2.3
Lymphangioma

10.2.3.1
Definition

Lymphangiomas resemble hemangiomas, since they are also composed of endothelial lined spaces containing lymph instead of red blood cells (URRUTIA et al. 1996).

10.2.3.2
Clinical Manifestations

Although most commonly encountered in the neck and axillary region, lymphangiomas also (rarely) occur in the abdominal viscera (WARSHAUER and KOEHLER 1998). Splenic lymphangiomas may be single or multiple (lymphangiomatosis; AVIGAD et al. 1976). Lymphangiomas are usually asymptomatic or discovered as a left upper-quadrant mass.

10.2.3.3
Pathology

Three types have been reported: capillary, cavernous and cystic, depending on the size of the vascular channels (FERROZZI et al. 1996). Gross pathology classically shows a unilocular or multilocular cystic mass (TAYLOR et al. 1991).

10.2.3.4
Imaging

On US, lymphangioma appears as a well-defined, hypoechoic mass occasionally containing internal septations and intralocular, echogenic debris (URRUTIA et al. 1996) (Fig. 10.10). CT findings include sharply marginated, thin-walled, single or multiple areas of low attenuation that do not enhance on post-contrast images (PYATT et al. 1981) (Fig. 10.11). Small, linear, peripheral calcifications may be present (PISTOIA and MARKOWITZ 1988). On MRI, lymphangiomas resemble cysts with homogeneously low signal and high signal intensity on T1- and T2-weighted images, respectively (ITO et al. 1995). Areas of high signal intensity on T1-weighted images may result from large amounts of proteinaceous fluid in internal hemorrhage (Fig. 10.12).

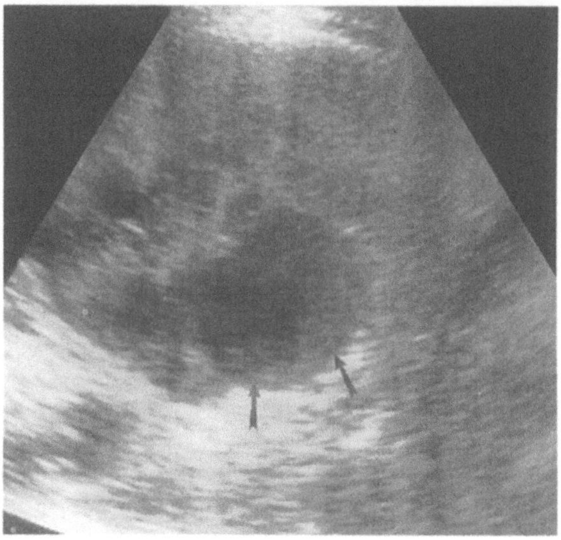

Fig. 10.10. Multiple lymphangiomas in a 74-year-old woman. A sagittal ultrasound shows multiple hypoechoic, rounded masses of different sizes. The largest mass contains low-level echoes (*arrows*) due to the proteinaceous nature of its contents

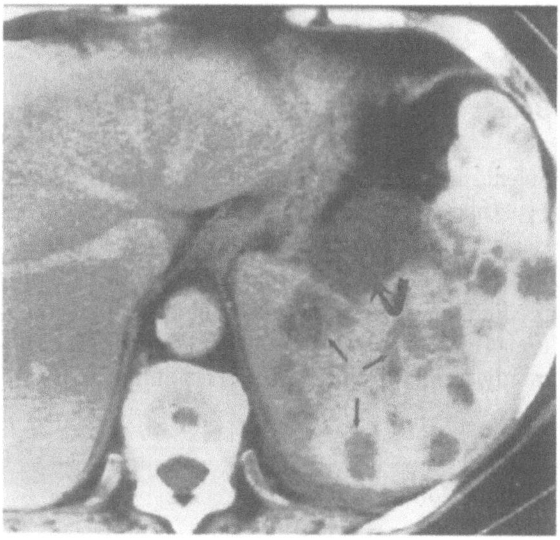

Fig. 10.11. Multiple lymphangiomas in a 74-year-old woman. A contrast-enhanced computed-tomography image depicts multiple non-enhancing lesions (*straight arrows*) throughout the spleen, with the normal splenic architecture being almost completely replaced. The largest focus is subcapsular in location (*curved arrow*)

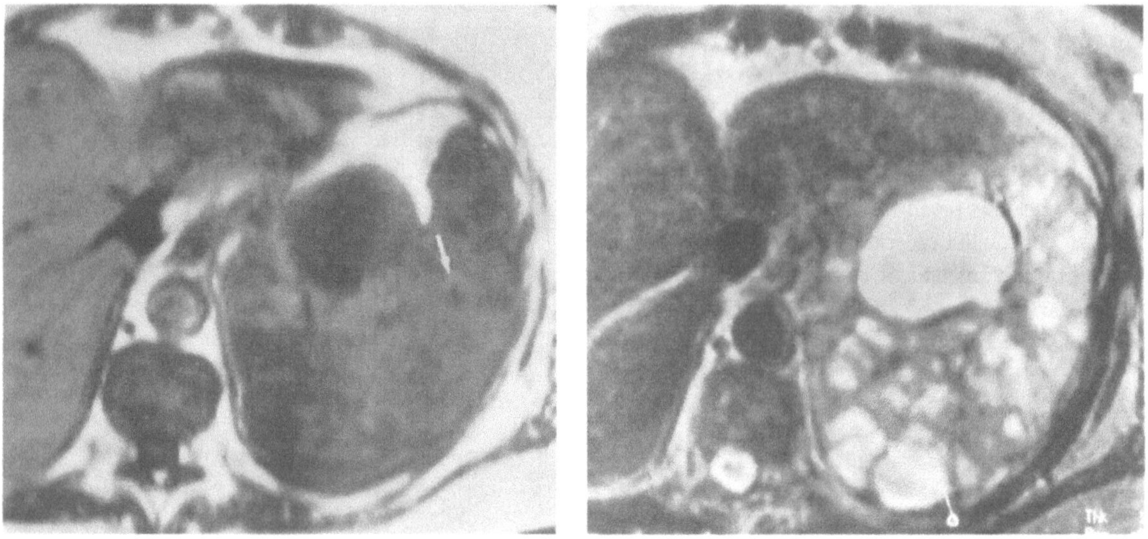

a b

Fig. 10.12. Multiple lymphangiomas in a 74-year-old woman. **a** A T1-weighted magnetic resonance (MR) image reveals variably sized foci of low signal intensity (*arrows*). **b** A T2-weighted MR image shows multiple lesions of variable size, with marked hyperintensity

10.2.4 Hamartoma

10.2.4.1 Definition

Splenic hamartoma (also called splenoma, nodular hyperplasia of the spleen) is a rare, benign tumor classically composed of anomalous mixtures of normal elements of splenic tissue, with red pulp predominating (Morgenstern et al. 1985). Hamartomas usually present as a solitary lesion or, less commonly, as multiple nodules (Steinberg et al. 1985).

10.2.4.2 Clinical Manifestations

Like most other benign splenic lesions, they are usually discovered incidentally or because of a mass-related symptomatology (Morgenstern et al. 1985). There are a few well-documented reports of symptomatic splenic hamartoma associated with hematological disturbances, marked splenomegaly or spontaneous rupture (Zissin et al. 1992).

10.2.4.3 Pathology

Hamartomas are usually solid lesions and occasionally contain cystic or necrotic components (Brinkley and Lee 1981). Minute speckled calcifications are rarely present (Ferrozzi et al. 1996).

10.2.4.4 Imaging

Sonography appears to be a more sensitive modality than CT in demonstrating the lesion (Norowitz and Morehouse 1989). In US studies, a hamartoma usually appears to be hyperechoic relative to the normal spleen and sometimes features cystic components (Spalding et al. 1980; Fig. 10.13). On non-enhanced *CT* images, they usually appear isoattenuating, causing only an abnormality of the contour of the spleen (Zissin et al. 1992). Hyperattenuation due to hemosiderin deposition, however, is occasionally seen (Ohtomo et al. 1992). *MRI* may show a well-delineated mass of isointensity on T1-weighted images and moderately high signal intensity on T2-weighted images (Ohtomo et al. 1992; Fig. 10.14). If the composition of fibrous tissue is substantial, hamartomas may have regions of low signal intensity on T2-weighted images (Pinto et al. 1995). Following administration of Gd chelates, immediate post-contrast images show an intense, diffuse, heterogeneous enhancement of hamartomas. This early diffuse, heterogeneous enhancement pattern permits distinction from hemangioma (Ramani et al. 1997). Due to stagnation of contrast material within the sinusoids of the red pulp, prolonged enhancement similar to that seen with hemangiomas may be seen on both delayed post-contrast CT and MR images (OHTOMO et al. 1992).

10.2.5 Miscellaneous Rare Benign Tumors

Other extremely rare primary benign splenic tumors encountered in autopsy series include dermoid, fibroma, chondroma, leiomyoma, osteoma and lipoma (BOSTICK 1945; EASLER and DOWLIN 1969). The imaging appearances of these tumors (except lipoma) have not been characterized (WARSHAUER and KOEHLER 1998)(Fig. 10.15).

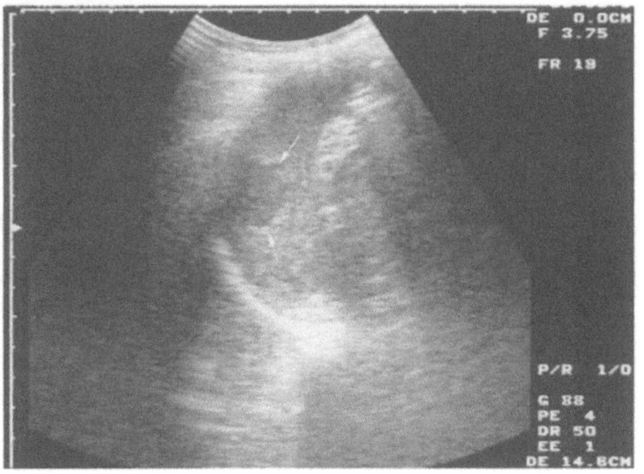

Fig. 10.13. Hamartoma of the spleen in a 27-year-old woman. A sagittal ultrasound reveals a homogeneous hypoechoic mass well demarcated from surrounding splenic parenchyma (*arrows*). The patient underwent splenectomy, which revealed a hamartoma

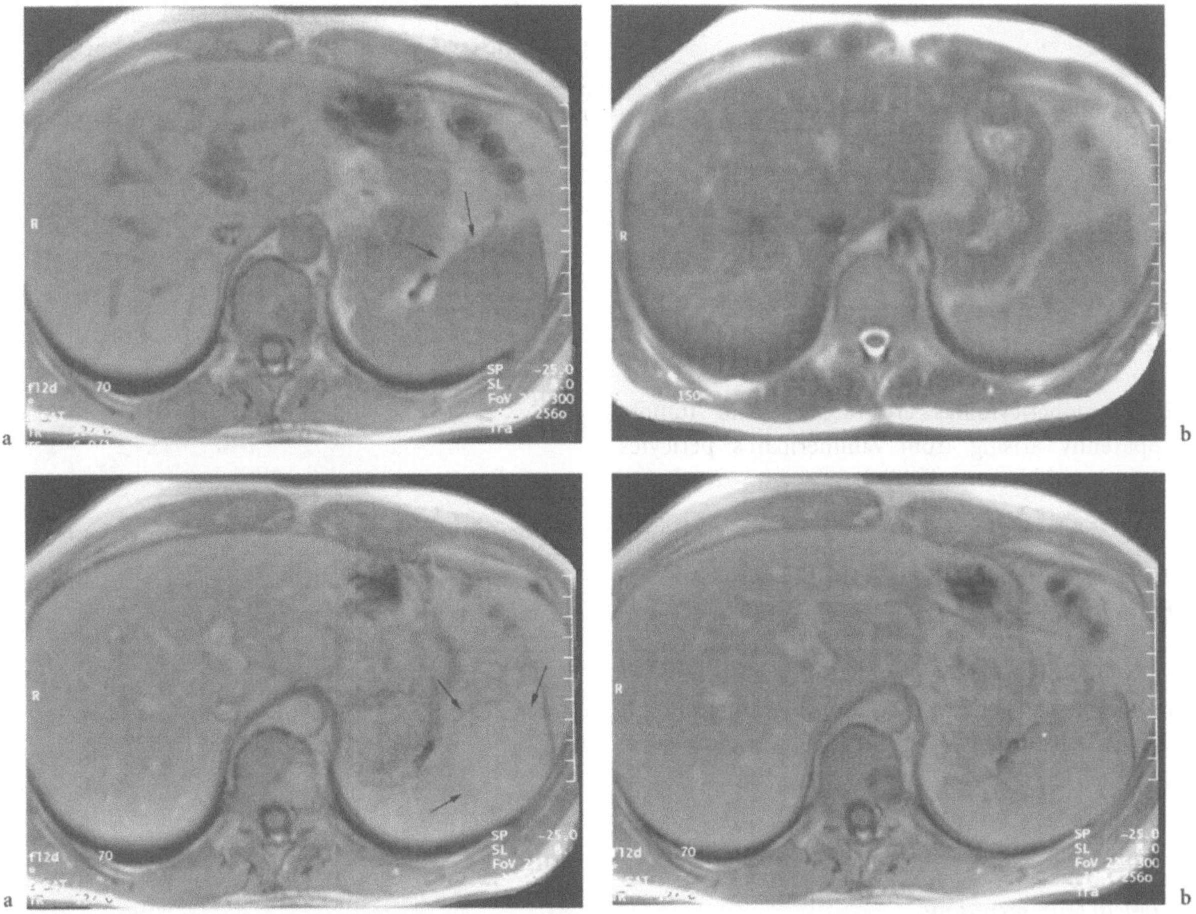

Fig. 10.14. Hamartoma of the spleen in a 39-year-old-man with a 4-month history of left upper-quadrant pain. (**a**) T1-weighted fast low-angle shot [FLASH; repetition time/echo time (TR/TE) = 127/6, 70°] and (**b**) T2-weighted half-Fourier single-shot turbo spin-echo images show a 5-cm lesion arising from the anterior aspect of the midportion of the spleen, with bulging of the medial splenic contour (*arrows*). The signal intensity of the hamartoma is very similar to that of background spleen on both imaging sequences. On the 90-s (**c**) and 3-min post-gadolinium (**d**) T1-weighted FLASH images (TR/TE = 130/6, 70°), the tumor shows intense and slightly heterogeneous enhancement on the early image (*arrows*) and persistent homogeneous enhancement greater than background spleen on the delayed image

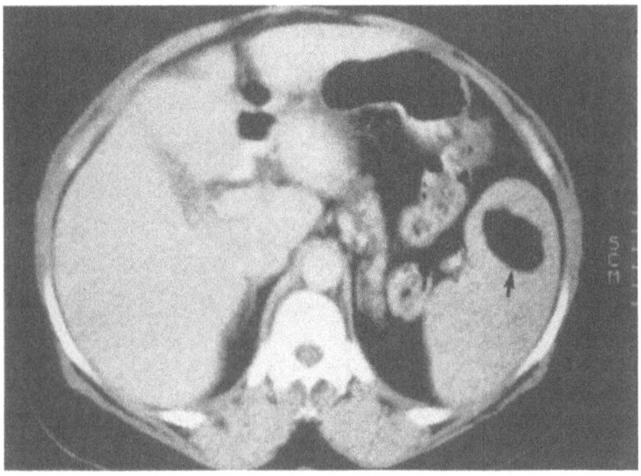

Fig. 10.15. Splenic lipoma. A contrast-enhanced computed-tomography scan shows a well-delineated fat-density mass consistent with a splenic lipoma (Warshauer and Koehler 1998)

10.3 Neoplasms with Variable Biologic Behavior

10.3.1 Hemangiopericytoma

10.3.1.1 Definition

Hemangiopericytomas are rare vascular tumors apparently arising from Zimmerman's pericytes (Stout and Murray 1942).

10.3.1.2 Pathology

Histologically, hemangiopericytomas are composed of spindle cells or ovoid cells proliferating around vascular channels lined with epithelium (Jurado et al. 1989).

10.3.1.3 Clinical Manifestations

They are most frequently found in the muscles of the lower extremities and subcutaneous tissue, with parenchymatous origin being extremely infrequent (Stout and Lattes 1967). The biologic behavior and prognosis of hemangiopericytomas are variable. The high rate of local recurrence (36%) and the malignant potential confirm the initial reports of biologic aggressiveness (Ferrozzi et al. 1996). The tumors arising in the abdomen, with the exception of stomach and uterus, behave especially aggressively, with the lung the most frequent site of metastases (Binder et al. 1973). Enzinger and Smith (1986) observed histologic findings associated with a bad prognosis in terms of recurrence or metastases; these are: the presence of hypercellularity, anisocytosis, hyperchromatism, important mitotic activity, necrosis and hemorrhage.

10.3.1.4 Imaging

Reported CT findings include the presence of a large mass with polylobular contours, along with numerous other smaller lesions disseminated throughout the whole spleen. Hyperdensity of the solid portions and internal septations on post-contrast images reflect the vascularity of the tumor (Ferrozzi et al. 1996) (Fig. 10.16).

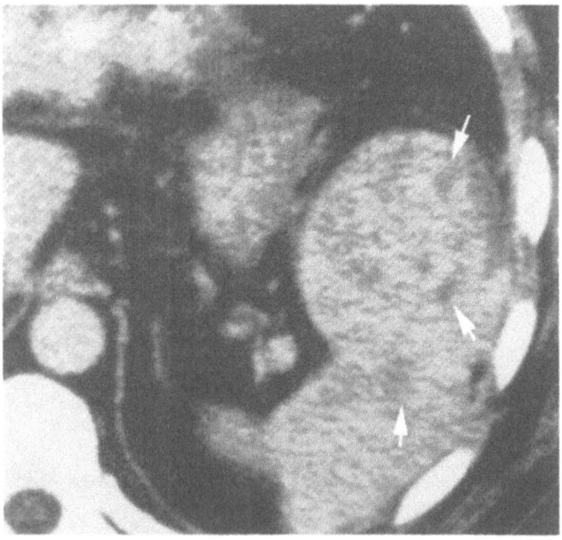

Fig. 10.16. Splenic hemangiopericytoma. A contrast-enhanced computed-tomography scan demonstrates an enlarged spleen with a large bulge in the anterior pole. The spleen is replete with numerous nodules of varying size (*arrows*) (Ferrozzi et al. 1996)

10.3.2 Epithelioid Vascular Tumors

10.3.2.1 Definition and Histology

Epithelioid vascular tumors are characterized by the proliferation of epithelioid (histiocytoid) endothelial cells accompanied by an infiltrate of lymphocytes and eosinophils (Tsang and Chan 1993). The range of this broad spectrum of unusual vascular neoplasms is from epithelioid hemangioma (histiocytoid hemangioma, angiolymphoid hyperplasia with eosinophilia) to malignant epithelioid angiosarcoma (Tsang and Chan 1993).

10.3.2.2 Clinical Manifestations

Symptoms include abdominal pain, left upper-quadrant mass, fever, weight loss, anemia and consumptive coagulopathy (Warshauer and Koehler 1998). Splenic rupture is reported to occur in approximately one-third of the patients.

10.3.2.3 Imaging

Non-specific radiologic findings make interpretation difficult, especially when fibrosis, calcification, thrombosis or necrosis is present (Vilanova et al. 1994). On CT, these tumors classically appear as focal, rounded or irregular areas of heterogeneous low attenuation (Tiu et al. 1992). Occasionally, cystic or necrotic portions may be demonstrated. Reported MR findings include a mass with well-defined borders, a heterogeneous texture and hypointense radial streaks representing fibrosis on both T1- and T2-weighted images (Vilanova et al. 1994) (Fig. 10.17).

10.3.3 Littoral Cell Angioma

10.3.3.1 Definition

Littoral cell angioma, first described by Falk et al. (1991), is a very rare splenic tumor that arises from splenic sinus-lining cells or littoral cells.

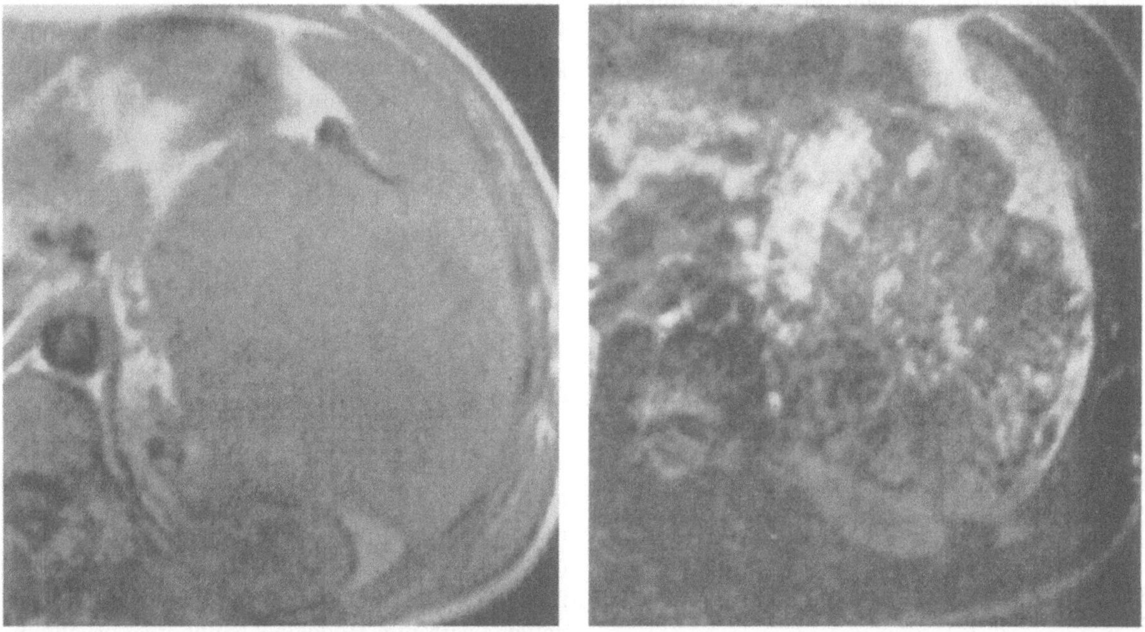

a b

Fig. 10.17. Splenic epithelioid hemangioma. (**a**) T1 and (**b**) T2-weighted magnetic-resonance images show a heterogeneous splenic mass with hypointense radial streaks (Vilanova et al. 1994)

10.3.3.2
Clinical Manifestations

Littoral cell angioma presents most commonly with constitutional symptoms, such as fatigue and low-grade fever, and with signs of hypersplenism (Falk et al. 1991).

10.3.3.3
Pathology

At gross pathology, an enlarged spleen containing multiple small nodules is usually seen. These nodules are histologically characterized by the presence of multiple vascular spaces similar to the venous sinuses of the spleen and covered by high endothelial cells that show hematophagocytosis. With the typical littoral cell angioma, no recurrent or metastatic disease was demonstrated. A case reported by Rosso et al. (1995), however, described a malignant form with intraluminal proliferation of tumor cells and increased mitotic activity; thus, the term "littoral cell angiosarcoma" was coined.

10.3.3.4
Imaging

On US, the lesions appear mainly isoechogenic, with anechogenic foci representing prominent, cavernous blood-filled spaces (Oliver-Goldaracena et al. 1998). On CT, an enlarged spleen containing multiple low-attenuation nodular masses reflecting the gross pathology has been described (Grantham et al. 1998) (Fig. 10.18). The signal of the lesions on MRI is very characteristic, showing markedly hypointense signal on both T1- and T2-weighted images. The reason for this classical appearance on MR is the presence of hemosiderin in these entities due to the hematophagocytic capacity of the neoplastic cells (Oliver-Goldaracena et al. 1998) (Fig. 10.19).

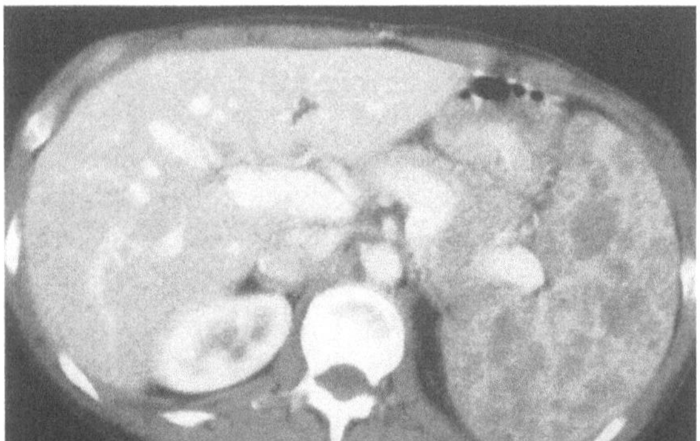

Fig. 10.18. Littoral cell angioma. A contrast-enhanced computed-tomography scan in a 39-year-old woman with splenomegaly and a decreasing platelet count shows an enlarged spleen that contains multiple low-attenuation nodular lesions (Grantham et al. 1998)

10.4
Malignant Tumors

10.4.1
Lymphoma

10.4.1.1
Incidence

Lymphoma constitutes the most common primary malignant splenic neoplasm and involves the spleen in both Hodgkin's and non-Hodgkin's disease (Urrutia et al. 1996). Laparotomy with splenectomy reveals clinically unsuspected splenic involvement in 23–34% of patients with Hodgkin's lymphoma (Strijk et al. 1985). Similarly, 30–40% of patients with non-Hodgkin's lymphoma have splenic involvement when they are initially seen.

10.4.1.2
Clinical Manifestations

Although splenomegaly is found in 80% of cases, the presence of splenomegaly alone does not establish the diagnosis of splenic involvement, because splenectomy series have shown that one third of enlarged spleens are uninvolved; also, one third of normal-sized spleens exhibit tumors in patients with Hodgkin's disease (Grumbach and McDowell 1994).

10.4.1.3
Classification

Splenic lymphoma may be classified as either primary splenic lymphoma or lymphomatous involvement as part of diffuse systemic involvement (Rabushka et al. 1994). Primary splenic lymphoma is uncommon and occurs in approximately 1% of all patients with non-Hodgkin's lymphoma, usually in older patients (Meyer et al. 1983). When it occurs, it is usually non-Hodgkin's lymphoma of the small

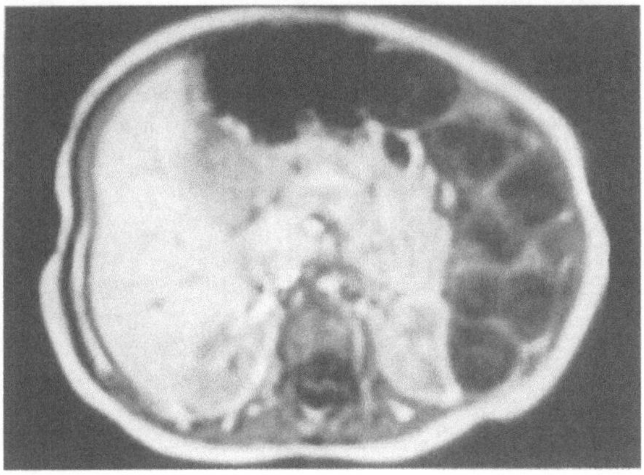

a

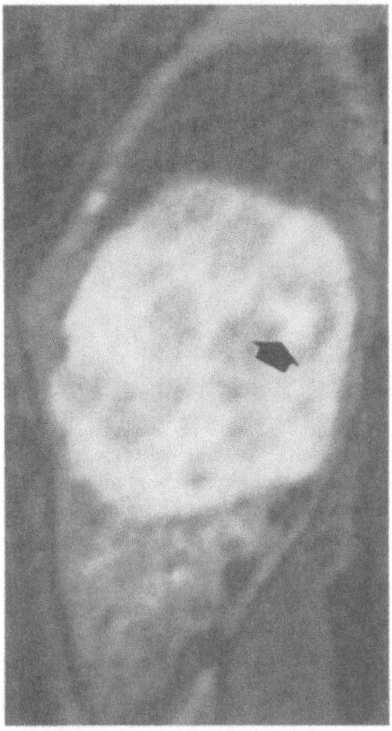

b

Fig. 10.19. Littoral cell angioma. **a** An axial, unenhanced T1-weighted gradient recalled-echo magnetic-resonance (MR) image shows multiple nodular lesions that replace the splenic parenchyma. These present a markedly hypointense signal compared with those of the hepatic parenchyma and paraspinal musculature. **b** A sagittal T2-weighted MR image shows multiple hypointense nodular lesions. The hyper-intense area (*arrow*) corresponds with that of the vascular spaces inside the lesion (Oliver-Goldaracena et al. 1998)

cell type, with evidence of B-cell origin (Spier et al. 1985). With the increasing prevalence of acquired immune deficiency syndrome (AIDS)-related lymphoma, however, the incidence of primary splenic lymphoma is growing; it occurs in 10% of patients with AIDS-related Hodgkin's lymphoma and 26% of those with non-Hodgkin's lymphoma (Nyberg et al. 1986).

10.4.1.4 Pathology

Three different macroscopic types of lymphomatous involvement are described: (a) infiltrative, without definite masses (45–70%); (b) miliary, with small (<2 cm) deposits of lymphomatous cells; and (c) massive, in which one or multiple large lymphomatous masses can be identified (Ahmann et al. 1966). As a general rule, large cell lymphomas produce either solitary or multiple masses of small cleaved and mixed cell types. Lymphocytic lymphomas commonly produce a miliary pattern, and low-grade lymphomas typically cause homogeneous involvement (Warshauer and Koehler 1998).

10.4.1.5 Imaging

US imaging features reflect the spectrum of the pathologic types of involvement: (a) diffuse heterogeneity; (b) small, nodular, hypoechoic lesions (<2 cm diameter); and (c) large, focal, hypoechoic lesions (Goerg et al. 1991) (Fig. 10.20). The CT appearances of splenic lymphoma also correspond well to the pathologic types, ranging from splenomegaly (over miliary multifocal lesions) to a solitary mass (Urrutia et al. 1996) (Figs. 10.21, 10.22). Splenic lesions, only detectable when larger than 1 cm in diameter, usually appear as low-attenuation masses (Strijk et al. 1985). Because the abnormal lymphoid foci are, however, usually less than 1 cm in diameter and beyond the resolution of CT scanning, the overall accuracy of CT in depicting splenic lymphoma is approximately 58–65% (Rabushka et al. 1994). Infarction of the spleen involved in lymphoma is not uncommon and classically appears as a peripheral wedge-shaped area of low attenuation (Rabushka et al. 1994) (Fig. 10.23). Calcifications in splenic lymphoma are rare and probably represent dystrophic calcifications following necrosis, hemorrhage and fibrosis (Rabushka et al. 1994). Necrosis of large lesions has been reported and can result in an irregular cystic appearance of the lesion (Harris et al. 1984). Primary splenic lymphoma may be

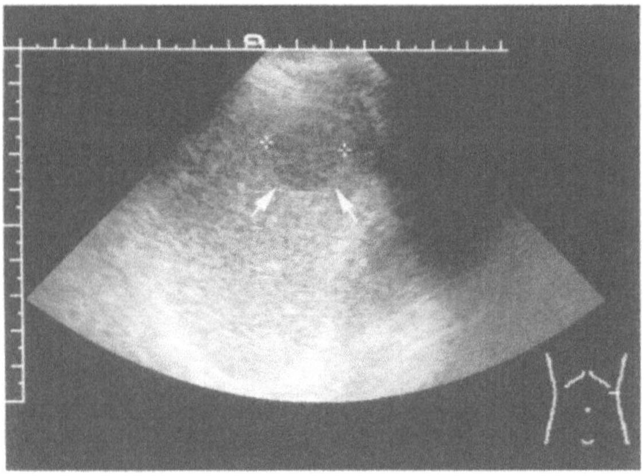

Fig. 10.20. Splenic lymphoma. An axial ultrasound image shows a 2.3-cm, well-delineated, hypoechoic mass in the spleen, consistent with focal splenic lymphoma

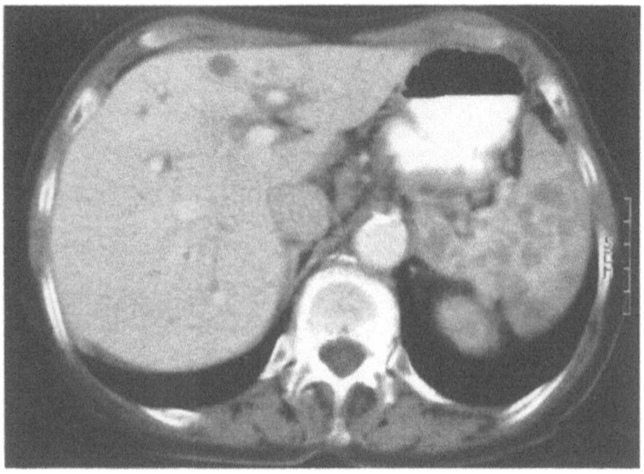

Fig. 10.21. Advanced Hodgkin's lymphoma in a 55-year-old-woman with fever and hepatosplenomegaly. A contrast-enhanced computed-tomography scan shows multiple hypodense nodules of varying size in the spleen, liver and pancreatic tail

a

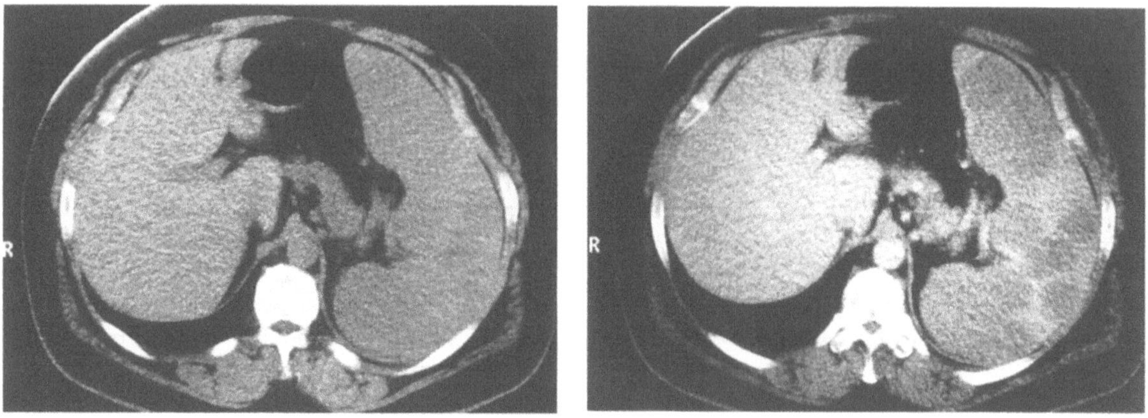

b

Fig. 10.22. Large cell type of B-cell non-Hodgkin's lymphoma. Non-enhanced (**a**) and contrast-material-enhanced (**b**) computed-tomography images reveal splenomegaly and multiple, faint, hypodense splenic nodules, which are better visualized after intravenous contrast administration

bulky, transgress the splenic capsule and involve adjacent organs, such as the diaphragm, stomach, pancreas and abdominal wall (Meyer et al. 1983).

Contrary to initial MRI expectations, detection of splenic lymphomatous involvement is often unreliable, since both normal splenic tissue and lymphoma may have similar T1 and T2 relaxation times and proton densities (Nyman et al. 1987). The sensitivity of conventional MRI for detection of splenic lymphoma in a focal or diffuse pattern varies from 10% to 87% in the reported literature, reflecting the variability of this tumor in appearance on MRI (Grumbach and McDowell 1994). On MRI, depending on the amount of cystic, hemorrhagic or necrotic foci of lymphoma, portions of the lesions may appear as hypointense and hyperintense areas on T1- and T2-weighted images, respectively (Nyman et al. 1987) (Fig. 10.24). However, due to their high cellularity, focal lymphomatous deposits may be low in signal intensity compared with background spleen on T2-weighted images; this feature distinguishes lymphomas from metastases. The latter are rarely low in signal intensity and usually present as isointense to hyperintense masses (Kelekis et al. 1997). The use of contrast material in MR may improve the detection rate of focal splenic lesions (Mirowitz et al. 1991). It is critical to acquire spoiled gradient echo (SGE) images within the first 30 s after contrast administration, because foci of lymphoma equilibrate early, becoming isointense with normal splenic tissue within 2 min or even earlier (Kelekis et al. 1997). Agents specific for reticu-

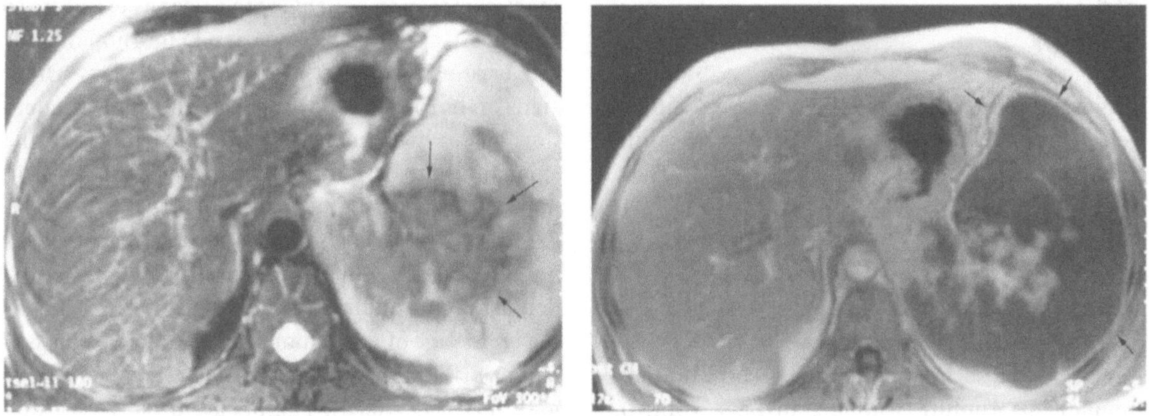

a b

Fig. 10.23. Diffuse infiltration with lymphoma complicated by hyperacute splenic infarction. (**a**) Fat-saturated, T2-weighted turbo spin echo (repetition time/echo time = 3000/99) and (**b**) post-gadolinium T1-weighted fast low-angle-shot images demonstrate inhomogeneous signal intensity on both sequences. On T2-weighted images, the intensity of the spleen is markedly increased, with a medial low-signal-intensity area with hemosiderin deposits consistent with a coexistent hemorrhage (*arrows*). The post-gadolinium T1-weighted image shows the acute intrasplenic contrast extravasation and the massive infarction of the remaining spleen (with the exception of the smooth capsular surface; *arrows*). This finding is helpful in distinguishing global infarction from large necrotic tumors. Splenectomy revealed a diffuse, infiltrated spleen complicated by complete splenic infarction

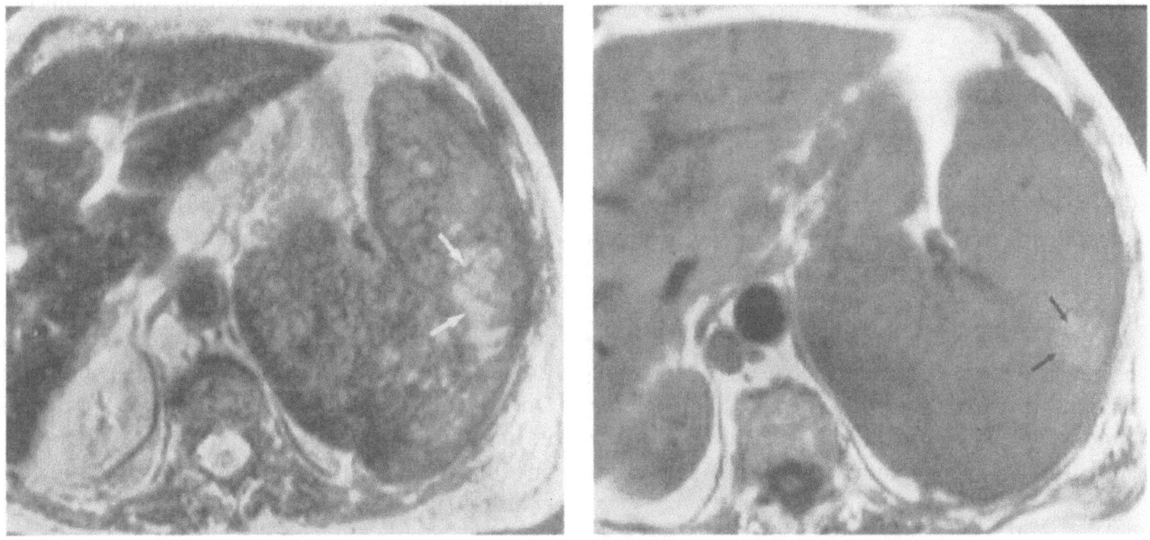

a b

Fig. 10.24. Lymphoma. **a** A T2-weighted magnetic-resonance image in a patient with diffuse, histiocytic lymphoma shows a peripheral area of hyperintensity (*arrows*), which was consistent with a focal area of necrosis in a lymphomatous splenic deposit. The entire spleen has heterogeneous increased signal intensity on T2-weighted images, which is secondary to the diffuse involvement. **b** The cystic area seen in **a** is hyperintense (*arrows*) on the T1-weighted image, which is secondary to the proteinaceous nature of the necrotic material

loendothelial tissue, such as superparamagnetic iron oxide, have been shown to significantly improve the ability of MR to differentiate normal splenic tissue from diffuse splenic lymphoma (Weissleder et al. 1989). Because superparamagnetic particles are not taken up by malignant lymphoid cells, splenic lymphoma remains hyperintense compared with normal enhancing splenic tissue, thus improving tumor-spleen contrast (Kelekis et al. 1997).

10.4.2 Angiosarcoma

10.4.2.1 Incidence

Although splenic angiosarcoma is exceedingly rare, it is the most common non-lymphoid primary malignant tumor of the spleen (Chen et al. 1979).

10.4.2.2
Pathology

Angiosarcoma of the spleen may present either as well-defined hemorrhagic nodules or as diffuse splenic involvement.

10.4.2.3
Clinical Manifestations

Angiosarcoma is frequently (30%) complicated by spontaneous rupture with hemorrhage (Mahony et al. 1982). Prognosis is very poor (20% survival rate at 6 months), with early and widespread metastases, most commonly to the liver (Sondenaa et al. 1993). The survival rate increases significantly when splenectomy is performed before rupture occurs (Ha et al. 1994). It appears to be associated with synchronous malignant lesions, such as non-Hodgkin's lymphoma and carcinomas of the breast and colon (Ferrozzi et al. 1996).

10.4.2.4
Imaging

CT may demonstrate an enlarged spleen with hypoattenuating areas having generally irregular and poorly defined contours (Mahony et al. 1982) (Fig. 10.25). Hyperattenuation on unenhanced scans may represent acute hemorrhage or hemosiderin deposits (Ha et al. 1994). Enhancement of angiosarcoma may be similar to that of hepatic hemangioma, although the pattern of filling is variable (Rabushka et al. 1994). Since angiosarcomas of the spleen are more common in patients with previous exposure to thorotrast, a colloidal suspension of thorium dioxide was used as a contrast agent until the 1950s. Other signs of thorotrast exposure, including high attenuation of the liver or densely opacified nodes in the splenic hilum or porta hepatis, may be helpful in making the correct diagnosis with CT (Findley and Childress 1987). On MRI, angiosarcoma shows nodular masses with hypointense rims, representing hemorrhagic nodules (Kaneko et al. 1992). Depending on the age of the hemorrhage and the presence of necrosis, the signal intensity on T1-weighted images may vary (Fig. 10.26). Tumors are usually very vascular and enhance intensively with Gd (Kelekis et al. 1997).

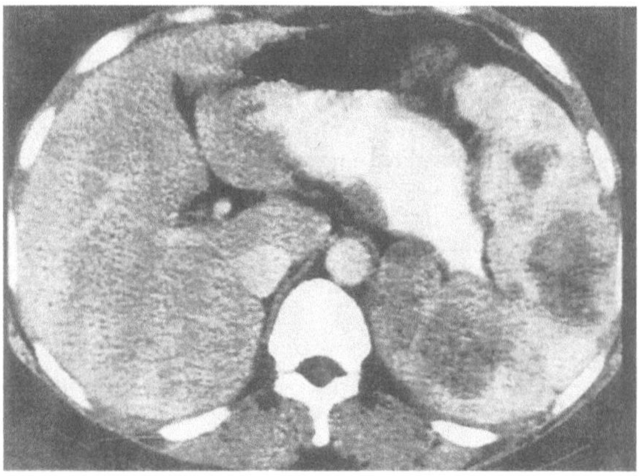

Fig. 10.25. Angiosarcoma. A contrast-enhanced computed-tomography image shows multiple hypodense masses in the enlarged spleen (Ha et al. 1994)

10.4.3
Miscellaneous

Other primary, malignant, mesenchymal neoplasms reported in the spleen include malignant fibrous histiocytoma, fibrosarcoma, leiomyosarcoma and malignant teratoma, the imaging appearances of which are non-characteristic (Wick et al. 1982; Morgenstern et al. 1985). Malignant fibrous histiocytoma has been described as a large mass with areas of necrosis (Bruneton et al. 1988).

Mucinous cystadenocarcinoma has also been reported in the spleen and is thought to arise either from invaginated capsular mesothelium of the spleen or from heterotopic pancreatic or enteric tissue within the spleen (Morinaga et al. 1992). On CT, mucinous cystadenocarcinoma resembles its hepatic or pancreatic variants, having the appearance of a large, multilocular, cystic mass (Morinaga et al. 1992).

10.4.4
Metastases

10.4.4.1
Incidence

Although the spleen contains abundant lymphoid tissue and manifests as a hematological barrier, metastatic splenic disease is relatively uncommon; it is only seen in 4–7% of patients with widespread malignancy (i.e. metastasis to three or more organs; Berge 1974). This phenomenon has been adapted to the lack of afferent lymphatics, the presence of some pulsatility of the spleen, or the anti-neoplastic prop-

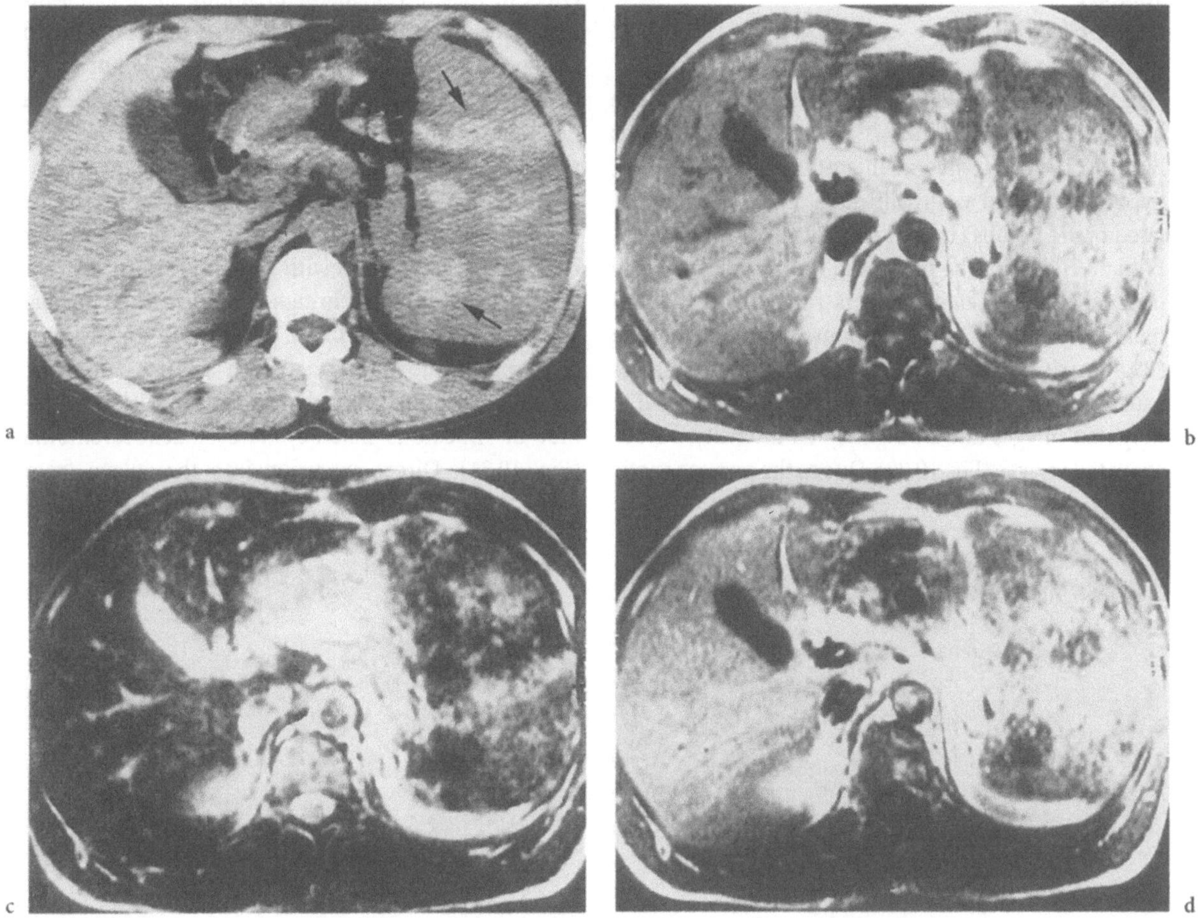

Fig. 10.26. Angiosarcoma. **a** Unenhanced computed tomography shows multiple high-attenuation masses (*arrows*) in a markedly enlarged spleen. **b** A T1-weighted magnetic-resonance (MR) image shows multiple hypointense nodules. Numerous tiny, hypointense spots throughout the spleen represent Gamna-Gandy nodules. **c** On T2-weighted MR at the same level, the spleen is heterogeneous in signal intensity, and the multiple masses are hypointense. The tiny, hypointense spots are also well demonstrated. **d** A gadolinium-enhanced T1-weighted image reveals inhomogeneous enhancement of the splenic parenchyma (Ha et al. 1994)

erties of the lymphoid-rich splenic parenchyma (Warshauer and Koehler 1998).

10.4.4.2
Clinical Manifestations

Small lesions are usually asymptomatic, although larger lesions may cause left upper-quadrant pain (Urrutia et al. 1996). Almost half of the splenic metastases are due to malignant melanoma, and the remaining 50% are predominantly due to adenocarcinoma of the breast (21%), lung (18%), ovary, prostate, colon and stomach (Marymont and Gross 1963).

10.4.4.3
Pathology

Many metastases in the spleen are cystic due to rapid growth and subsequent autoinfarction (Urrutia et al. 1996). One third of the splenic metastases observed at autopsy are microscopic aggregates of tumor and are not visible on imaging (Warren and Davis 1981). Splenic metastases most frequently appear as multiple nodules, although diffuse involvement occurs in 8–10% of affected patients (Warshauer and Koehler 1998).

10.4.4.4
Imaging

Due to internal necrosis, splenic metastases (97%) are hypoechoic on US images (GOERG et al. 1991; Fig. 10.27). At CT, splenic metastases are ill-defined, hypodense foci or well-delineated, unilocular or septated cystic lesions (URRUTIA et al. 1996) (Fig. 10.28). Enhancement may be present in the periphery and in internal septae. Calcification is rare unless the primary tumor is a mucinous adenocarcinoma (RABUSHKA et al. 1994). On MRI, splenic metastases usually appear as areas of low signal intensity on T1-weighted images and of high signal intensity on T2-weighted images (Fig. 10.29). Due to the paramagnetic effect of melanin or methemoglobin, high-signal-intensity lesions can be demonstrated on T1-weighted images in metastases of melanoma or hemorrhagic metastases (TORRES et al. 1995) (Fig. 10.30). Lesion detection is improved by acquiring post-Gd SGE images, because metastases remain hypointense compared with enhancing normal splenic tissue (MIROWITZ et al. 1991). Due to the lack of Kuppfer cells, image acquisition with iron oxide particles renders metastases higher in signal intensity than normal spleen (KELEKIS et al. 1997). Direct tumor invasion is uncommon but may occur from a large pancreatic cancer including ductal adenocarcinoma, islet-cell tumor or mucinous macrocystic cystadenocarcinoma (Fig. 10.31). Direct extension into the spleen from

a 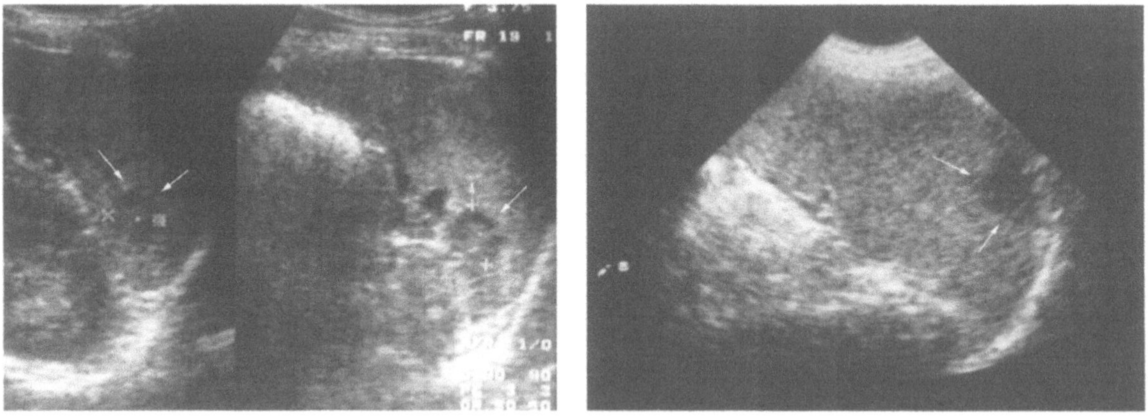 b

Fig. 10.27. Splenic metastases. **a** An axial sonogram in a patient with malignant melanoma shows an isoechoic splenic lesion with a hypoechoic rim (*arrows*). A biopsy revealed splenic metastasis (courtesy of F. Vanhoenacker). **b** An axial ultrasound image in a patient with colon cancer shows a round, well-delineated splenic lesion (*arrows*). Splenectomy revealed a solitary metastasis of the spleen

a 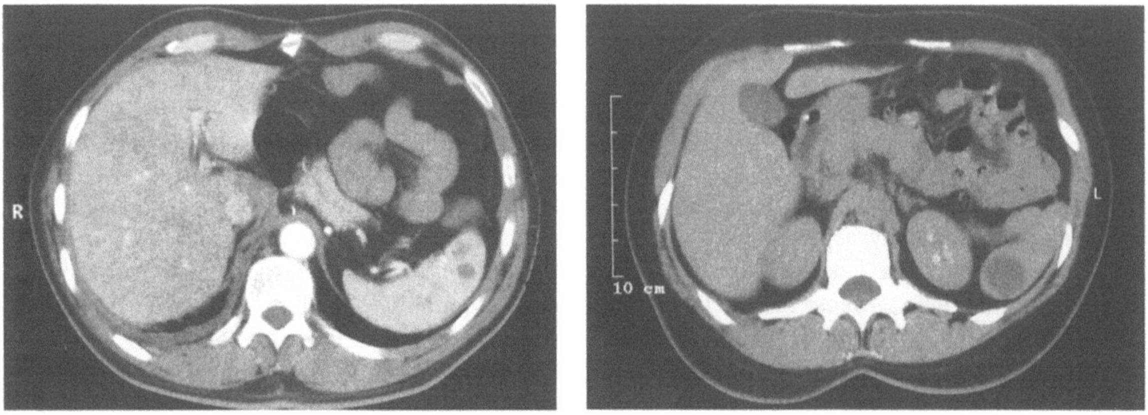 b

Fig. 10.28. Splenic metastasis. **a** A contrast-enhanced computed-tomography (CT) scan in a patient with esophageal cancer shows multiple low-attenuation masses. **b** An unenhanced CT image in a patient with breast carcinoma demonstrates a solitary hypodense lesion that is well demarcated from the splenic parenchyma lymphoma or tumors of gastric, colonic, renal and adrenal origin is also reported (Kelekis et al. 1997). Capsular implantation of metastatic deposits is particularly seen in patients with ovarian cancer, since ovarian metastases commonly spread by peritoneal seeding rather than hematogenously. Therefore, metastatic deposits will appear on imaging as cystic serosal implants on the visceral peritoneal surface. This is in contradiction to most other splenic lesions, which are intraparenchymal (Fig. 10.32).

10.5 Conclusion

Although, in general, tumoral involvement of the spleen is relatively uncommon, a vast array of specific neoplastic disorders may be encountered. Many of the neoplasms affecting the spleen have a similar appearance on radiological studies and exhibit substantial overlap in their imaging findings. In a gamut of cases, however, familiarity with the most relevant

a 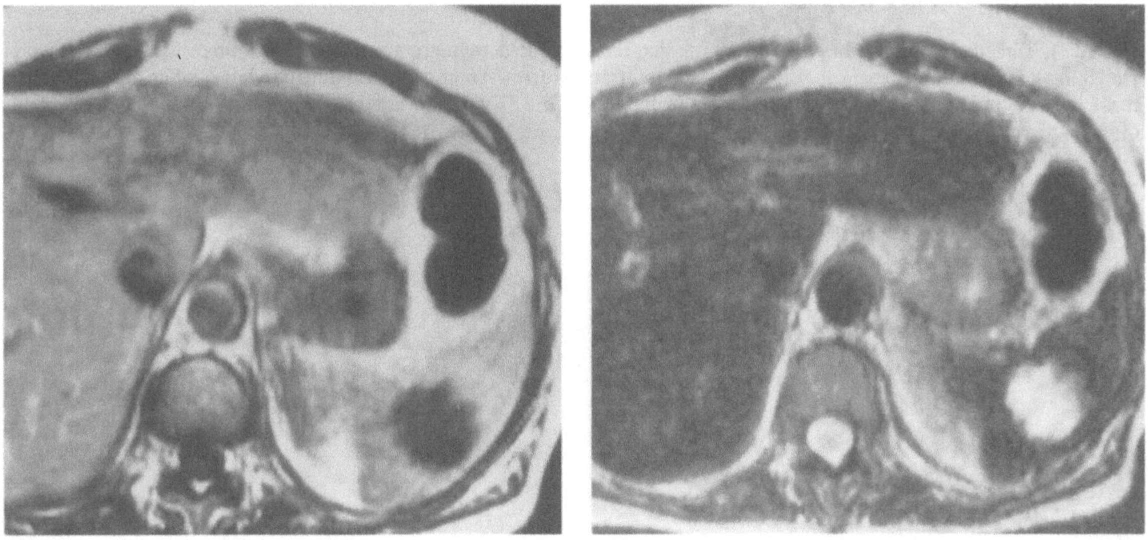 b

Fig. 10.29. Unknown primary adenocarcinoma metastatic to the spleen. (a) T1-weighted and (b) T2-weighted magnetic-resonance images show a solitary focal splenic lesion with low and high signal intensities, respectively

a 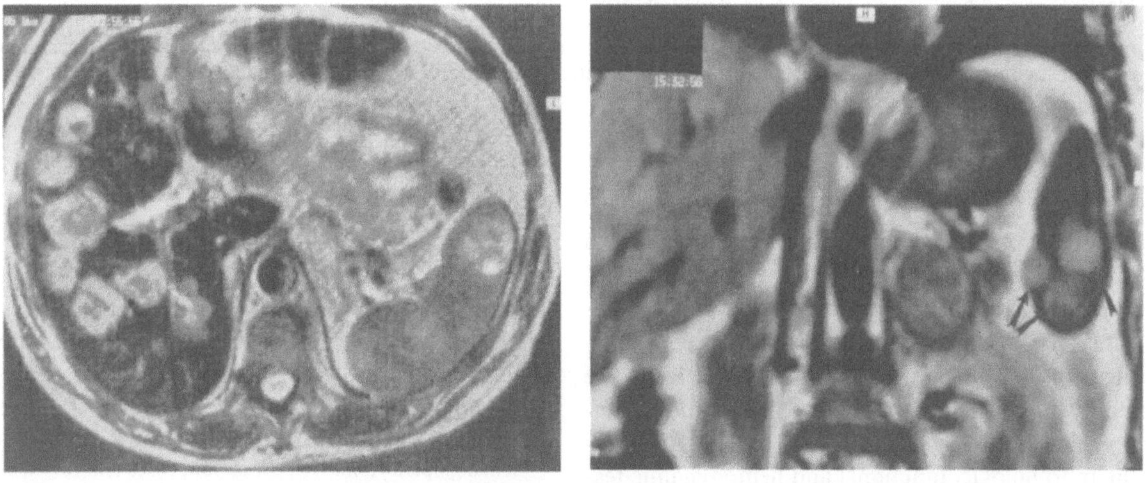 b

Fig. 10.30. Malignant melanoma metastatic to the spleen. **a** A T2-weighted magnetic-resonance image demonstrates multiple hyperintense lesions in the liver and spleen in this patient with metastatic melanoma. **b** A T1-weighted coronal image shows high signal intensity of several of the lesions due to the paramagnetic effect of melanin (*arrows*)

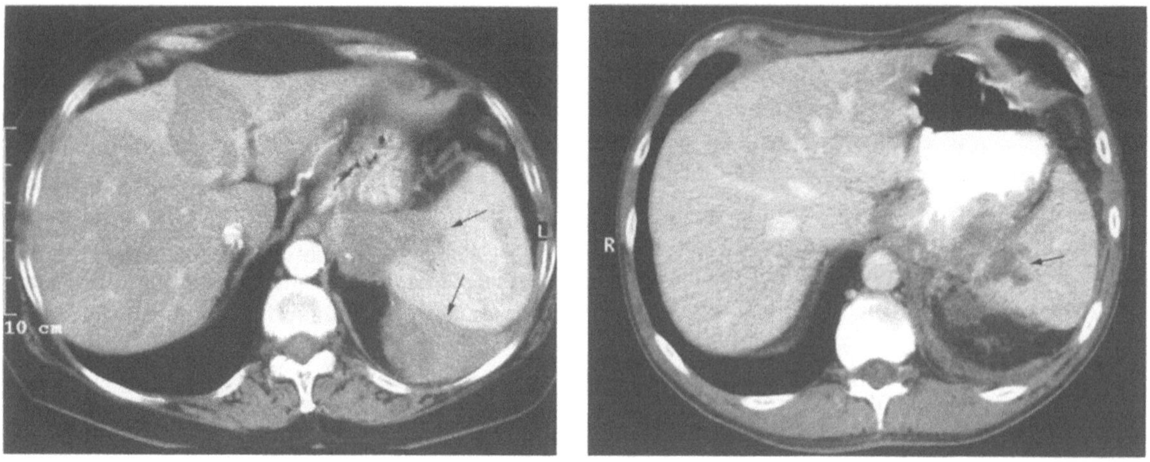

Fig. 10.31. Direct tumor invasion. **a** A contrast-enhanced computed tomography image in a woman with extensive non-Hodgkin's lymphoma and hepatic localization shows infiltration (*arrows*) of the splenic hilum by a large, infiltrative, perisplenic mass. **b** Direct invasion into the spleen, stomach and diaphragm in a 52-year-old woman with a mucinous cystadenocarcinoma of the pancreatic tail

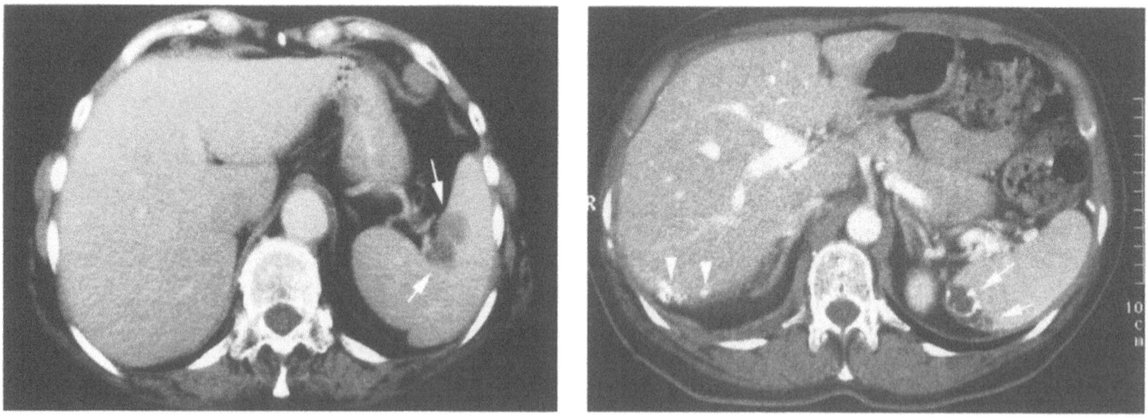

Fig. 10.32. Seeding metastasis. **a** A contrast-enhanced computed tomography (CT) image shows two hypoattenuating lesions with irregular margins (*arrows*) implanted on the splenic surface in a patient with ovarian carcinoma and widespread peritoneal metastatic disease. **b** A contrast-enhanced CT image in another patient treated for metastatic ovarian cancer shows partially calcified seeding metastases in the splenic (*arrows*) and hepatic (*arrowheads*) capsules

radiologic features, in combination with critical additional clinical information, provides enough information for adequate lesion characterization. Furthermore, due to the rapid technological advances in imaging techniques, including the refinement of both dynamic spiral CT and MRI and the ability to use tailored MR techniques and organ-specific contrast agents, it is now possible to assess the morphologic, functional and hemodynamic features of splenic tumors as useful tools in distinguishing the tumoral pathology of the spleen.

References

Ahmann DL, Kiely JM, Harrison EG, et al. (1966) Malignant lymphoma of the spleen: a review of 49 cases in which the diagnosis was made at splenectomy. Cancer 19:461–469

Avigad S, Jaffe R, Frand M, et al. (1976) Lymphangiomatosis with splenic involvement. JAMA 236:2315–2317

Berge T (1974) Splenic metastases: frequencies and patterns. Acta Pathol Microbiol Scand [A] 82:499–506

Binder SC, Wolfe HJ, Deterling RA (1973) Intra-abdominal hemangiopericytoma. Report on four cases and review of the literature. Arch Surg 107:536–543

Bostick WL (1945) Primary splenic neoplasm. Am J Pathol 21:1143–1165

Brinkley AA, Lee JK (1981) Cystic hamartoma of the spleen: CT and sonographic findings. J Clin Ultrasound 9:136–138

Bruneton JN, Drouillard J, Rogopoulos A, et al. (1988) Extraretroperitoneal abdominal malignant fibrous histiocytoma. Gastrointest Radiol 13:299–305

Chen KT, Bolles CG, Gilbert EF (1979) Angiosarcoma of the spleen. Arch Pathol Lab Med 103:122–128

Dachman AH, Ros PR, Marari PJ, et al. (1986) Non-parasitic splenic cysts: a report of 52 cases with radiologic–pathologic correlation. AJR Am J Roentgenol 147:537–542

Dawes LG, Malangoni MA (1986) Cystic masses of the spleen. Am Surg 52:333–336

Disler DG, Chew FS (1991) Splenic hemangioma. AJR Am J Roentgenol 157:44

Duddy MJ, Calder CJ (1989) Cystic hemangioma of the spleen: findings on ultrasound and computed tomography. Br J Radiol 62:180–182

Easler RE, Dowlin WM (1969) Primary lipoma of the spleen. Arch Pathol 88:557–559

Enzinger FM, Smith B (1976) Hemangiopericytoma: an analysis of 106 cases. Hum Pathol 7:61–82

Falk S, Stutte HJ, Frizzera G (1991) Littoral cell angioma. A novel splenic vascular lesion demonstrating histiocytic differentiation. Am J Surg Pathol 15:1023–1033

Ferrozzi F, Bova D, Draghi F, et al. (1996) CT findings in primary vascular tumors of the spleen. AJR Am J Roentgenol 166:1097–1101

Findley A, Childress MH (1995) Computed tomography of thorotrastosis. J Comput Assist Tomogr 11:188–189

Freeman JL, Jafri SZ, Roberts JL, Mezwa DG, Shirkhoda A (1993) CT of congenital and acquired abnormalities of the spleen. Radiographics 13:597–610

Garvin DF, King FM (1981) Cysts and non-lymphomatous tumors of the spleen. Pathol Annu 16:61–80

Gilmartin D (1978) Familial multiple epidermoid cyst of the spleen. Conn Med 42:297–300

Goerg C, Schwerk WB, Goerg K (1991) Sonography of focal lesions of the spleen. AJR Am J Roentgenol 156:949–953

Grantham M, Einstein D, McCarron K, et al. (1998) Littoral cell angioma of the spleen. Abdom Imaging 23:633–635

Griscom NT, Hargreaves HK, Schwartz MZ, et al. (1977) Huge splenic cyst in a newborn: comparisons with 10 cases in later childhood and adolescence. AJR Am J Roentgenol 129:889–891

Grumbach K, McDowell R (1994) The spleen. In: Haaga JR, Lanzieri CF, Sartoris DF, Zerhouni ED (eds) Computed tomography and magnetic resonance imaging of the whole body, 3rd edn. Mosby Year Book, St Louis, pp 1136–1147

Ha HK, Kim HH, Kim BK, et al. (1994) Primary angiosarcoma of the spleen. CT and MR imaging. Acta Radiol 35:455–458

Harris RD, Simpson W (1989) MRI of splenic hemangioma associated with thrombocytopenia. Gastrointest Radiol 14:308–310

Harris NL, Aisenberg AC, Meyer JE, et al. (1984) Diffuse large cell (histiocytic) lymphoma of the spleen: clinical and pathological characteristics of ten cases. Cancer 54:2460–2467

Husni EA (1961) The clinical course of splenic hemangioma. Arch Surg 83:681–688

Ito K, Murata T, Nakanishi T (1995) Cystic lymphangioma of the spleen: MR findings with pathologic correlation. Abdom Imaging 20:82–84

Jurado JG, Turégano F, Garcia C, et al. (1989) Hemangiopericytoma of the spleen. Surgery 106:575–577

Kaneko K, Onitsuka H, Murakami J, et al. (1992) MRI of primary spleen angiosarcoma with iron accumulation. J Comput Assist Tomogr 16:298–300

Kelekis NL, Burdeny DA, Semelka RC (1997) Spleen. In: Semelka RC, Ascher SM, Reinhold C (eds) MRI of the abdomen and pelvis. A text atlas. Wiley-Liss, New York, pp 239–256

Mahony B, Jeffrey RB, Federle MP (1982) Spontaneous rupture of hepatic and splenic angiosarcoma demonstrated by CT. AJR Am J Roentgenol 138:965–966

Manor A, Starinsky R, Garfinkel D, et al. (1984) Ultrasound features of symptomatic splenic hemangioma. J Clin Ultrasound 12:95–97

Marymont JGJ, Gross S (1963) Patterns of metastatic cancer in the spleen. Am J Clin Pathol 40:58–66

Meyer JE, Harris NL, Elman A, et al. (1983) Large-cell lymphoma of the spleen: CT appearance. Radiology •:199–201

Mirowitz SA, Brown JJ, Lee JKT, et al. (1991) Dynamic gadolinium-enhanced MR imaging of the spleen: normal enhancement patterns and evaluation of splenic lesions. Radiology 179:681–686

Morgenstern L, Rosenberg J, Geller SA (1985) Tumors of the spleen. World J Surg 9:468–476

Morinaga S, Ohyama R, Koizumi J (1992) Low-grade mucinous cystadenocarcinoma in the spleen. Am J Surg Pathol 16:903–908

Niizawa M, Ishida H, Morikawa P, et al. (1991) Color doppler sonography in a case of splenic hemangioma: value of compressing the tumor. AJR Am J Roentgenol 157:965–966

Norowitz DG, Morehouse HT (1989) Isodense splenic mass: hamartoma, a case report. Comput Med Imaging Graph 13:347–350

Nyberg DA, Jeffrey RB Jr, Federle MP, Bottles K, Abrams DI (1986) AIDS-related lymphomas: evaluation by abdominal CT. Radiology 159:59–63

Nyman R, Rehn S, Glimelius B, et al. (1987) Magnetic resonance imaging, chest radiography, computed tomography, and ultrasonography in malignant lymphoma. Acta Radiol 28:253–262

Ohtomo K, Fukuda H, Mori K, et al. (1992) CT and MR appearances of splenic hamartoma. J Comput Assist Tomogr 16:425–428

Oliver-Goldaracena JM, Blanco A, Miralles M, et al. (1998) Littoral cell angioma of the spleen: US and MR imaging findings. Abdom Imaging 23:636–639

Pakter RL, Fishman EK, Nussbaum A, et al. (1987) CT findings in splenic hemangiomas in the Klippel-Trenaunay-Weber syndrome. J Comput Assist Tomogr 11:88–91

Peene P, Wilms G, Stockx L, et al. (1991) Splenic hemangiomatosis: CT and MR features. J Comput Assist Tomogr 15:1070–1073

Pines B, Rabinovitch J (1942) Hemangioma of the spleen. Arch Pathol 33:487–503

Pinto PO, Avigado P, Garcia H, et al. (1995) Splenic hamartoma: a case report. Eur Radiol 5:93–95

Pistoia F, Markowitz SK (1988) Splenic lymphangiomatosis: CT diagnosis. AJR Am J Roentgenol 150:121–122

Pyatt RS, Williams ED, Clark M, et al. (1981) CT diagnosis of splenic lymphangiomatosis. J Comput Assist Tomogr 5:446–448

Rabushka LS, Kawashima A, Fishman EK (1994) Imaging of the spleen: CT with supplemental MR examination. Radiographics 14:307–332

Ramani M, Reinhold C, Semelka RC, et al. (1997) Splenic hemangiomas and hamartomas: MR imaging characteristics of 28 lesions. Radiology 202:166–172

Ros PR, Moser RP, Dachman AH, et al. (1987) Hemangioma of the spleen: radiologic-pathologic correlation in ten cases. Radiology 162:73–77

Rosenthal T, Adar R, Wolfstein I, et al. (1973) Cavernous hemangioma of the spleen: angiographic observations. Angiology 24:430–433

Rosso R, Paulli M, Gianelli U, et al. (1995) Littoral cell angiosarcoma of the spleen. Case report with immunohistochemical and ultrastructural analysis. Am J Surg Pathol 19:1203–1208

Shanberge JN, Tanaka K, Gruhl MC (1971) Chronic consumption coagulopathy due to hemangiomatous transformation of the spleen. Am J Clin Pathol 56:723–729

Shirkhoda A, Freeman J, Armin AR, et al. (1995) Imaging features of splenic epidermoid cyst with pathologic correlation. Abdom Imaging 20:449–451

Sondenaa K, Heikkilä R, Nysted A, et al. (1993) Diagnosis of brain metastases from a primary hemangiosarcoma of the spleen with magnetic resonance imaging. Cancer 71:138–141

Spalding RM, Jennings CV, Yam LT (1980) Splenic hamartoma. Br J Radiol 53:1197–1200

Spier CM, Kjeldsberg CR, Eyre HJ, et al. (1985) Malignant lymphoma with primary presentation in the spleen: a study of 20 patients. Arch Pathol Lab Med 109:1076–1080

Steinberg JJ, Suhrland MJ, Valensi QJ (1985) The association of splenoma with disease. Lab Invest 52:65A

Stout AP, Lattes R (1967) Tumors of soft tissues. Armed Forces Institute of Pathology, Washington, pp 67–72

Stout AP, Murray MR (1942) Hemangiopericytoma: a vascular tumor featuring Zimmerman's pericytes. Ann Surg 16:26–33

Strijk SP, Wagener DJT, Bogman MJJT, et al. (1985) The spleen in Hodgkin disease: diagnostic value of CT. Radiology 154:753–757

Taylor AJ, Dodds WJ, Erickson SJ, et al. (1991) CT of acquired abnormalities of the spleen. AJR Am J Roentgenol 157: 1213–1219

Tiu CM, Chou YH, Wang HT, et al. (1992) Epithelioid hemangioendothelioma of the spleen with intrasplenic metastasis: ultrasound and computed tomography appearance. Comput Med Imaging Graph 16:287–290

Torres GM, Terry NL, Mergo PJ, et al. (1995) MR imaging of the spleen. Magn Reson Imaging Clin N Am 3:39–50

Tsang WYW, Chan JKC (1993)The family of epithelioid vascular tumors. Histol Histopathol 8:187–212

Urrutia M, Mergo PJ, Ros LH, et al. (1996) Cystic masses of the spleen: radiologic-pathologic correlation. Radiographics 16:107–129

Vilanova JC, Capdevila A, Aldoma et al. (1994) Splenic epithelioid hemangioma: MR findings. AJR Am J Roentgenol 163:747–748

Warren S, Davis AH (1981) Studies on tumor metastasis: the metastases of carcinoma to the spleen. Am J Cancer 21:517–533

Warshauer DM, Koehler RE (1998) Spleen. In: Lee JK, Sagel SS, Stanley RJ, Heiken JP (eds) Computed body tomography with MR correlation, 3rd edn. Lippencott-Raven, Philadelphia, pp 845–872

Weissleder R, Elizondo G, Stark DD, et al. (1989) Diagnosis of splenic lymphoma by MR imaging: value of superparamagnetic iron. AJR Am J Roentgenol 152:175–180

Wick MR, Smith SL, Scheithauer BW, et al. (1982) Primary non-lymphoreticular malignant neoplasm of the spleen. Am J Pathol 6:229–242

Younger KA, Hall CM (1990) Epidermoid cyst of the spleen: a case report and review of the literature. Br J Radiol 63:652–653

Zissin R, Lishner M, Rathaus V (1992) Case report: unusual presentation of splenic hamartoma. Computed tomography and ultrasound findings. Clin Radiol 45:410–411

11 Pseudotumors of the Spleen

H. Irie, H. Honda, T. Kuroiwa, K. Yoshimitsu, H. Aibe, T. Tajima, and K. Masuda

CONTENTS

11.1 Introduction

There are many disorders, either neoplastic or non-neoplastic, that give rise to focal splenic tumoral lesions. Since most of these disorders are discussed extensively in other chapters of this book, the main topic of this chapter is inflammatory pseudotumors of the spleen. Miscellaneous disorders (other than neoplastic, infectious, vascular or systemic disorders) that may cause tumoral lesions in the spleen (thus mimicking primary splenic neoplasm, metastatic disease or lymphomatous infiltration) are also discussed briefly.

H. Irie, H. Honda, T. Kuroiwa, K. Yoshimitsu, H. Aibe, T. Tajima, K. Masuda; Department of Radiology, Faculty of Medicine, Kyushu University, 3-1-1 Maidashi, Higashi-ku Fukuoka, 812-8582, Japan

11.2 Inflammatory Pseudotumors of the Spleen

11.2.1 Epidemiology and Pathogenesis

Inflammatory pseudotumors are rare benign masses composed of a localized area of inflammatory and reparative fibroblastic changes and granulomatous components. This entity, which has the gross appearance of a malignant tumor but has a benign histologic appearance and course, has mostly been observed in tissues of the respiratory tract and, rarely, in the gastrointestinal tract, orbit, soft tissue, lymph nodes, liver and central nervous system (Honda et al. 1996). Inflammatory pseudotumor is rarely seen in the spleen and, since the first two reported cases (Cotelingam and Jaffe 1984), less than 40 cases have been reported in the English language literature. Extremely rarely, inflammatory pseudotumor can arise within the accessory spleen. There is no gender predominance in inflammatory pseudotumor of the spleen, and the condition usually affects adults who are over 50 years of age, although inflammatory pseudotumor of the spleen in a 5-year-old boy has been reported (Aru et al. 1997).

Although inflammatory pseudotumor is considered by most pathologists to represent a reparative process of an inflammatory lesion, the cause of inflammatory pseudotumor is unknown (Safran et al. 1991). Histologic findings are consistent with a polymorphous inflammatory cell infiltration occurring in response to some unidentified stimulus. For pulmonary inflammatory pseudotumors, previous respiratory infection was once thought to be an important etiologic factor, but respiratory infection has been shown to be associated with less than one third of affected patients (Berardi et al. 1983). For hepatic inflammatory pseudotumors, some reports have suggested that the inflammatory process originating from micro-organic infection may cause inflammatory pseudotumors, and cholangitis of various causes is thought to be the most likely etiology (Horiuchi et al. 1990). In the case of inflammatory pseudotumors of the spleen, regions of parenchymal necrosis and microscopic evidence of previous hemorrhage have been associated with polymorphous cellular infiltrate, implicating trauma-induced cell death as a possible stimulus for subsequent inflammation. However, cultures and histochemical stains of involved splenic parenchyma have failed to isolate any infectious source (Safran et al. 1991). Someron (1978) has discussed the possibility of an autoimmune mechanism underlying inflammatory pseudotumor formation, while Perrone et al. (1988) have suggested that the cytokine interleukin-1 may play a central role in the pathogenesis of inflammatory pseudotumors. Herman et al. (1994) have considered inflammatory pseudotumor a neoplasm of myofibroblasts related to myofibromatoses, and they have proposed calling them "inflammatory myofibroblastic tumors". Overall, it would seem that inflammatory pseudotumor formation may be the result of an exaggerated, non-specific inflammatory or immune reactions that can occur in response to many different stimuli.

11.2.2 Pathology

Grossly, inflammatory pseudotumors arise within the substance of the spleen as discrete, well-circumscribed, sometimes lobulated masses. They are generally solitary lesions, although multiple nodules have been reported. Individual tumor size has varied from less than 1.5 cm to 17 cm. When multiple tumor nodules have been found, they have been smaller than solitary lesions, suggesting that larger tumor masses might form via the coalescence of smaller lesions. Small multiple nodules and large singular masses may therefore represent two points in the temporal spectrum of inflammatory pseudotumor pathogenesis. On a cut section, inflammatory pseudotumors can appear gray, tan, pink, white or yellow, with the predominant color reflecting the more prominent aspects of the underlying histologic composition (Safran et al. 1991).

Microscopically, inflammatory pseudotumor is composed of a mixture of inflammatory cells, including plasma cells, lymphocytes, foreign-body giant cells, histiocytes, foam cells, numerous vascular elements, fibrous stroma and spindle cells that are sometimes associated with a granulomatous reaction (Honda et al. 1996). A number of histologic patterns have been described, all sharing the theme of an inflammatory–reparative cycle. Someron (1978) has classified inflammatory pseudotumors into three histologic types based on the predominant cellular component: xanthogranulomas (prominent histiocytic cellular component), plasma cell granulomas (prominent plasma cell component) and sclerosing pseudotumors (obvious sclerotic features). Within the spleen, granuloma formation with multinucleated giant cells has commonly been described. Such formation is accompanied by an abundant polymorphous leukocytic infiltrate, and zones of bland or caseous cell necrosis are usually found near the core of this dense cellular reaction. Occasionally, deposits of erythrocyte breakdown products are seen, including hemosiderin, hematoidin and cellular debris. Often, there is a fibroblastic reaction with hyalinization of the connective tissue matrix. Fibroblastic, reparative changes may be found centrally and peripherally, often leading to the formation of a well-defined, fibrous capsule. Encapsulation, absence of dysplastic elements and the polyclonal character of the involved lymphocyte populations confirm the non-neoplastic nature of the process.

11.2.3 Clinical Findings

The symptoms related to inflammatory pseudotumors of the spleen include fever, epigastralgia, vomiting, general malaise and weight loss; these symptoms are almost the same as those seen in cases of inflammatory pseudotumors of other organs, such as the lung and the liver. Laboratory data sometimes show the presence of leukocytosis. These symptoms have been reported to represent a non-specific, systemic reaction to the underlying process (Safran et al. 1991). Symptoms usually disappear after complete excision of the mass. More than half of the patients with inflammatory pseudotumors of the spleen are symptomatic; however, the rest of the patients are asymptomatic (Irie et al. 1996). Approximately one half of the lesions have been discovered incidentally during work-up for other malignancies (Aru et al. 1997).

11.2.4 Imaging

As discussed in the pathology section, inflammatory pseudotumors have a wide spectrum of pathologic findings, and there seem to be no specific radiologic findings. These radiologic findings may vary according to the extent of the inflammatory process and the fibrotic reaction (IRIE et al. 1996).

The sonographic appearance of inflammatory pseudotumor of the spleen is usually hypoechoic (Fig. 11.1a), although it may be hyperechoic. Occasionally, calcification within the mass causes an acoustic shadow, either centrally or peripherally (FRANQUET et al. 1989). There has been one report in which Doppler ultrasonography revealed a hypovascular mass in the spleen (HAYASAKA et al. 1998).

On plain computed tomography (CT), inflammatory pseudotumor of the spleen shows a discrete, hypodense mass compared with the normal splenic parenchyma; this finding, however, is nonspecific. Calcification may be seen in the central or peripheral portions of the mass. In the early phase of CT after the contrast-medium injection, the inflammatory pseudotumor is usually observed to be hypodense (Fig. 11.1b), either homogeneously or heterogeneously, in relation to the normal spleen. The delayed-phase CT usually demonstrates enhancement of the mass (Fig. 11.1c) (IRIE et al. 1996). This pattern of delayed enhancement corresponds to the hypovascular and fibrotic nature of the lesion. YAMAKADO et al. (1994) have reported that CT performed 1 h after angiography reveals the central stellate area to be markedly hyperdense, corresponding to the prominent fibroblastic proliferation in the center of the mass. This central stellate area (Fig. 11.2a) has been reported to be suggestive of an inflammatory pseudotumor (FRANQUET et al. 1989), but the results were not definitive. Occasionally, a non-enhanced area that corresponds microscopically to the central necrosis is noted within the center of the mass.

On T1-weighted magnetic-resonance (MR) images, inflammatory pseudotumors are usually isointense or hypointense compared with the normal spleen (Fig. 11.1d) (IRIE et al. 1996), although hyperintense inflammatory pseudotumors of the spleen (for which the etiology is unknown) have been reported (GLAZER et al. 1992). A gradient-echo image may show very hypointense, minute nodules within the mass; these correspond histologically to hemosiderin (Fig. 11.1e). On T2-weighted MR images, most of the reported cases have revealed a heterogeneously hypointense mass in comparison with the normal spleen (Fig. 11.1f; IRIE et al. 1996). This finding corresponds to the fibrotic stroma within inflammatory pseudotumor and is relatively characteristic. However, isointense or hyperintense inflammatory pseudotumors of the spleen on T2-weighted images have also been reported (GLAZER et al. 1992). The varying appearances on T2-weighted images probably depend on the relative amount of fibrous stroma and cellular material in the inflammatory pseudotumor (IRIE et al. 1996). We have encountered an inflammatory pseudotumor of the accessory spleen, and the mass was slightly hyperintense to the spleen on the T2-weighted images (Fig. 11.3). Occasionally, central necrosis is demonstrated as a hyperintense area on a T2-weighted image. A dynamic MR study after bolus injection of contrast material is also useful in evaluating inflammatory pseudotumors of the spleen (Fig. 11.1g–j). The findings on dynamic MR imaging are similar to those on dynamic CT; however, because of their higher contrast resolution, dynamic MR images may demonstrate internal architecture, such as fibrous septa of the mass, more clearly than dynamic CT (IRIE et al. 1996). The delayed phase of a contrast-enhanced T1-weighted image may demonstrate the central stellate area as a hyperintense region more clearly than CT (Fig. 11.2b).

Angiography usually shows a non-specific hypovascular or avascular mass in the spleen (HAYASAKA et al. 1998; Fig. 11.1k). There has been only one report concerning a radio-isotopic study of inflammatory pseudotumor. Single-photon emission computed tomography imaging using labeled red blood cells has shown the inflammatory pseudotumor to be avascular (GLAZER and SAGAR 1993).

The differential diagnosis of inflammatory pseudotumor of the spleen includes malignant lymphoma, hemangioma, metastatic lesion and hamartoma (IRIE et al. 1996). The radiologic characteristics of these tumors are limited, because only a few isolated cases have been reported in the literature. However, malignant lymphoma usually demonstrates a bulky mass, transgresses the splenic capsule to involve adjacent organs and does not show delayed enhancement (MEYER et al. 1983). Gallium scintigraphy is thought to be useful in differentiating inflammatory pseudotumor from malignant lymphoma. Autopsy series have shown that metastases to the spleen almost never occur in patients older than 50 years of age without evidence of widespread disease (HAHN et al. 1988). Hemangioma

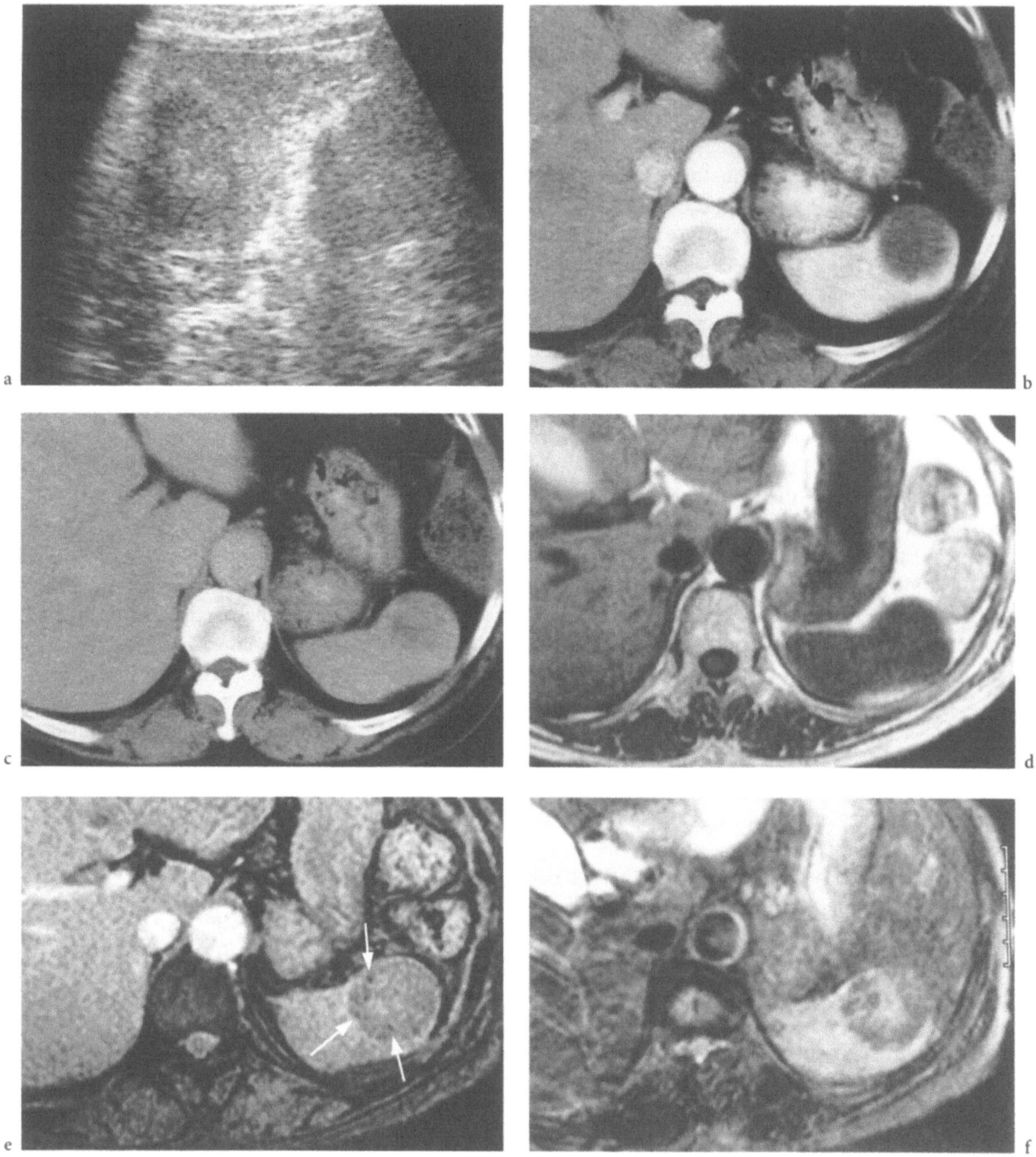

Fig. 11.1. Inflammatory pseudotumor of the spleen. **a** Ultrasound demonstrates a well-defined, slightly hypoechoic mass in the spleen. **b** An early phase of computed tomography (CT) after contrast injection shows a homogeneous hypodense mass in the spleen. **c** A delayed phase of CT reveals delayed enhancement of the mass. **d** The mass in the spleen is almost isointense to the normal spleen, and is difficult to detect on a T1-weighted magnetic-resonance (MR) image. **e** On the gradient-echo MR image, minute hypointense nodules that histologically correspond to hemosiderin (*arrows*) are noted within the mass. **f** On T2-weighted MR images, the peripheral portion of the mass is hypointense, and the central portion is almost isointense in relation to the surrounding spleen.

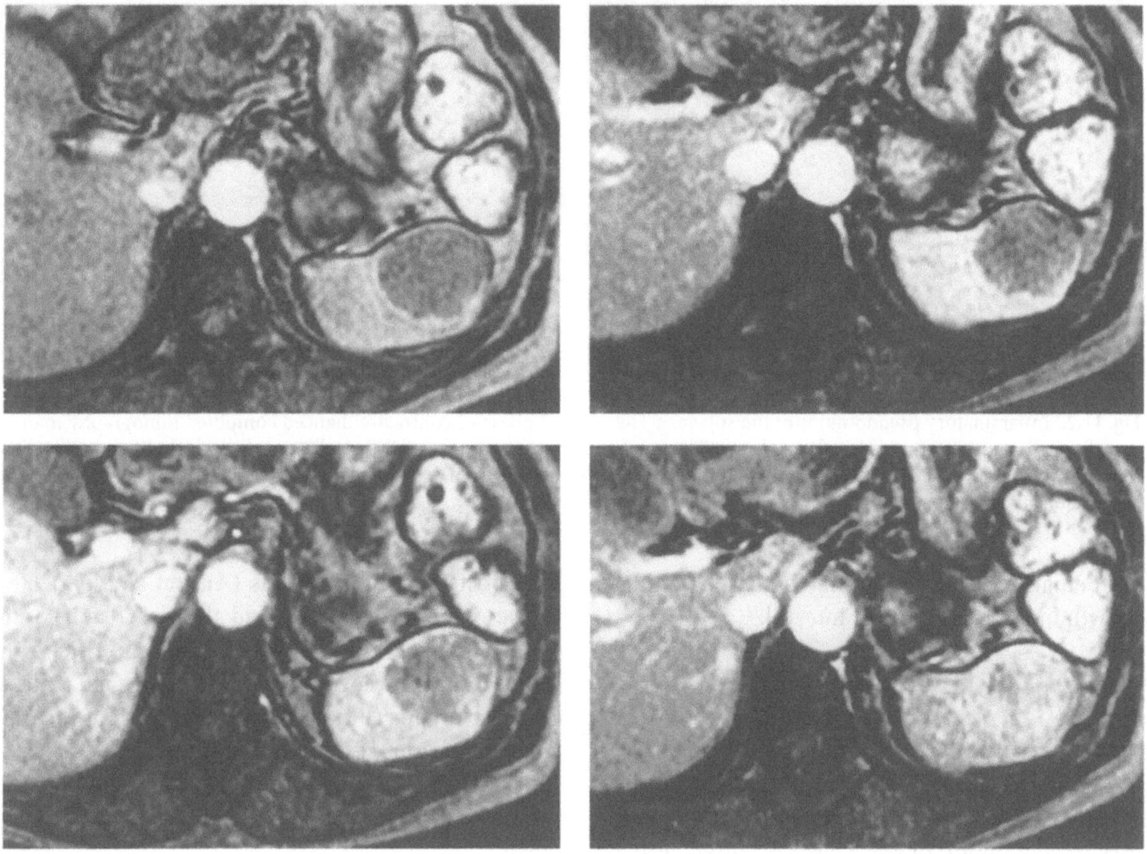

g h i j

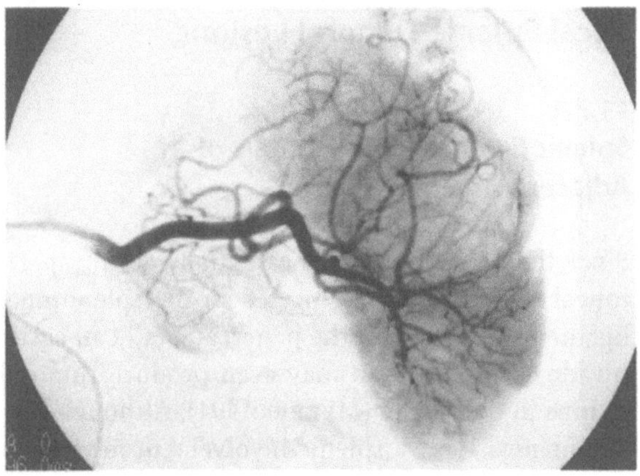

k

Fig. 11.1. Inflammatory pseudotumor of the spleen (*Continued*) **g, h, i, j** Dynamic MR study after bolus injection of contrast material (g:30 s; h:60 s; i:90 s; j:360 s after contrast injection) clearly demonstrates inhomogeneous delayed enhancement of the mass. **k** Digital subtraction angiography of the splenic artery shows displacement of the splenic arteries and reveals the mass to be hypovascular

and hamartoma of the spleen may show delayed enhancement on dynamic study, but they usually show hyperintensity on T2-weighted images, which may differentiate these conditions from inflammatory pseudotumor (Ramani et al. 1997). However, hyperintense inflammatory pseudotumors of the spleen on T2-weighted images have been reported, and hypointense hemangioma and hamartoma on T2-weighted images have also been reported (Ramani et al. 1997). Differentiation among these disorders, therefore, is thought to be impossible using current methods.

11.2.5 Natural History

Spontaneous regression of inflammatory pseudotumors of the liver has been reported (Irie et al. 1988); there has been no report, however, concerning the natural history of inflammatory pseudotumors of the spleen. We have observed two cases of inflammatory pseudotumors of the spleen that were followed-up and demonstrated an increase in size during a period of less than 1 year (Fig. 11.4). Although inflammatory pseudotumors of the spleen

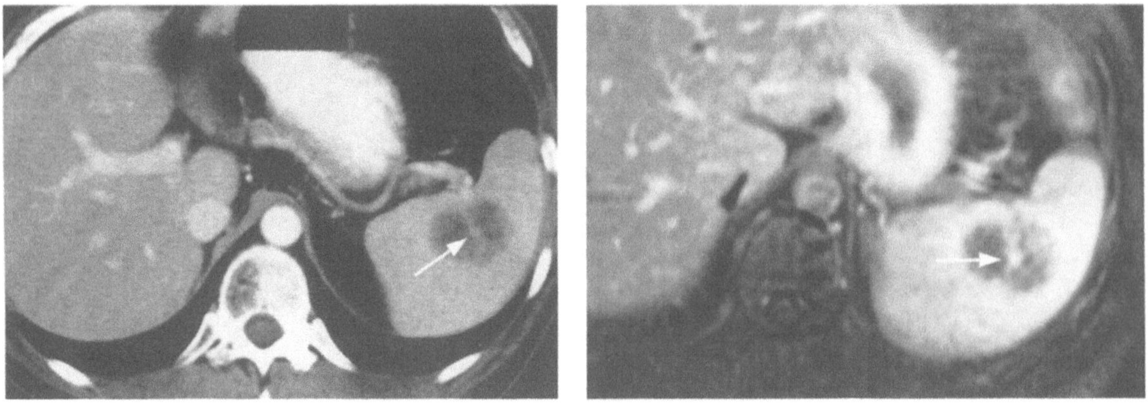

a b

Fig. 11.2. Inflammatory pseudotumor of the spleen. **a** The delayed phase of contrast-enhanced computed tomography mainly reveals a hypodense mass in the spleen. The mass demonstrates a central stellate area of slight hyperdensity (*arrow*). **b** A contrast-enhanced T1-weighted image with fat suppression clearly demonstrates a central stellate area of hyperintensity (*arrow*)

are benign disorders, they may undergo significant growth in a relatively short interval.

11.2.6 Treatment

Because correct radiologic diagnosis of inflammatory pseudotumor of the spleen is often difficult, splenectomy has been performed in all reported cases. Malignant transformation, local invasion or metastatic spread of inflammatory pseudotumors arising from any organ has never been reported; therefore, splenectomy is considered to be a complete curative procedure (Safran et al. 1991). If possible, partial splenectomy may be preferable, because it can preserve splenic function and avoid a rare postsplenectomy sepsis (Aru et al. 1997). Because of poor specificity and the risk of bleeding (Aru et al. 1997) fine-needle aspiration, which can be used in the preoperative work-up of such a mass in other organs (Fukuya et al. 1994), is not recommended for masses within the spleen.

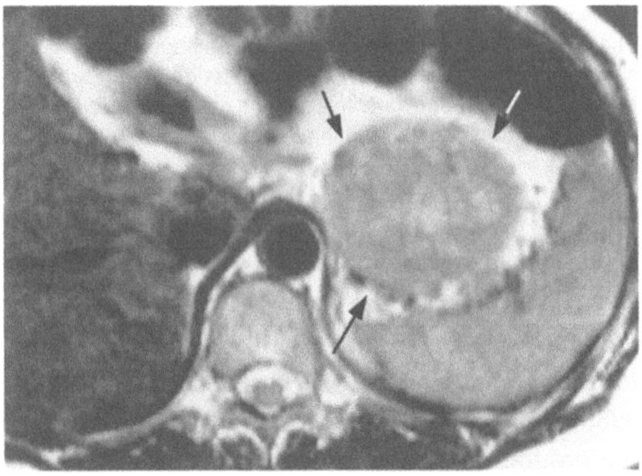

Fig. 11.3. Inflammatory pseudotumor of an "accessory" spleen. The T2-weighted magnetic-resonance image demonstrates a slightly hyperintense, inhomogeneous mass (*arrows*) in the splenic hilum

11.3 Miscellaneous Disorders that Give Rise to Focal Splenic Tumoral Lesions

11.3.1 Splenic Extension of Disorders of Adjacent Organs

Since the pancreatic tail is essentially an intraperitoneal structure and is located in the splenorenal ligament, disorders of the pancreatic tail can easily invade the spleen and may even produce tumoral lesions in the spleen (Myeres 1994). Although rare (frequency: 1–5%), splenic involvement in pancreatitis can include intrasplenic pseudocyst, abscess, hemorrhage, infarction, splenic rupture and vascular injury (Fishman et al. 1995). Intrasplenic pancreatic pseudocyst (Fig. 11.5) without communication with the main pancreatic duct may be misdiagnosed as a splenic tumor (Gaia et al. 1992). In addition, pancreatic-tail cancer can directly invade the spleen and may cause a mass in the spleen (Fig. 11.6).

The gastrosplenic ligament extends from the greater curvature of the stomach to the spleen, and this ligament may be a pathway to the spleen for gastric malignancies, such as carcinoma (Fig. 11.7)

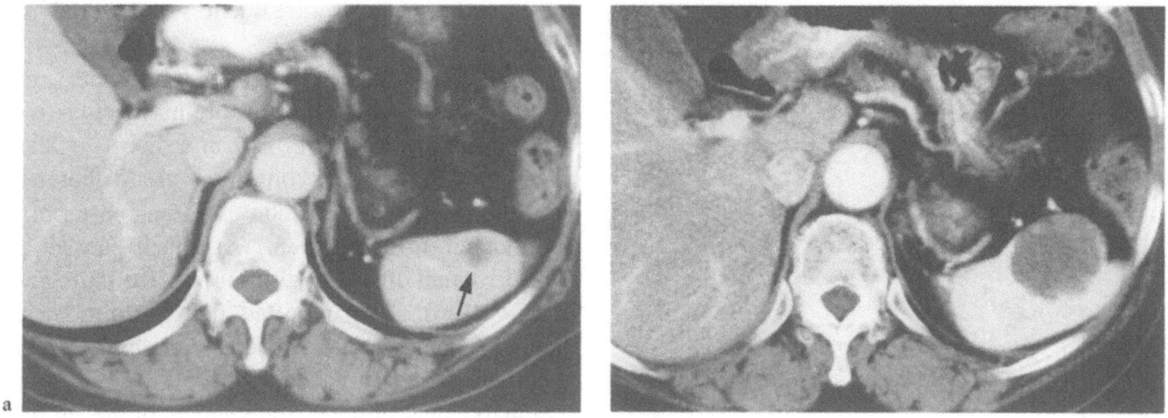

Fig. 11.4. Inflammatory pseudotumor of the spleen; the tumor exhibited enlargement on follow-up examination (same case as Fig. 11.1). **a** The splenic mass of less than 1 cm in diameter (*arrow*) is seen on initial computed tomography (CT). **b** The CT obtained 10 months after the image shown in **a** demonstrates that the mass has apparently increased in size

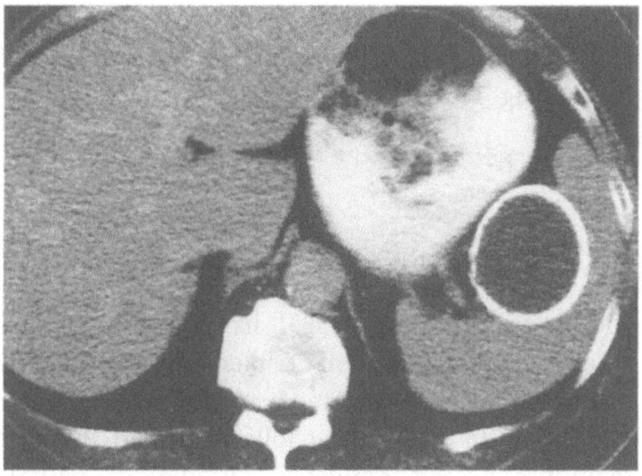

Fig. 11.5. Pancreatic pseudocyst in the spleen. Computed tomography demonstrates a nearly water-density mass with ring-like calcification within the splenic hilum. The presence of a pancreatic pseudocyst was confirmed through surgery

and lymphoma. A tract may be formed in the gastrosplenic ligament to enable spread from the stomach, enabling the development of a splenic mass (Myeres 1994). Very rarely, benign gastric ulcers may penetrate into the spleen, and Killeen et al. (1997) have reported that CT is useful for correct diagnosis. According to their report, CT revealed both a gastric ulcer projecting from the greater curvature of the stomach into the spleen and a splenic cavity filled with debris, and prone scanning revealed gas within the splenic cavity, confirming communication with the stomach. Colonic perforation may also result in an invasion of the spleen, leading to the formation of an abscess mass. Chun et al. (1997) have reported colosplenic fistula due to colonic rupture caused by side effects of interleukin-2.

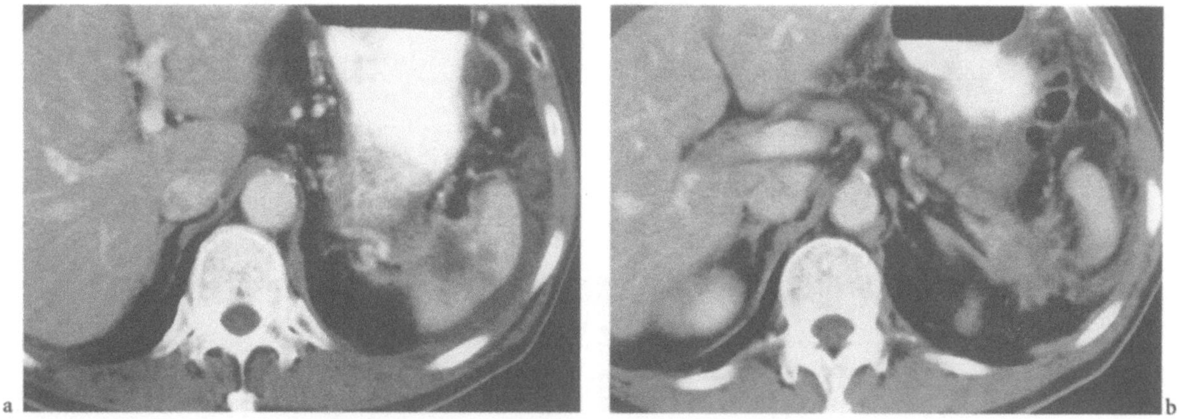

Fig. 11.6. Direct invasion of pancreatic-tail cancer to the spleen. **a** An irregularly shaped hypodense mass is seen in the splenic hilum on computed tomography (CT). **b** On a slightly caudal level on CT, the pancreatic-tail tumor is demonstrated. The pancreatic cancer was verified during surgery, and the splenic mass was composed of pancreatic cancer cells

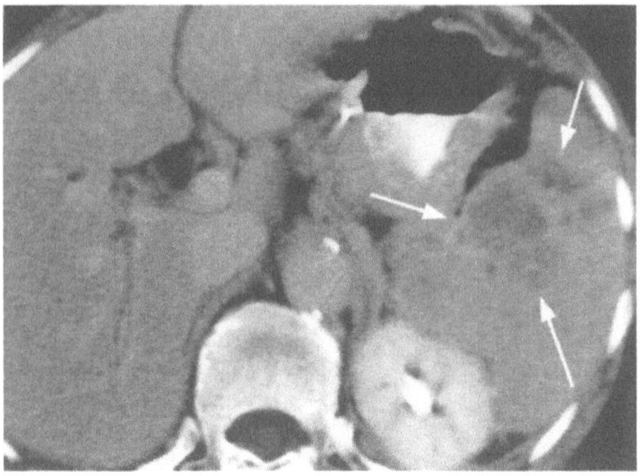

Fig. 11.7. Direct invasion of gastric cancer into the spleen. Computed tomography demonstrates ill-defined hypodense masses in the spleen (*arrows*). Wall thickening of the greater curvature of the stomach is also demonstrated

11.3.2 Pseudo-Lesions Caused by Disorders of Other Tissues

Ectopic splenic tissue simulating renal, pancreatic, hepatic and even pelvic tumors have been reported, and HOLLOWAY et al. (1997) have reported a case of an accessory spleen markedly enlarged by portal hypertension and presenting as a splenic pseudotumor. An accessory spleen in the splenic hilum is usually isodense in relation to the spleen and is less than 4 cm in diameter on CT; therefore, its diagnosis is easily obtained in most cases. However, in this particular case, a 14 × 12 × 7-cm, enlarged, hypodense mass displaced the medial aspect of the spleen, mimicking a splenic tumor. The marked enlargement of the accessory spleen and the hypodensity of the mass that corresponded histologically to prominent areas of necrosis were due to severe portal hypertension.

Enlargement of the left hepatic lobe, either congenital or due to liver cirrhosis, may simulate a splenic abnormality. DUNLOP and EVANS (1996) have reported a case of a congenital variant of the left lobe of the liver. The left lobe, extending posteriorly and lateral to the spleen, was misdiagnosed as splenic hematoma on ultrasound (DUNLOP and EVANS 1996). They reported that a contrast-enhanced sequential CT scan made it possible to make a correct diagnosis.

Enlargement of the lateral segment of the left hepatic lobe is often seen in patients with cirrhosis. When a part of the enlarged lateral segment of the liver is located in the left lateral upper abdomen separate from the liver, that enlarged segment may resemble an enlarged spleen on CT or MR. In addition, when a hepatic tumor exists in an enlarged lateral segment, it may be misinterpreted as a splenic tumor (Fig. 11.8; ITO et al. 1996).

11.3.3 Others

GAREL and HASSAN (1995) have reported seven cases of small, asymptomatic splenic cysts diagnosed by ultrasound in fetuses and neonates. None of these cysts grew in size during follow-up, and three of them disappeared completely. Although the pathology of these cysts was unknown, it was emphasized in the report that they were asymptomatic and were discovered in fetuses (during the prenatal survey) or in neonates by chance and that they might regress completely. It was proposed that they be called

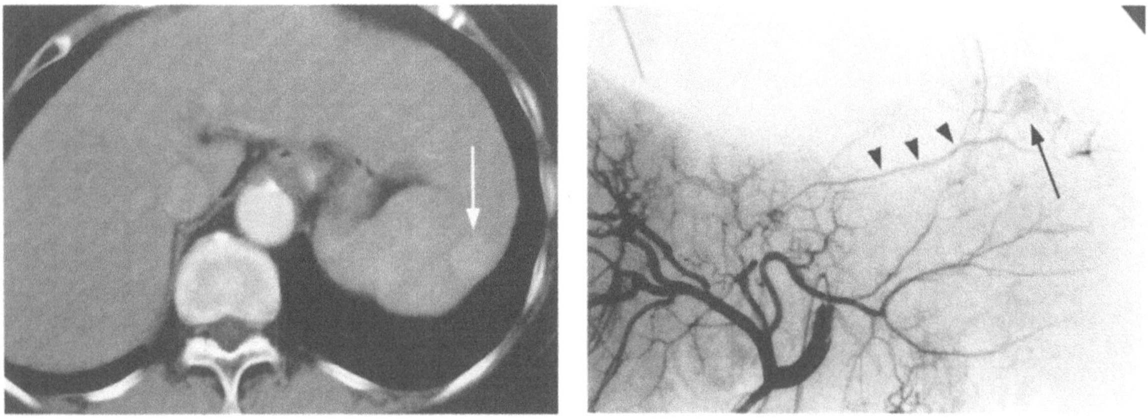

a b

Fig. 11.8. Hepatocellular carcinoma mimicking a splenic tumor. **a** Computed tomography shows an enlarged lateral segment of the liver and a hyperdense mass (*arrow*) mimicking a splenic tumor. **b** Digital subtraction angiography of the common hepatic artery reveals that the hypervascular mass (*arrow*) is fed by the left hepatic artery (*arrowheads*) splenic cyst-like lesions (CLL), and the authors suggested that, since they may spontaneously regress, asymptomatic splenic CLL in neonates can be followed-up without interventional therapy.

Patients with sickle cell anemia are prone to both infective and infarctive crises, and splenic abscess and splenic infarction are well-known complications of the spleen in hematologic disorders, both of which are discussed in detail in Chap. 5. Occasionally, round masses may be noted within the otherwise calcified spleen, and these have been a source of clinical confusion when diagnosed as abscess or infarction, particularly in the setting of sickle cell crises with pain and fever. These masses have been found to represent areas of preserved splenic tissue (Heck and Brittin 1989). Levin et al. (1996) have reported six patients with sickle cell disease in whom rounded intrasplenic masses have proven to be preserved, functioning splenic tissue. According to their report, the masses exhibit hypodensity in an otherwise calcified spleen on CT, are hypoechoic relative to the echogenic spleen on ultrasound and have the imaging characteristics of normal spleen on MR. The masses fail to accumulate ^{99m}Tc-methylene disphosphonate but do demonstrate an uptake of ^{99m}Tc–sulfur colloid. They concluded that, in patients with sickle cell disease and intrasplenic masses, the proper correlation of multiple imaging modalities can establish a diagnosis of functioning splenic tissue and avoid a mistaken diagnosis of splenic abscess or infarction.

Chronic expanding hematoma is an entity that was first described by Reid and Kommareddi (1980). In contrast to the ordinary hematoma that resolves rapidly, chronic expanding hematoma persists for long periods as a slowly expanding, space-occupying mass. The mechanism whereby exudation or bleeding continues within a fibrous capsule remains unknown, but experimental evidence favors an inflammatory cause. Histopathologically, the outer zone of a chronic expanding hematoma is composed of dense collagenous tissue with deposits of hemosiderin and many clusters of iron-laden macrophages. The midzone is composed of loose connective tissue, and the inner lining is composed of granulation tissue; some parts are overlain by eosinophilic fibrinoid material, others by red blood cells and fibrin, into which new capillaries sprout. The best known of these chronic expanding hematomas are subdural hematomas and pseudotumors of bone in hemophiliacs; however, chronic expanding hematoma has been reported in a variety of locations, and there have been five reported cases of chronic expanding hematoma in the spleen (Asayama et al. 1998). The most common cause of the initial hemorrhage of chronic expanding hematoma is trauma, and four of five cases of splenic expanding hematoma were secondary to trauma. Asayama et al. (1998) have reported a case of chronic expanding hematoma of the spleen in which a small splenic angiomyolipoma associated with tuberous sclerosis, too small to be detected radiologically, was considered to be the cause. According to their report, the CT features of the splenic chronic expanding hematoma were as follows: a hypodense splenic mass that contained the area of contrast enhancement and the foci of calcification in the peripheral portion of the mass. Contrast enhancement appeared minimal in the central portion (Fig. 11.9a). A follow-up CT examination 16 months

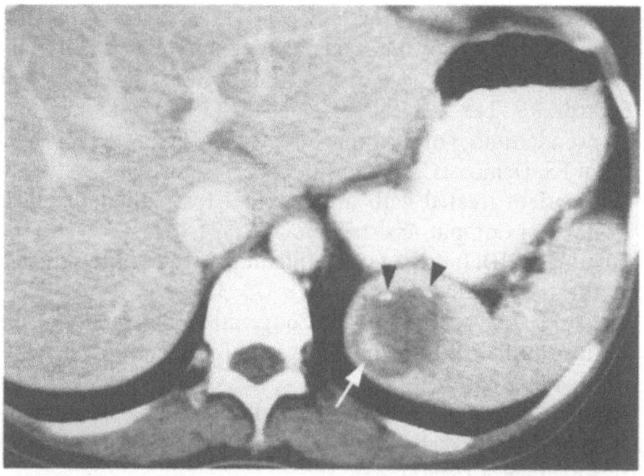
a

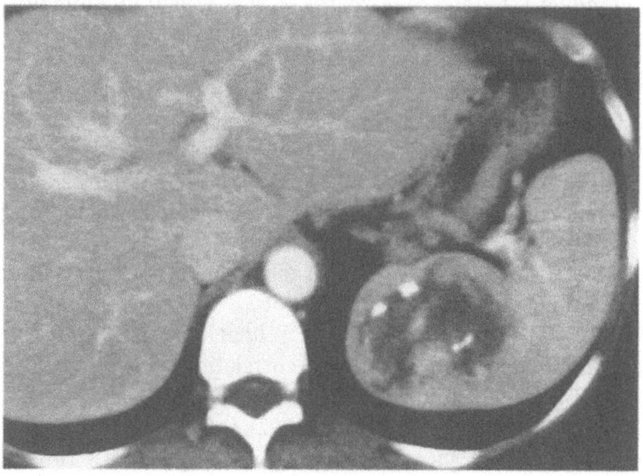
b

Fig. 11.9. Chronic expanding hematoma of the spleen. **a** Computed tomography (CT) shows a hypodense mass in the spleen. Note the area of enhancement (*arrow*) and the foci of calcifications (*arrowheads*) within the mass. **b** The CT obtained 16 months after the image shown in **a** shows that the mass has increased in size. Areas of contrast enhancement and calcifications have become more prominent after the initial CT showed that the splenic mass had increased in size, and the areas of contrast enhancement and the foci of calcification in the peripheral portion had become more prominent (Fig. 11.9b). MR imaging demonstrated a splenic mass that was hypointense on T1-weighted images and slightly hyperintense on T2-weighted images. There were small areas of hyperintensity on both T1- and T2-weighted images within the splenic mass, suggesting a hematoma. Radiologists should be aware of this rare entity in the spleen, which might be misdiagnosed as a neoplasm due to its noted increase in size at the follow-up examination.

References

Aru GM, Abramowsky CR, Ricketts RR (1997) Inflammatory pseudotumor of the spleen in a young child. Pediatr Surg Int 12:299–301

Asayama Y, Fukuya T, Honda H, et al. (1998) Chronic expanding hematoma of the spleen by angiomyolipoma in a patient with tuberous sclerosis. Abdom Imaging 23:527–530

Berardi RS, Lee SS, Chen HP, et al. (1983) Inflammatory pseudotumors of the lung. Surg Gynecol Obstet 156:89–96

Chun ES, Demos TC, Gaynor ER (1997) Colosplenic fistula in a patient treated with interleukin-2 for malignant melanoma. J Comput Assist Tomogr 21:674–676

Cotelingam JD, Jaffe ES (1984) Inflammatory pseudotumor of the spleen. Am J Surg Pathol 8:375–380

Dunlop DG, Evans RM (1996) Congenital abnormality of the liver initially misdiagnosed as splenic haematoma. J R Soc Med 89:702–704

Fishman EK, Soyer P, Bliss DF, et al. (1995) Splenic involvement in pancreatitis: spectrum of CT findings. AJR Am J Roentgenol 164:631–635

Franquet T, Montes M, Aizcorbe M, et al. (1989) Inflammatory pseudotumor of the spleen: ultrasound and computed tomographic findings. Gastrointest Radiol 14:181–183

Fukuya T, Honda H, Matsumata T, et al. (1994) Diagnosis of inflammatory pseudotumor of the liver: value of CT. AJR Am J Roentgenol 163:1087–1091

Gaia E, Babini G, Dughera L, et al. (1992) Intrasplenic penetration of a pancreatic pseudocyst: early ultrasonographic detection. J Clin Ultrasound 20:608–611

Garel C, Hassan M (1995) Foetal and neonatal splenic cyst-like lesions. Pediatr Radiol 25:360–362

Glazer M, Sagar V (1993) SPECT imaging of the spleen in inflammatory pseudotumor: correlation with ultrasound, CT and MRI. Clin Nucl Med 18:527–529

Glazer M, Lally J, Kanzer M (1992) Inflammatory pseudotumor of the spleen: MR findings. J Comput Assist Tomogr 16:980–983

Hahn PH, Weissleder R, Stark DD, et al. (1988) MR imaging of focal splenic tumors. AJR Am J Roentgenol 150:823–827

Hayasaka K, Soeda S, Hirayama M, et al. (1998) Inflammatory pseudotumor of the spleen: US and MRI findings. Radiat Med 16:47–50

Heck LL, Brittin GM (1989) Splenic uptake of both technetium-99m diphosphonate and technetium-99m-sulfur colloid in sickle cell beta thalassemia. Clin Nucl Med 14:557–563

Herman TE, Shackelford GD, Ternberg JL, et al. (1994) Inflammatory myofibroblastic tumor of the spleen: report of a case in an adolescent. Pediatr Radiol 24:280–282

Holloway BJ, Pei L, Pfister R (1997) Portal hypertension causing massive enlargement of an accessory spleen: a rare cause of splenic pseudotumor. Clin Radiol 52:882–884

Honda H, Fukuya T, Kaneko K, et al. (1996) Inflammatory pseudotumor of the liver: radiologic diagnosis. J Hep Bil Pancr Surg 3:133–141

Horiuchi R, Uchida T, Kojima T, et al. (1990) Inflammatory pseudotumor of the liver: clinicopathological study and review of the literature. Cancer 65:1583–1590

Irie H, Muranaka T, Nanjo T, Hanada K, Oshiumi Y (1988) Inflammatory pseudotumor of the liver. Radiat Med 7:217–219

Irie H, Honda H, Kaneko K, et al. (1996) Inflammatory pseudotumors of the spleen: CT and MRI findings. J Comput Assist Tomogr 20:244–288

Ito K, Mitchell DG, Honjo K, et al. (1996) Gadolinium-enhanced MR imaging of the spleen: artifacts and potential pitfalls. AJR Am J Roentgenol 167:1147–1151

Killeen KL, DeMeo JH, Mullaney JM (1997) Splenic penetration by a benign gastric ulcer: preoperative computed tomographic diagnosis. Emerg Radiol 4:91–93

Levin TL, Berdon WE, Haller JO, et al. (1996) Intrasplenic masses of "preserved" functioning splenic tissue in sickle cell disease: correlation of imaging findings (CT, ultrasound, MRI, and nuclear scintigraphy). Pediatr Radiol 26:646–649

Meyer JE, Harris NL, Elman A, et al. (1983) Large-cell lymphoma of the spleen: CT appearance. Radiology 148: 199–201

Meyers MA (1994) Dynamic radiology of the abdomen, 4th edn. Springer, Berlin Heidelberg New York

Perrone T, DeWolf-Peeters C, Frizzera G (1988) Inflammatory pseudotumor of lymph nodes. Am J Surg Pathol 12:351–361

Ramani M, Reinhold C, Semelka RC, et al. (1997) Splenic hemangiomas and hamartomas: MR imaging characteristics of 28 lesions. Radiology 202:166–172

Reid JD, Kommareddi S (1980) Chronic expanding hematomas: a clinicopathological entity. JAMA 244:2241–2242

Safran D, Welch J, Resuke W (1991) Inflammatory pseudotumors of the spleen. Arch Surg 126:904–908

Someron A (1978) Inflammatory pseudotumor of liver with occlusive phlebitis: report of a case in a child and review of the literature. Am J Clin Pathol 69:176–181

Yamakado K, Matsuda A, Katoh N, et al. (1994) Inflammatory pseudotumor of the spleen: CT and MRI findings. Eur Radiol 4:271–273

12 Splenic Pathology in Infancy and Childhood

E.C. Benya

CONTENTS

12.1 Introduction

The spleen, normally situated in the left upper quadrant of the abdomen, is fixed in position by the gastrosplenic and splenorenal ligaments. The splenorenal ligament, in addition to providing structural support, also carries the splenic artery. The spleen contains interspersed lymphatic follicles, reticuloendothelial cells and vascular sinusoids, which act in concert to produce antibodies and filter particulate matter, cells and bacteria from the blood stream (Boles 1991). In this chapter, the normal and abnormal imaging appearances of the spleen in children will be discussed.

12.2 Developmental Abnormalities

A variety of developmental malformations of the spleen may be detected in infancy and childhood, including congenital absence of the spleen (asplenia), the presence of multiple spleens (polysplenia), splenogonadal fusion and absent or improper splenic fixation (wandering spleen). These congenital developmental lesions of the spleen are discussed more fully in Chap. 3.

The wandering spleen is a rare but important developmental lesion, which may be the cause of acute splenic torsion, a pediatric abdominal emergency. The classic clinical presentation of torsion of the wandering spleen is the acute onset of abdominal pain and a palpable lower-abdominal mass in children ranging from 3 months to 10 years of age (Emery 1997). However, children with wandering spleens may also present with an abdominal mass or with episodic abdominal pain due to intermittent splenic torsion (Herman and Siegel 1991). Plain abdominal radiographs may reveal a soft-tissue mass in the lower abdomen but are often nonspecific. Cross-sectional imaging can help confirm or clarify the diagnosis of a wandering spleen with or without torsion. Ultrasound (US) images may reveal absence of normal splenic tissue in the left upper-abdominal quadrant and a soft-tissue mass compatible with ectopic splenic tissue in the lower abdomen or pelvis. If splenic infarction secondary to torsion has occurred, color and pulsed Doppler interrogation of this abnormally positioned spleen will show an absence of internal blood flow (Nemcek et al. 1991; Emery 1997). Since overlying air-filled bowel loops can interfere with abdominal US evaluation, it has been suggested that computed tomography (CT) should be the study of choice for this condition (Herman and Siegel 1991). CT features of a wandering spleen with acute splenic torsion include detection of a soft-tissue mass in the lower abdomen or pelvis (with decreased attenuation compared with that expected of normal splenic tissue) and absence of normal splenic tissue in the left upper quadrant (Fig. 12.1) (Herman and Siegel 1991).

12.3 Splenic Size

The spleen grows throughout childhood, reaching maximal size in adulthood. Normally, the splenic tip is visualized above the lower pole of the left kidney

E.C. Benya; 157 Scottswood Road, Riverside, IL 60546-2221, USA

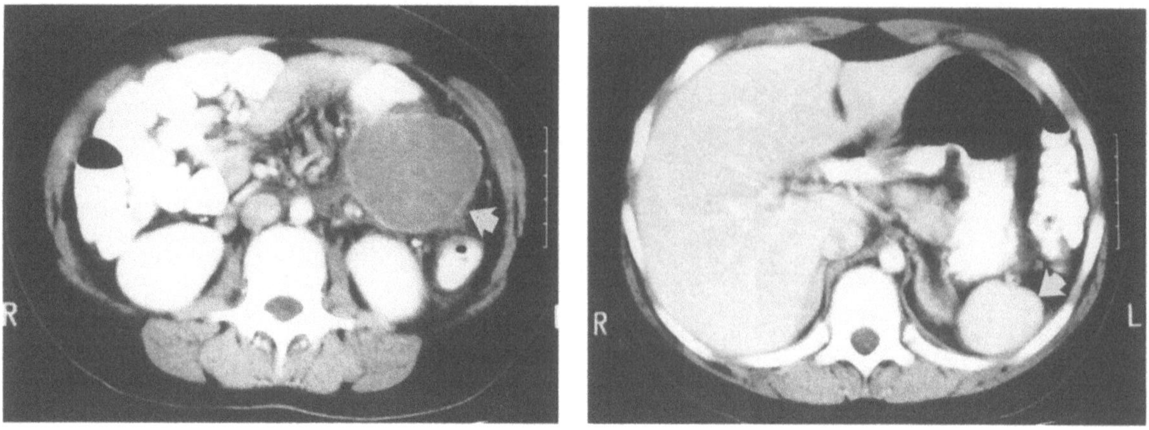

a b

Fig. 12.1. Splenic torsion of a residual accessory spleen. **a** A contrast-enhanced computed-tomography (CT) image through the mid-abdomen in a child with acute abdominal pain reveals a low-attenuation mass with peripheral enhancement and surrounding inflammatory changes (*arrow*) caused by infarction of the torsed wandering spleen. **b** In this unusual case, a CT image through the upper abdomen shows a small, enhancing accessory spleen (*arrow*) rather than absence of splenic tissue (courtesy of J. K. Zawin)

on cross-sectional imaging studies (Teele and Share 1991). Standard splenic measurements have been determined, guiding the assessment of splenic size (Dittrich et al. 1983; Rosenberg et al. 1991; Schlesinger et al. 1993). Rosenberg et al. (1991) reported the normal expected values for a single sonographic measurement of the greatest splenic length in patients newborn to 20 years of age. Normal standard splenic-volume measurements on CT scans as a function of body weight have also been determined (Schlesinger et al. 1993). Since altered splenic size most often indicates the presence of disease, knowledge of the normal expected splenic size in children is important.

Splenomegaly frequently occurs in infants with intrauterine infections, such as toxoplasmosis, syphilis and cytomegalovirus and in older children with viral infections. Children with hemolytic diseases, including hereditary spherocytosis, thalassemia and sequestration crisis in sickle cell disease, all may develop splenic enlargement. Additionally, splenomegaly can be detected as a result of splenic infiltration with neoplastic disease and storage disorders, such as Gaucher's disease, and is associated with portal hypertension in children with liver disease. Occasionally, medical therapy rather than disease affects splenic size, as occurs in neonates placed on extracorporeal membrane oxygenation for treatment of respiratory failure, who may have associated enlargement of the spleen (Klippenstein et al. 1994).

12.4 Imaging Appearance of the Normal Spleen in Children

In children, the normal spleen should appear as a homogeneous soft-tissue-density structure in the left upper quadrant of the abdomen on plain abdominal radiographs, without a significant mass effect on the adjacent stomach, small bowel or large bowel loops. At sonography, the normal spleen demonstrates a homogeneous echotexture hyperechoic to the adjacent left kidney and similar or increased in echogenicity to the liver. With color and pulsed Doppler imaging, the splenic artery and vein can be interrogated to ensure their patency. In children, as in adults undergoing helical CT examination after dynamic, intravenous contrast administration, a heterogeneous pattern of enhancement of the red and white pulp of the spleen may be seen during the early arterial phase of imaging. A homogeneous pattern of enhancement should subsequently be seen on delayed CT imaging through the normal spleen.

The magnetic-resonance-imaging (MRI) appearance of the spleen changes dramatically between infancy and childhood. The relative signal intensity of the spleen in older children mirrors that of adults, with the spleen hypointense relative to the liver on T_1-weighted images and hyperintense relative to the liver on T_2-weighted images. However, the MRI appearance of the spleen in neonates less than 8 months of age may differ significantly from that in older children and adults (Donnelly et al. 1996).

In infants, the splenic signal intensity is typically isointense to the liver on T_1-weighted images and isointense to hypointense to the liver on T_2-weighted images. This alteration in signal intensity in neonates is believed to be related to the histologic changes in the spleen, which occur in the first year of life and should not be mistaken for splenic pathology (Donnelly et al. 1996). In neonates, the spleen is predominantly composed of red pulp and, with increasing age, the volume of white pulp increases relative to the volume of red pulp, likely accounting for the change in the signal intensity of the spleen as seen on MRI.

12.5 Imaging Appearance of the Abnormal Spleen in Children

12.5.1 Splenic Infections

In children, as in adults, bacterial, viral and fungal infections can occur in the spleen. Children who are immunocompromised due to human immunodeficiency virus infection or anti-neoplastic or immunosuppressive therapies have an increased likelihood of developing splenic infection, particularly with fungal organisms. *Candida* and *Aspergillus* are the most frequent fungal infections of the spleen; they may result in numerous splenic microabscesses, which are hypoechoic on US images. Sometimes, these hypoechoic foci contain a central hyperechoic focus, producing a "target" appearance. The corresponding appearance of splenic fungal microabscesses on CT is numerous, low-attenuation foci in the spleen (Fig. 12.2). Since some lesions may be better detected on non-contrast-enhanced CT (Freeman et al. 1993), images prior to and after contrast may be helpful. Coexistent lesions in the liver and kidney may be identified. Fungal infection of the spleen may not always be detectable in imaging studies.

Bacterial infection can lead to the development of larger abscesses, which may be amenable to image-guided drainage. Typical features of splenic abscesses include central low attenuation, often with peripheral enhancement on CT examination (Freeman et al. 1993), and hypoechoic foci lacking central Doppler vascularity on US (Goerg et al. 1991). MRI is not usually performed for evaluation of splenic abscesses.

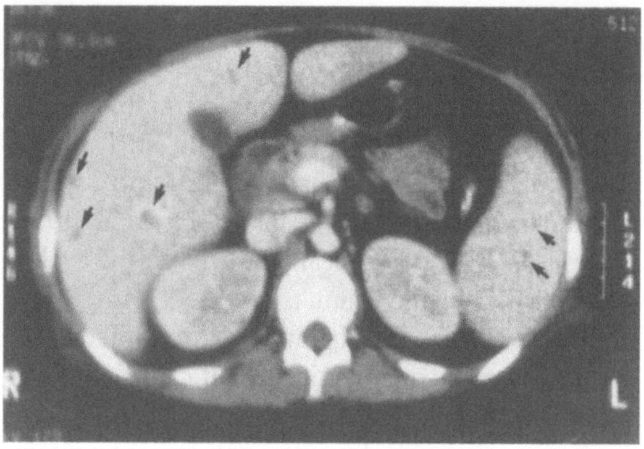

Fig. 12.2. Candida microabscesses of the spleen and liver. Small, low-attenuation foci detected in the spleen and liver in an immunosuppressed child with systemic Candida infection on contrast-enhanced computed tomography (*arrows*)

Viral infections of all types in children may lead to splenomegaly (Teele and Share 1991). Infectious mononucleosis caused by Epstein-Barr virus causes splenomegaly in approximately 50% or more of cases. This enlargement has been attributed to lymphocytic infiltration of the spleen (Schooley 1995). Rarely, affected children and adolescents can develop rupture of the spleen following minor trauma, with sudden onset of left upper-quadrant pain, peritonitis and/or shock. Because of this rare but potentially life-threatening complication of infectious mononucleosis, restriction of physical activities in children (particularly contact sports) is recommended until resolution of splenomegaly (Miller et al. 1992).

12.5.2 Trauma

The spleen is the second most frequently injured abdominal organ in children suffering blunt trauma (Sivit and Bulas 1993). The imaging appearance of splenic trauma in children resembles that seen in adults; for a more detailed discussion of splenic trauma, refer to Chap. 8. The mode of initial evaluation following blunt trauma has undergone significant change in the last several decades. This has occurred due in part to the shift towards non-operative management of splenic injuries in children in an effort to preserve the spleen and prevent the increased risk of post-splenectomy sepsis. In the United States, CT remains the technique of choice to evaluate splenic injury in hemodynamically stable children (Taylor and Kaufman 1993; Sivit and

Kaufman 1995). However, in Europe, Canada and Japan, US imaging is often used in the evaluation of blunt abdominal trauma (Luks et al. 1993; Filiatrault and Garel 1995). The MRI appearances of subcapsular hematomas and splenic lacerations have been described (Ito et al. 1997); however, MRI is not typically utilized in the evaluation of acute splenic trauma.

Plain abdominal radiographs are of limited use in the detection of splenic injuries but can identify associated rib fractures. Contrast-enhanced CT reveals linear or rounded, low-attenuation, intrasplenic foci with lacerations or hematomas of the spleen (Fig. 12.3a). Perisplenic or free peritoneal fluid caused by hemoperitoneum is frequently (but not always) detected in children with splenic injury (Taylor and Sivit 1995). At US examination, intrasplenic injuries may be detected as foci of increased, decreased or mixed echogenicity within the spleen. Subcapsular splenic hematomas typically appear as hypoechoic fluid collections beneath the splenic capsule (Fig. 12.3b) (Adler et al. 1986; Filiatrault et al. 1987). One recent study directly comparing US and CT for detection and grading of splenic injuries in children found that US had a sensitivity of only 69% compared with CT and that, in many cases, the degree of injury was underestimated by US (Krupnick et al. 1997).

Delayed complications following splenic trauma in children, including the development of splenic-artery pseudoaneurysms, splenic abscesses and cysts and delayed splenic rupture are rare (Fig. 12.4) (Cohen et al. 1982; Benya and Bulas 1996). Healing of splenic injuries in children can be documented on follow-up CT or US examinations, with the rate of healing on follow-up CT study related to the initial grade of splenic injury (Benya et al. 1995).

12.5.3 Benign Splenic Masses

Benign mass lesions occurring in the spleen, including cysts, lymphangiomas, hamartomas, hemangiomas and hemangioendotheliomas, may be detected in infants and children. Most often, these splenic lesions are asymptomatic and unsuspected, discovered during abdominal examination performed for other indications. Splenic cysts are generally categorized histologically as true epidermoid cysts with an inner endothelial lining and as false cysts or pseudocysts, which lack an endothelial lining, most commonly the result of prior splenic injury (Dachman et al. 1986). True and false splenic cysts are indistinguishable on imaging studies, appearing as rounded unilocular or multilocular lesions that are of low-attenuation on CT examination. There may be enhancement of internal septations seen on contrast-enhanced CT (Dachman et al. 1986). Occasionally, calcification of the cyst wall may be present. On US imaging, splenic cysts are generally hypoechoic, with or without internal septations. Echogenic material, if seen on US, is caused by deposition of cholesterol crystals within the cyst (Urrutia et al. 1996).

Splenic lymphangiomas are rare, multicystic lesions containing numerous endothelium-lined channels filled with proteinaceous fluid (Ros et al. 1987). On US, lymphangiomas are hypoechoic masses, often with internal septations and echoic

a

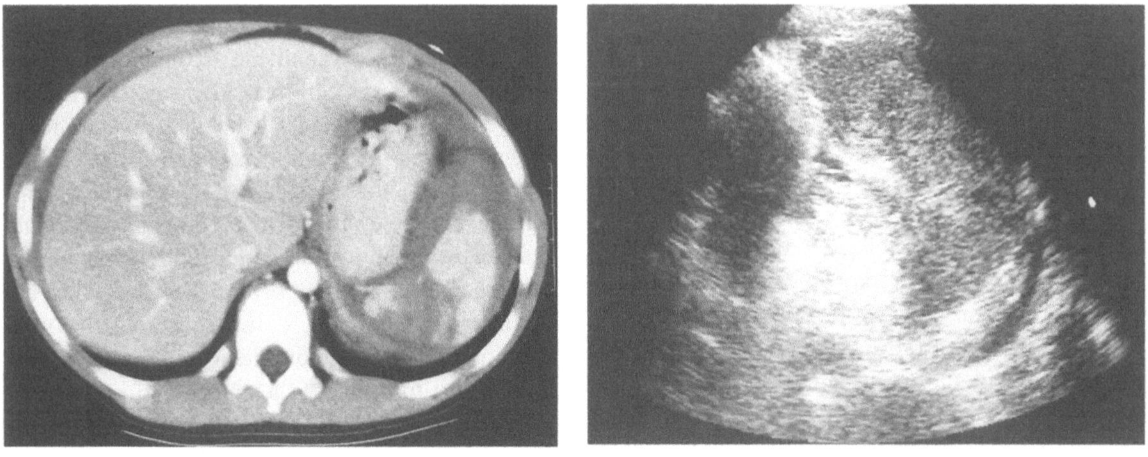

b

Fig. 12.3. Splenic trauma. **a** Contrast-enhanced computed tomography reveals a low-attenuation splenic hematoma with perisplenic blood in a child with blunt abdominal injury. **b** Ultrasound examination reveals inhomogeneity of the splenic echotexture due to splenic injury (courtesy of A. Shkolnik)

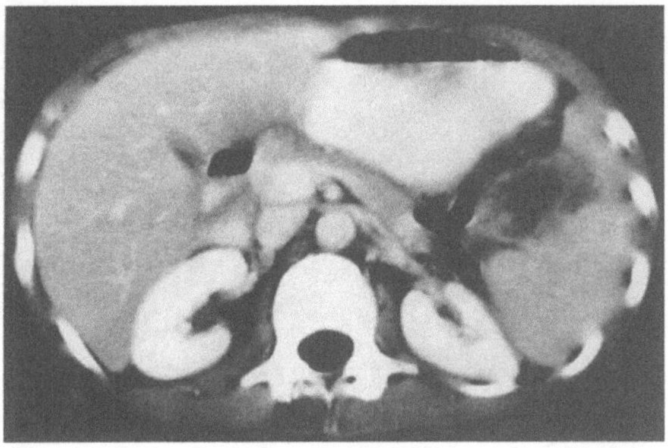

Fig. 12.4. Splenic cyst following injury. A post-traumatic splenic cyst is detected on follow-up computed-tomography study in a child with a history of prior splenic injury (courtesy of D. J. PENNINGTON)

debris. On CT, they are visualized as cystic mass lesions without central contrast enhancement and may contain thin septa and peripheral calcification (URRUTIA et al. 1996). Differentiating multilocular splenic lymphangiomas from splenic cysts, hydatid cysts and other cystic mass lesions on imaging studies alone may not be possible due to the overlapping appearances of these lesions (Fig. 12.5) (FERROZZI et al. 1996). Diffuse involvement of the spleen, with or without extrasplenic soft-tissue or bone lymphangiomas, is termed splenic lymphangiomatosis. The US, CT and MRI features of splenic lymphangiomatosis in children have recently been described (WADSWORTH et al. 1997).

Hemangiomas of the spleen have a variable solid, cystic or mixed appearance. As a result, the sonographic and CT appearance is nonspecific. These vascular lesions may reveal homogeneous or heterogeneous enhancement on contrast-enhanced CT examinations (Fig. 12.6) (FERROZZI et al. 1996). CT may detect calcifications when present. In three reported cases of pediatric splenic hemangioma, the CT appearance varied with both solid enhancing and cystic lesions, with peripheral enhancement noted (PANUEL et al. 1992). On US examination, hemangiomas may be seen as single or multiple hyperechoic foci in the spleen with internal vascularity on color and pulsed Doppler imaging (GOERG et al. 1991; SCANDERBEG et al. 1997) or as complex heterogeneous cystic lesions (PANUEL et al. 1992).

12.5.4 Malignant Splenic Masses

Primary splenic malignancy in children is exceedingly rare. The spleen is much more frequently the site of metastatic disease in children, most commonly lymphoma and leukemia. Lymphoma involving the spleen has a variety of presentations. Contrast-enhanced CT examination may demonstrate heterogeneous splenic enhancement, single or multiple focal, low-attenuation mass lesions, or splenomegaly alone, without visible focal lesions (Fig. 12.7). US imaging may detect lymphoma in the spleen as small or large hypoechoic lesions (GOERG et al. 1991). Additional US signs of lymphoma in the spleen include heterogeneous splenic echotexture with or without splenomegaly (URRUTIA et al. 1996). However, US and CT imaging may fail to detect lymphomatous lesions. On MRI, lymphoma lesions in the spleen may appear hypointense on T1-weighted images and hyperintense on T2-weighted images. However, lesions may not be visualized on conventional spin-echo MRI, and ITO and colleagues have

a

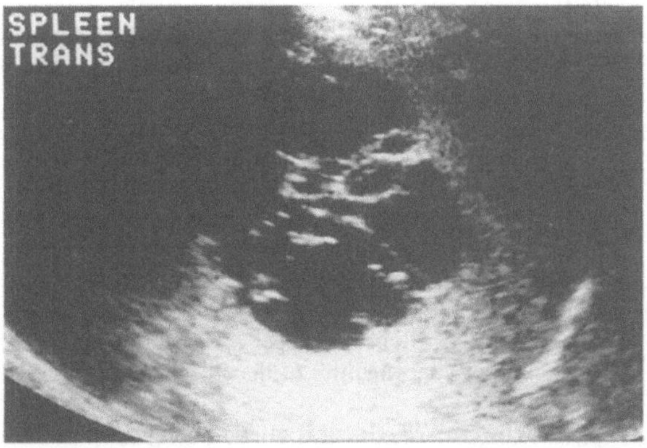

b

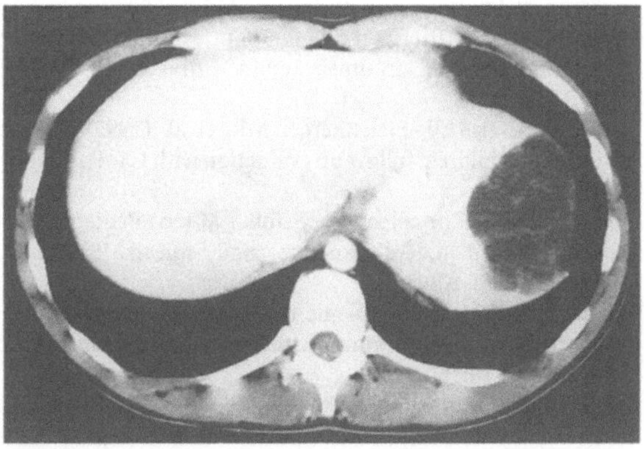

Fig. 12.5. Splenic lymphangioma. a A transverse ultrasound image of the spleen reveals a multiloculated cystic lesion. b A contrast-enhanced computed-tomography image demonstrates a low-attenuation lesion in the spleen with multiple, fine, enhancing septations (courtesy of D. J. PENNINGTON)

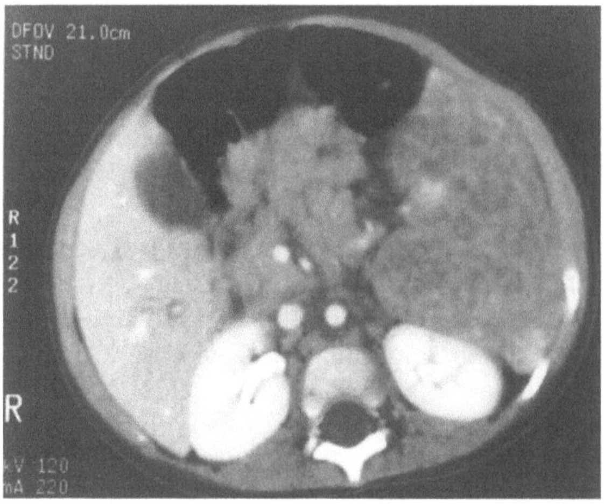

Fig. 12.6. Splenic hemangiomatosis. A contrast-enhanced computed-tomography image reveals an enlarged, heterogeneously enhancing spleen in this child with Kasabach-Merritt syndrome

recommended double-phase, multisection dynamic MRI with contrast enhancement (Ito et al. 1997).

12.6 Conclusion

In summary, this chapter has reviewed the imaging appearance of the normal spleen in children, as well as a variety of splenic pathologies that occur in infancy and childhood.

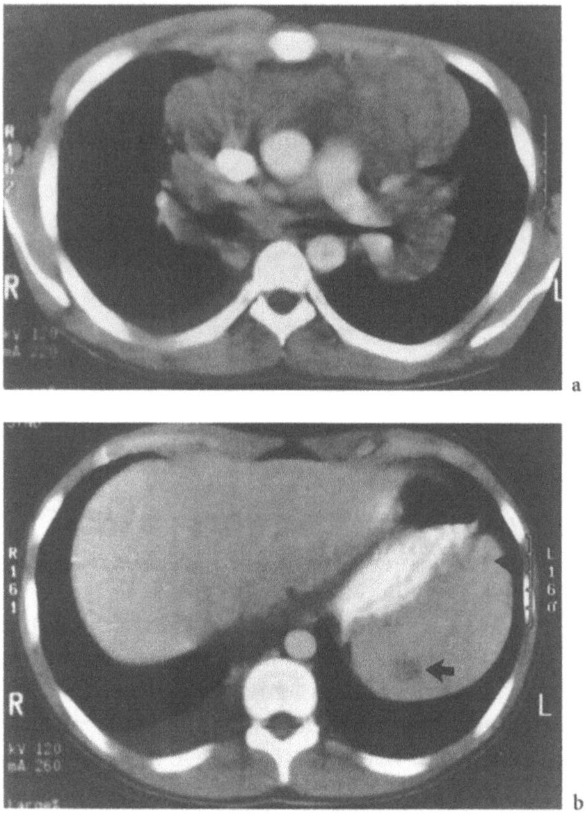

Fig. 12.7. Lymphoma. **a** A computed-tomography (CT) image through the chest, showing extensive anterior mediastinal and hilar masses due to Hodgkin's lymphoma with an associated right pleural effusion. **b** A CT image through the upper abdomen revealing rounded, low-attenuation lesions (*arrows*) related to lymphomatous deposits. The right pleural effusion is again visualized

References

Adler DD, Blane CE, Coran AG, et al. (1986) Splenic trauma in the pediatric patient: the integrated roles of ultrasound and computed tomography. Pediatrics 78:576–580

Benya EC, Bulas DI (1996) Splenic injuries in children after blunt abdominal trauma. Semin Ultrasound CT MR 17:170–176

Benya EC, Bulas DI, Eichelberger MR, et al. (1995) Splenic injury in children: follow up evaluation with CT. Radiology 195:685–688

Boles ET (1991) The spleen. In: Schiller M (ed) Pediatric surgery of the liver, pancreas and spleen. Saunders, Philadelphia, p 205

Cohen RC (1982) Blunt splenic trauma in children: a retrospective study of non-operative management. Aust Paediatr J 18:211–215

Dachman AH, Ros PR, Murari PJ, et al. (1986) Nonparasitic splenic cysts: a report of 52 cases with radiologic pathologic correlation. AJR Am J Roentgenol 147:537–542

Dittrich M, Milde S, Dinkel E, et al. (1983) Sonographic biometry of liver and spleen size in childhood. Pediatr Radiol 13:206–211

Donnelly LF, Emery KH, Bove KE, et al. (1996) Normal changes in the MR appearance of the spleen during early childhood. AJR Am J Roentgenol 166:635–639

Emery KH (1997) Splenic emergencies. Radiol Clin North Am 35:4

Ferrozzi F, Bova D, Draghi F, et al. (1996) CT findings in primary vascular tumors of the spleen. AJR Am J Roentgenol 166:1097–1101

Filiatrault D, Garel L (1995) Commentary: pediatric blunt abdominal trauma – to sound or not to sound? Pediatr Radiol 25:329–331

Filiatrault D, Longpre D, Patriquin H, et al. (1987) Investigation of childhood blunt abdominal trauma: a practical approach using ultrasound as the initial diagnostic modality. Pediatr Radiol 17:373–379

Freeman JL, Jafri SZ, Roberts JL, et al. (1993) CT of congenital and acquired abnormalities of the spleen. Radiographics 13:597–610

Goerg C, Schwerk WB, Goerg K (1991) Sonography of focal lesions of the spleen. AJR Am J Roentgenol 156:949–953

Herman TE, Siegel MJ (1991) CT of acute splenic torsion in children with wandering spleen. AJR Am J Roentgenol 156:151–153

Ito K, Mitchell DG, Honjo K, et al. (1997) MR imaging of acquired abnormalities of the spleen. AJR Am J Roentgenol 168:697–702

Klippenstein DL, Zerin JM, Hirschl RB, et al. (1994) Splenic enlargement in neonates during ECMO. Radiology 190:411–412

Krupnick AS, Teitelbaum DH, Geiger JD, et al. (1997) Use of abdominal ultrasonography to assess pediatric splenic trauma: potential pitfalls in diagnosis. Ann Surg 225:408–414

Luks FI, Lemire A, St.-Vil D, et al. (1993) Blunt abdominal trauma in children: practical value of ultrasonography. J Trauma 34:604–607

Miller G, Katz BZ, Niederman JC (1992) Epstein-Barr virus infections. In: Krugman S, Katz SL, Gershon AA, Wilfert CM (eds). Infectious disease in children, 9th ed. Mosby Year Book, St. Louis, pp 87–104

Nemcek AA, Miller FH, Fitzgerald SW (1991) Acute torsion of a wandering spleen: diagnosis by CT and duplex Doppler and color flow sonography. AJR Am J Roentgenol 157:307–309

Panuel M, Ternier F, Michel G, Schneiner C, et al. (1992) Splenic hemangioma - report of three pediatric cases with pathologic correlation. Pediatr Radiol 22:213–216

Ros PR, Moser RP, Dachman AH, et al. (1987) Hemangioma of the spleen: radiologic–pathologic correlation in ten cases. Radiology 162:73–77

Rosenberg HK, Markowitz RI, Kolberg H, et al. (1991) Normal splenic size in infants and children: sonographic measurements. AJR Am J Roentgenol 157:119–121

Scanderbeg AC, Mingarelli R, Sacco M, et al. (1997) Splenic hemangioma in Turner syndrome: a case report. Pediatr Radiol 27:894

Schlesinger AE, Edgar KA, Boxer LA (1993) Volume of the spleen in children as measured on CT scans: normal standards as a function of body weight. AJR Am J Roentgenol 160:1107–1109

Schooley R (1995) Epstein-Barr Virus (infectious Mononucleosis) in Principles and Practice of Infectious Diseases, eds Mondell GL, Benaett JE and Dolin R. Churchill Civiugston New York

Sivit CJ, Bulas DI (1993) Diagnostic imaging. In: Eichelberger MR (ed) Pediatric trauma: prevention, acute care and rehabilitation. Mosby, St. Louis pp 226–288

Sivit CJ, Kaufman RA (1995) Commentary: sonography in the evaluation of children following blunt trauma: is it to be or not to be? Pediatr Radiol 25:326–328

Taylor GA, Kaufman RA (1993) Commentary: emergency department sonography in the initial evaluation of blunt abdominal injury in children. Pediatr Radiol 23:161–164

Taylor GA, Sivit CJ (1995) Posttraumatic peritoneal fluid: is it a reliable indicator of intraabdominal injury in children? J Pediatr Surg 33:39–43

Teele RU, Share JC (1991) The spleen. In: Ultrasonography of infants and children. Saunders, Philadelphia, p 405

Urrutia M, Mergo PJ, Ros LH, Torres GM, Ros PR (1996) Cystic Masses of the spleen: radiologic pathologic correlation. Radiographics 16:107–129

Wadsworth DT, Newman B, Abramson SJ, et al. (1997) Splenic lymphangiomatosis in children. Radiology 202:173–176

13 Interventional Radiology of the Spleen

H. Vereycken, R. Van Hee, E. Totté and L. Hendrickx

CONTENTS

13.1 Introduction

Interventional radiological techniques have been used increasingly in the management of splenic disorders during recent decades. This attitude went along with a more conservative approach that surgeons and traumatologists adopted in dealing with splenic trauma and hypersplenism. When it became obvious that a correlation existed between splenectomy and increased risk for life-threatening sepsis (*Pneumococcus*, *Hemophilus influenza*, *Meningococcus*, *Staphylococcus aureus*, *Streptococcus* and *Pseudomonas*), especially in children and adolescents, a progressive shift was noted from an aggressive and resectional type of management to a more conservative, possibly spleen-saving therapy (Greco and Alvarez 1981). Moreover, greater understanding has been reached concerning not only the immunological role of the spleen and its diseases, but also the definition and classification of hypersplenic syndromes, thereby reducing the number of splenectomies performed for such syndromes (King and Schumacker 1952; O'Neal and McDonald 1981; Green et al. 1986; Pickhardt et al. 1989; Van Hee 1997).

H. Vereycken, R. Van Hee, E. Totté, L. Hendrickx; Department of Radiology, Academic Surgical Center, Stuivenberg, Lange Beeldekensstraat 267, B-2060 Antwerp, Belgium

There are many interventional radiological procedures. Percutaneous biopsy of splenic lesions is performed for cytological or histological diagnosis but still carries a substantial morbidity that is directly related to the technique. Indications for biopsy are also limited due to more performant and less dangerous alternatives in medical imaging and diagnosis. Accidental puncture of the spleen during biopsy or during drainage of abdominal processes may occur and should be considered a severe complication that needs careful follow-up. Splenic abscesses may be drained successfully using a percutaneous approach. Embolization of the splenic artery in trauma aims to achieve a quick peripheral occlusion of the lacerated vessel in these often critically ill patients. Peripheral embolization as the sole treatment in hypersplenism may be performed in selected patients but has an important complication rate. Combined peripheral and main splenic-artery embolization, as a procedure before laparoscopic splenectomy, yields favorable results by decreasing perioperative complications and increasing the comfort and ease of the surgeons.

13.2 Percutaneous Biopsy of the Splenic Parenchyma

Percutaneous puncture of the spleen has been proposed, for diagnostic purposes, in cases of hematological or oncological disorders. Recently, O'Malley et al. (1999) defined the indications for percutaneous biopsy of the spleen:

1. The presence of a single lesion or multiple lesions without characteristics on medical imaging in a patient without known primary tumor and with a normal immune status
2. The presence of a splenic mass in a patient with a known primary malignancy
3. More rarely, the presence of a splenic lesion in an immunocompromised patient for whom the re-

sults of clinical, imaging and blood culture findings are inconclusive

Preparation for the procedure consists of coagulation studies, a conscious sedation, an intravenous line and informed consent. The risk of bleeding must be minimized by identifying an underlying coagulopathy (prothrombin time, partial thromboplastin time and platelet count), avoiding biopsy of hilar lesions, using 20- to 22-gauge needles, having a cytopathologist who can limit the number of passes in the examination room, performing the procedure under ultrasound (US) guidance instead of computed tomography (CT) and embolizing the needle track with autologous blood cloths or gelfoam particles. Monitoring of vital functions during and after the procedure and follow-up after discharge will decrease the morbidity rate of splenic aspiration biopsies.

Accidental puncture of the spleen during US- or CT-guided diagnostic or therapeutic percutaneous maneuvers may occur. Bleeding often results. Careful intensive care observation with regular clinical and US controls is mandatory to evaluate intra-abdominal bleeding or hematoma formation that may need surgical intervention.

Percutaneous drainage of splenic abscesses has been performed successfully in many instances. The same precautions as for percutaneous biopsy are taken. A trocar or Seldinger technique can be used with a success rate of 70–80%. The splenic abscess is evacuated via an anterolateral of posterolateral approach, and antibiotic therapy is administered. Post-puncture pleural effusion may occur (Berkman et al. 1983; Quinn et al. 1986).

13.3 Endovascular Embolization as a Sole Treatment in the Splenic Trauma Patient

In view of the spleen's well-documented importance in the immune response of the body, surgeons increasingly tend to treat splenic trauma in a conservative, non surgical-manner if possible (Kreuzfelder et al. 1991). Adequate clinical, biological and radiological examinations are mandatory to select patients for conservative treatment (Traub and Perry 1981; Buntain et al. 1988). Angiography, particularly with embolization, should not be performed without careful monitoring the general condition of a potentially instable patient. Therefore, some prerequisites for treatment by embolization should be taken into account (Getrajdman and Sclafani 1997).

1. The patient must be hemodynamically stable without signs of hollow viscus perforation.
2. A CT scan should demonstrate non-splenic lesions that may need urgent operation or require immediate treatment; in such a case, a careful balance of priorities must be made and may turn in favor of immediate surgery.
3. In smaller hospitals, especially at night, the unavailability of an experienced interventional radiologist may preclude an embolization procedure.

However, coagulopathy may be only a relative contraindication, since a vascular sheath can be left in place until the coagulopathy is corrected. Taking the cited prerequisites into account, the ultimate goal may also be to save the patient's splenic parenchyma.

Concerning the embolization technique, a celiac trunk angiography is initially performed not only to detect possible additional lesions but to obtain a complete anatomical cartography. Subsequently, selective catheterization of the splenic artery is performed at a point distal to the dorsal pancreatic artery, an important collateral-supply artery. Diagnostic angiography in one or two incidences is then obtained. If no extravasation is seen, the procedure is ended. Some teams perform another series after intra-arterial vasodilatation (with tolazoline) to overcome false-negative results due to vasospasm.

In cases of extravasation, selective catheterization and embolization of the artery is obtained with relatively large hand-cut gelfoam particles, to which a small coil may be added. If this "superselective" embolization cannot be achieved within a reasonable time span and using a reasonable amount of contrast medium, the distal splenic artery is embolized just before the hilus with one or more bigger (5–8 mm) coils. Generally, a complete embolization may be achieved. Even when extravasation is not completely stopped, the procedure (in most instances) results in clinical success. Extra care is given to sterility during the whole procedure. Preventive antibiotics are generally administered, which virtually annihilates infectious complications. As already mentioned, no embolization is performed if there is no active extravasation. A patchy "starry-night" appearance of the spleen is not considered an extravasation and is not treated by embolization (Chap. 8 Fig. 8.12). If, at the end of the procedure, a tolerable contrast dose has not been exceeded, a control angiography of the celiac trunk is performed to illustrate collateral vascular supply to the spleen.

The patient is generally kept in an intensive care unit for a couple of days; in most cases, if his/her general condition permits, he/she can be discharged after 1 week following a control CT scan (Dondelinger and Kurdziel 1990; Getrajdman and Sclafani 1997). The spleen normally has an excellent capacity to regenerate, so up to 80% of the parenchyma may be sacrificed without jeopardizing immunological function.

Results of splenic embolization for trauma have been very rewarding. More than 95% of patients with arterial extravasation may be managed conservatively and do not re-bleed or require operation. Combining CT scan, peritoneal lavage and angiography with arterial-splenic embolization allowed Sclafani et al. (1991) to non-operatively manage a great number of patients with splenic trauma with success.

13.4. Embolization of the Spleen as a Treatment of Hypersplenism

Hypersplenism is a condition occurring in several diseases and is characterized by severe pancytopenia, splenomegaly and reactive, hyperplastic bone marrow. The term hypersplenism was first used by Chauffard in 1907. There are primary and secondary forms of hypersplenism. The primary form consists of depression of one or more of the blood cell lines. This form is associated with clear-cut splenomegaly and is successfully treated by splenectomy (Schwartz et al. 1971). Secondary hypersplenism refers to a condition of pancytopenia that is associated with either portal hypertension of intra- or extrahepatic origin, or splenic-vein obstruction. In contrast to hepatically induced portal hypertension, splenic-vein obstruction (characterized by gastric variceal bleeding) responds well to splenectomy.

To avoid a surgical intervention and its complications, radiological catheter embolization of the spleen has been proposed. Initial failures included frequent abscess formation, splenic rupture, sepsis and pneumonia. Antibioprophylaxis and repeated treatment, with occlusion of different arterial branches at each session, have improved the final outcome (Papadimitriou et al. 1976; Wholey et al. 1978; Spigos et al. 1979). Splenic artery embolization represents a most attractive alternative option, especially in patients with hypersplenism after renal transplantation or due to immunosuppressive diseases (Gerlock et al. 1982).

The technique of embolization is essentially the same as the one used in trauma patients. However, in patients with hypersplenism, the procedure is frequently divided into different sessions to avoid major complications (Dondelinger and Kurdziel 1990).

Data published between 1975 and 1985 reported an overall complication rate of 18%, with a mortality rate of 7.5% (O'Neal and McDonald 1981). However, dividing the series into two 5-year time periods shows a significant reduction in complications and mortality rate. In particular, the complication rate was reduced by following the multistage protocol advocated by Spigos et al. (1980) or by limited peripheral embolization, as proposed by Delcour et al. (1982). Minor complications may still occur and include left upper-quadrant abdominal pain, fever, paralytic ileus with nausea and vomiting and pleural effusions (Kumpe et al. 1985). Nevertheless, even with the use of these protocols, embolization in patients with hypersplenism remains hazardous, and careful selection of patients should be considered.

13.5 Embolization of the Spleen as a Preoperative Measure in Laparoscopic Splenectomy

Splenic-artery embolization as a preoperative adjunct to laparoscopic splenectomy was first described by Poulin et al. (1993) in an attempt to reduce intraoperative bleeding during the laparoscopic procedure. Indeed, bleeding frequently occurred in early cases of laparoscopic splenectomy, when the operation was performed by means of an anterior approach (Carrol et al. 1992; Delaitre and Maignien 1992; Lefor et al. 1993; Poulin et al. 1993; Flowers et al. 1996). Later laparoscopic splenectomy has mostly been performed by means of a lateral approach, the so called hanging-spleen technique introduced by Delaitre (1995). This operative technique allows an easy dissection of the avascular retrosplenic plane, starting at the lower pole attachments with the colon and going up to the phrenicosplenic ligament (Trias et al. 1996). Even with this lateral approach, anterior splenic-dissection bleeding may occur from small gastric vessels, the splenic capsule or the parenchyma during lifting of the spleen with laparoscopic instruments (Totté et al. 1988; Mitchell et al. 1993; Poulin et al. 1993).

To manage these hemorrhagic events, preoperative arterial embolization of the spleen has been proposed. The technique is identical to the one used in cases of post-traumatic splenic rupture. After embolization of the splenic parenchyma with large hand-cut gelfoam particles, the procedure is ended with the introduction of one or two coils (5–8mm) distal to the dorsal pancreatic artery. If anatomical variations are present, the embolization technique is adapted to the radiological findings, and additional catheterization and selective embolization of polar arteries may be performed (Figs. 13.1, 13.2).

Indications for laparoscopic splenectomy include various hematological disorders, such as immune thrombocytopenic purpura, autoimmune hemolytic anemia, hereditary spherocytosis and, to a lesser extent, non-Hodgkin lymphoma. In the reported series, the results of preoperative embolization techniques have been excellent, especially in moderately sized spleens not exceeding 20 cm in length. These results are shown in Table 1.

In larger spleens (>20cm), Poulin et al. (1998) found a higher frequency of blood loss despite of preoperative embolization of the spleen. As shown in Table 2, this was not confirmed in the series of Totté et al. (1988). Complications in both series included a case of mild pancreatitis not inducing clinical symptoms and occurring in one of 26

a

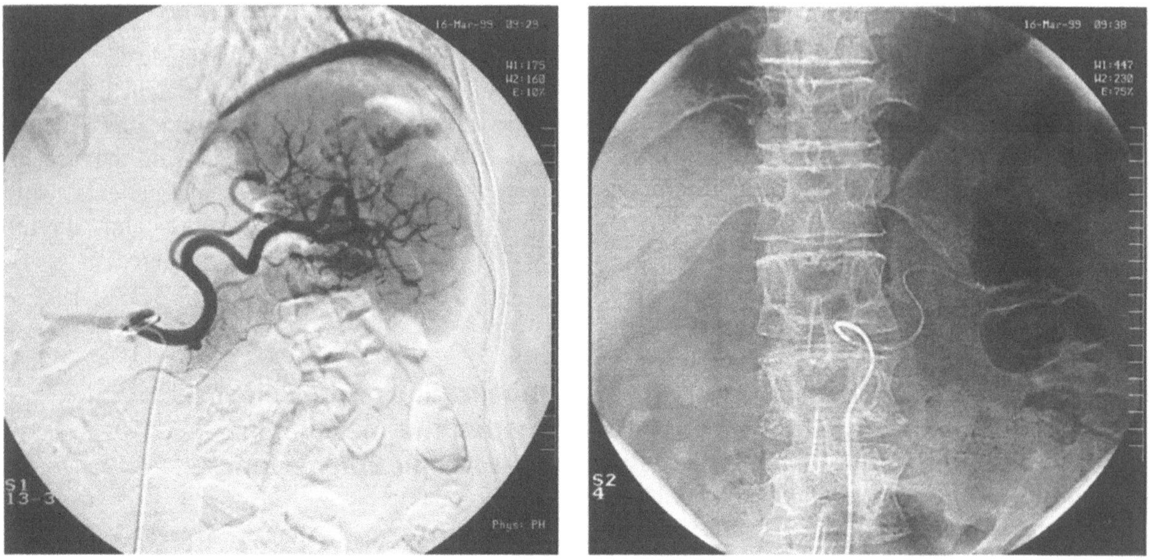

b

c

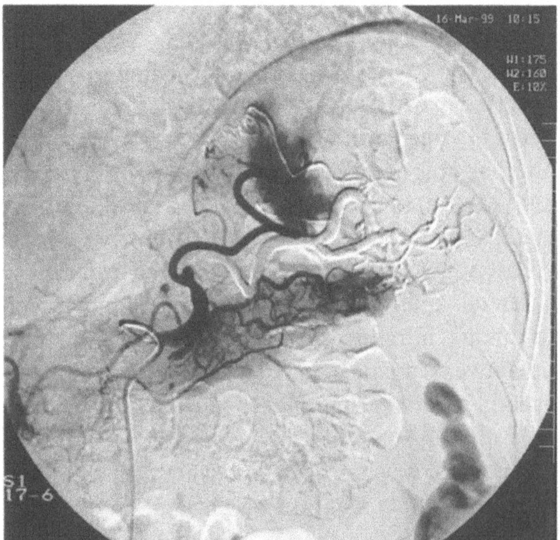

Fig. 13.1. Embolization of the splenic artery. **a** Angiography of the splenic artery before embolization. **b** Superselective catheterization of the splenic artery. **c** Angiography of the splenic artery after embolization, with sparing of the pancreatica magna artery

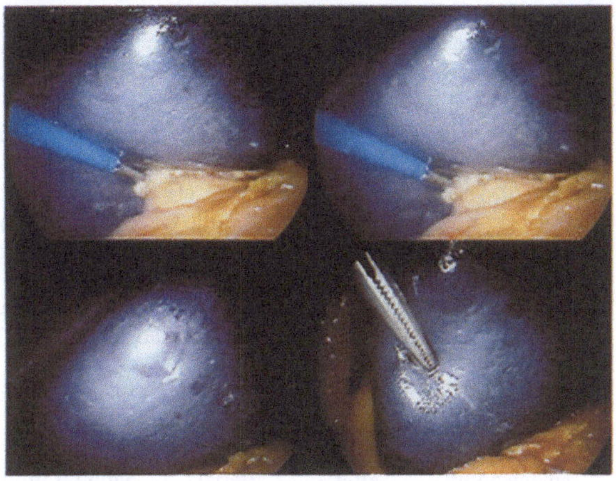

Fig. 13.2. Laparoscopic view of the spleen 24 h after embolization of the splenic artery. The spleen is enlarged and has a blueish discoloration

Table 1. Results after preoperative splenic-artery embolization of moderate-sized (<20 cm) spleens

Reference	Approach	Number of patients	Blood loss requiring transfusion
Poulin et al. 1993, 1998	Anterior	18	2
Totté et al. 1998	Lateral	18	0

Table 2. Results after preoperative splenic-artery embolization of large-sized (>20 cm) spleens

Reference	Approach	Number of patients	Blood loss requiring transfusion
Poulin et al. 1998	Anterior	8	7
Totté et al. 1998	Lateral	4	0

patients, and two of 22 patients in the respectively cited series. This complication may result from too proximal embolization that included the pancreatica magna artery or from using microsphere or gelatin particles that were too small and were thus capable of moving to the pancreatic vascular bed following backflow during injection (Poulin et al. 1998). As preoperative arterial embolization may be painful, an epidural infusion of 0.5% marcaine is used during embolization and during the early postoperative period.

Complications related to splenectomy have previously been documented and include pneumonia, overwhelming post-splenectomy sepsis and later forms of excessive infection (O'Neal and McDonald 1981; Green et al. 1986). As is the case after surgical splenectomy, these complications may occur after laparoscopic excision of the spleen, as experienced by Totté et al. (1988).

13.6 Conclusions

Interventional radiological techniques have taken an important place in splenic disease and surgery. In patients with hypersplenism, total or partial splenic-artery embolization may replace surgical splenectomy in selected patients. Results are comparable with those of surgical splenectomy series. However, in patients with hematological diseases, for whom laparoscopic splenectomy has become a standard (and very successful) procedure, preoperative splenic artery embolization has proven to be an excellent adjunct to the laparoscopic procedure. It is characterized by a minimal complication rate and offers great comfort to the patient and the surgeon.

References

Berkman WA, Harris SA Jr, Bernardino ME (1983) Nonsurgical drainage of splenic abscess. AJR Am J Roentgenol 141:395–396

Buntain WL, Gould HR, Maull KI (1988) Predictability of splenic salvage by computed tomography. J Trauma 28:24–34

Carrol BJ, Phillips DH, Semel DJ (1992) Laparoscopic splenectomy. Surg Endosc 6:183–185

Delaitre B (1995) Laparoscopic splenectomy: the "hanged-spleen" technique. Surg Endosc 9:528–529

Delaitre B, Maignien B (1992) Laparoscopic splenectomy: technical aspects. Surg Endosc 6:305–308

Delcour C, Spiegl G, Brion JP, et al. (1982) Complications in splenic embolization. Ann Radiol (Paris) 25:453–454

Dondelinger RF, Kurdziel JC (1990) Embolization of the spleen. In: Dondelinger RF, Rossi P, Kurdziel JC, Wallace S (eds) Interventional radiology. Thieme, Stuttgart, pp 505–512

Flowers JL, Lefor AT, Steers J, et al. (1996) Laparoscopic splenectomy in patients with hematologic diseases. Ann Surg 224:19–28

Gerlock AJ Jr, MacDonnell RC Jr, Muhletaler CA, et al. (1982) Partial splenic embolization for hypersplenism in renal transplantation. AJR Am J Roentgenol 138:451–456

Getrajdman GI, Sclafani SJA (1997) Transcatheter arterial embolization in the management of splenic trauma. In: Baum S, Pentecost MJ (eds) Abrams' angiography: vascular and interventional radiology, vol 3. Little, Brown and Company, Boston, pp 884–891

Greco RS, Alvarez FE (1981) Protection against pneumococcal bacteremia by partial splenectomy. Surg Gynecol Obstet 152:67–69

Green JB, Shackford SR, Sise MJ, et al. (1986) Late septic complications in adults following splenectomy for trauma: a prospective analysis in 144 patients. J Trauma 26:999–1004

King H, Schumacker HB Jr (1952) Splenic studies I: susceptibility to infection after splenectomy performed in infancy. Ann Surg 136:239–242

Kreuzfelder E, Obertacke U, Erhard J, et al. (1991) Alterations of the immune system following splenectomy in childhood. J Trauma 31:358–364

Kumpe DA, Rumack CM, Pretorius SH, et al. (1985) Partial splenic embolization in children with hypersplenism. Radiology 155:357–362

Lefor AT, Melvin WS, Bailey RW, et al. (1993) Laparoscopic splenectomy in the management of immune thrombocytopenic purpura. Surgery 114:613–618

Mitchell A, Dick R, Akle C (1993) Case report: an adjunct to laparoscopic splenectomy. A new role for interventional radiology. Clin Radiol 48:213–214

O'Malley ME, Wood BJ, Boland GW, et al. (1999) Percutaneous imaging-guided biopsy of the spleen. AJR Am J Roentgenol 172:661–665

O'Neal BJ, McDonald JC (1981) The risk of sepsis in the asplenic adult. Ann Surg 194:775–778

Papadimitriou J, Tritakis C, Karatzas G, et al. (1976) Treatment of hypersplenism by embolus placement in the splenic artery. Lancet 2:1268–1270

Pickhardt B, Moore EE, Moore FA, et al. (1989) Operative splenic salvage in adults: a decade perspective. J Trauma 29:1386–1391

Poulin EC, Thibault C, Mamazza J, et al. (1993) Laparoscopic splenectomy: clinical experience and the role of preoperative splenic artery embolization. Surg Laparosc Endosc 3:445–450

Poulin EC, Mamazza J, Schlachta CM (1998) Splenic artery embolization before laparoscopic splenectomy. Surg Endosc 12:870–875

Quinn SF, Van Sonnenberg E, Casola G, et al. (1986) Interventional radiology in the spleen. Radiology 161:289–291

Schwartz SI, Adams JT, Bauman AW (1971) Splenectomy for hematologic disorders. Curr Probl Surg 1971:1–57

Sclafani SJ, Weisberg A, Scalea TM, et al. (1991) Blunt splenic injuries: non-surgical treatment with CT, arteriography and transcatheter arterial embolization of the splenic artery. Radiology 181:189–196

Spigos DG, Jonasson O, Mozes M, et al. (1979) Partial splenic embolization in the treatment of hypersplenism. AJR Am J Roentgenol 132:777–782

Spigos DG, Tan WS, Mozes MF, et al. (1980) Splenic embolization. Cardiovasc Intervent Radiol 3:282–287

Totté E, Van Hee R, Kloeck I, et al. (1988) Laparoscopic splenectomy after arterial embolisation. Hepatogastroenterology 45:773–776

Traub AC, Perry JF Jr (1981) Injuries associated with splenic trauma. J Trauma 21:840–847

Trias M, Targarona EM, Balague C (1996) Laparoscopic splenectomy: an evolving technique. A comparison between anterior and lateral approach. Surg Endosc 10:389–392

Van Hee R (1997) Milt. In: Bruining HA, Broos PLO, Goris RJA, Van Hee R, Kootstra G, Van Schilfgaarde R, Terpstra OT (eds) Leerboek chirurgie, 5th edn. Bohn, Stafleu and Van Loghem, Houten, pp 518–525

Wholey MH, Chamorro HA, Rao G, et al. (1978) Splenic infarction and spontaneous rupture of the spleen after therapeutic embolization. Cardiovasc Radiol 1:249–253

14 Differential Diagnostic Tables

J.L. Bloem, A. Spilt, P. Vanhoenacker, B. Op De Beeck, J. Delanote, H. Rigauts, L. Steyaert, F. Vanhoenacker, A.M. De Schepper, and F. Deckers

Table 14.1. Splenomegaly (table by J.L. Bloem and A. Spilt)

	Common	Uncommon
Splenomegaly with abnormal portal or splenic blood flow	Congestive heart failure Hepatic cirrhosis	Cavernous transformation of the portal vein Splenic vein obstruction Hepatic echinococcosis Splenic artery aneurysm Hepatic vein obstruction Portal vein obstruction Other causes of portal hypertension Hepatic schistosomiasis
Splenomegaly without morphological abnormalities; hematologic disorders	Early sickle cell anemia Nutritional anemias Leukemias Hodgkin's disease Non-Hodgkin's lymphoma	Ovalocytosis Spherocytosis Thalassemia major Paroxysmal nocturnal hemoglobinuria Hemoglobinopathies Immune hemolytic anemias Immune thrombocytopenias Immune neutropenias Myelofibrosis Marrow damage Marrow infiltration Myeloproliferative syndromes Langerhans' cell histiocytosis
Splenomegaly without morphological abnormalities; infectious diseases	Infectious mononucleosis Acquired immune deficiency syndrome Viral hepatitis Cytomegalovirus Subacute bacterial endocarditis Malaria Sepsis Other infections (especially in children)	Congenital syphilis Bacterial septicemia Histoplasmosis Leishmaniasis Trypanosomiasis Tuberculosis
Splenomegaly without morphological abnormalities; miscellaneous	Rheumatoid arthritis Felty's syndrome Drug reactions	Systemic lupus erythematosus Sarcoidosis Angioimmunoblastic lymphadenopathy Thyrotoxicosis Serum sickness Gaucher's disease Metastatic tumors Lymphoma
Massive splenomegaly	Chronic congestive splenomegaly Chronic malaria Chronic myelogenous leukemia Myeloproliferative disorders	Sarcoidosis Leishmaniasis Gaucher's disease Niemann-Pick disease Longstanding thalassemia major Hairy cell leukemia Congenital syphilis

Table 14.2. Solitary focal lesions (table by P. Vanhoenacker)

	Common	Uncommon
Cystic lesions	Post-traumatic cyst Epidermoid Cystic degeneration of infarct Pancreatic pseudocyst Necrotic metastases Hematoma	Hydatid cyst Abscess Cavernous hemangioma Lymphangioma
Solid lesions	Malignant: • Metastases (melanoma, islet cell tumor, breast, lung, colon, renal cell, ovarium, pancreas) • Lymphoma Benign: • Hemangioma • Infarct • Hematopoietic • Hematoma	Malignant: • Angiosarcoma • Fibrosarcoma Benign: • Hamartoma • Lymphangioma • Myxoma • Chondroma • Osteoma
Calcified masses or cysts	Abscess • Tuberculous • Pyogenic Hematoma Vascular • Splenic artery • Splenic artery aneurysm • Infarct Calcified cyst • Congenital • Post-traumatic • Hydatid cyst • Cystic dermoid Neoplasm • Chondroma • Osteoma • Treated and aggressive lymphoma • Hemangioma/lymphangioma • Hamartoma	

Table 14.3. Multiple focal lesions (table by B. Op De Beeck)

	Common	Uncommon
Multiple splenic calcifications	Phleboliths Healed granulomas (tuberculosis, histoplasmosis) Acquired immune deficiency syndrome Healed *Pneumocystis* infection Hemangiomas	Infarcts Hamartomas Brucellosis Hemosiderosis Sickle cell anemia Echinococcal cysts Epidermoid cysts Post-traumatic cysts Healed abscesses *Armillifer armillatus* infestation Collagen vascular diseases Amyloidosis Gamna-Gandy bodies

Table 14.3. *(Continued)*

	Common	Uncommon
Multiple hypoechoic splenic masses	Lymphoma Infarcts Metastases Septic emboli Abscesses (pyogenic, fungal)	Granulomatous disease (tuberculosis, MAI, sarcoidosis, cat-scratch disease) Cysts (simple, epidermoid, hydatid, pancreatic) Hemangiomas Hamartomas Lymphangiomatosis Disseminated *Pneumocystis carinii* infection Langerhans' cell histocytosis
Multiple echogenic splenic masses	Calcified granulomas Metastases Chronic infarcts Hematomas	Plasmocytomas Abscesses with air bubbles Hereditary spherocytosis Schistosomiasis Hydatid "sand" in hydatid cysts Niemann-Pick disease
Multiple hypodense splenic lesions; non-contrast scan	Lymphoma Metastases Infarcts Abscesses Granulomatous disease (tuberculosis, MAI, sarcoidosis, cat-scratch disease)	Congenital or traumatic cysts Echinococcal cysts Hemangiomas Hamartomas Lymphangiomatosis Extramedullary hematopoiesis Niemann-Pick disease
Multiple hyperdense splenic lesions; non-contrast scan	Calcified granulomas Hemorrhagic acute infarcts Acute hemorrhage (post-traumatic, spontaneous)	Mucinous metastases (colon, stomach, pancreas) Hydatid infection Pneumocystis infection (healed) Calcified hematomas Hemangiomas complicated by rupture and hemorrhage Complicated cysts attributable to intracystic hemorrhage or infection
Multiple hyperintense splenic masses on T2-weighted images	Infarcts Metastases Septic emboli Abscesses (pyogenic, fungal) Subacute hemorrhage	Cysts (posttraumatic, epidermoid, hydatid) Acute granulomatous disease Hemangiomas Hamartomas Lymphangiomas Niemann-Pick disease
Multiple hypointense splenic masses on T2-weighted images	Gamna-Gandy bodies Healed granulomas Healed infarcts	Lymphoma Sarcoidosis Sickle cell disease
Multiple predominantly hypointense splenic masses on immediate post-gadolinium T1-weighted spoiled gradient-echo images	Lymphoma Infarcts Metastases Hematomas Septic emboli Abscesses (pyogenic, fungal) Healed granulomas	Cysts (posttraumatic, epidermoid, hydatid) Hemangiomas Lymphangiomatosis Sarcoidosis

MAI, mycobacterium avium intracellulare.

Table 14.4. Abnormal diffuse alteration of reflectivity on ultrasound (table by J. Delanote, H. Rigauts and L. Steyaert). For abnormal reflectivity in solitary focal lesions, see Table 14.2; for abnormal reflectivity in multiple focal lesions, see Table 14.3

	Common	Uncommon
Increased reflectivity		
Diffuse small nodules with deposition of calcium or iron	Phleboliths; calcified hemangioma Healed granulomas (tuberculosis, histoplasmosis)	Infectious (*Pneumocystis carinii*, hydatid cysts, brucellosis, hamartomas) Inflammatory (BBS) Hemosiderosis Gamna-Gandy bodies Transfusion related hemochromatosis Infarction Sickle cell anemia Thorotrast residuals Collagen vascular diseases (rheumatoid arthritis, systemic lupus erythematosus) Amyloidosis
Diffuse small nodules without deposition of calcium or iron	Metastases (ovary, thyroid) Inflammatory (BBS) Lymphoma	Storage disease [Gaucher's disease, Niemann-Pick disease (type B/C)] Hereditary spherocytosis
Diffuse or patchy	Hematoma Lymphoma	Opportunistic infections (*Pneumocystis*, cytomegalovirus, MAI, *Candida albicans*)
	Myelofibrosis (hypersplenism) Infarction (chronic) Portal vein thrombosis	Neoplasm (leukemia, metastases, angiosarcoma) Hemangioma (atypical) Punctate calcifications (sickle cell anemia, thorotrast, *Pneumocystis carinii*, malaria) Gaucher's disease (infarction) Spherocytosis, hereditary Intrasplenic gas Extramedullary hematopoiesis (myeloproliferative disease, aplastic anemia) Spontaneous splenic rupture (mononucleosis, sickle cell disease) Dysgammaglobulinemia
Multiple channel-like	Portal hypertension [cirrhosis, congestive splenomegaly (Banti syndrome)] Arterial calcifications	
Decreased reflectivity		
Diffuse small nodules	Lymphoma Myeloproliferative diseases	Sarcoidosis Infection - Bacterial (miliary tuberculosis, MAI, bacterial endocarditis) - Fungal (candidiasis, aspergillus, histoplasmosis) - Parasital (echinococcus, schistosomiasis, malaria) Metastases (melanoma, lung, breast) Storage disease (Gaucher's disease) Langerhans' cell histiocytosis Bacillary angiomatosis (cat-scratch disease)
Diffuse or patchy	Hematoma Lymphoma Myeloproliferative diseases Infarction Metastases	Acute infectious diseases (viral infections) Chronic infectious diseases (tuberculosis, malaria, brucellosis) Gaucher's disease Wegener's granulomatosis

BBS, Besnier Boeck Schaumann; *MAI*, *mycobacterium avium intracellulare.*

Table 14.5. Abnormal diffuse alteration of attenuation on CT (table by F. Vanhoenacker and A. M. De Schepper). For abnormal attenuation in solitary focal lesions, see Table 14.2; for abnormal attenuation in multiple focal lesions, see Table 14.3

	Common	Uncommon
High density before IV contrast administration	Calcifications (Table 14.3) Hemosiderosis Transfusion-related hemochromatosis	Thorotrast exposure Pseudo-thorotrast spleen (sickle cell disease) Lymphangiogram contrast Calcified hemangiomatosis Gamna-Gandy bodies
Low density before IV contrast administration	Hematoma, subcapsular or intrasplenic Infarction (atheromatosis, sickle cell disease) Lymphoma Metastases	Abscesses Angiosarcoma Peliosis
Intrasplenic gas		Necrosis (infarction, lymphoma, tumor, postembolization) Abscess
Heterogeneous attenuation on pre-contrast images	Hematoma (trauma)	Spontaneous splenic rupture (Table 14.8) Some angiosarcoma
Heterogeneous on post-contrast images (no splenomegaly)	Normal transient heterogeneity after bolus injection of contrast medium Lymphoma Infiltrating metastatic disease Direct tumor extension from tumors outside the spleen Multiple infarcts Multiple abscesses or septic emboli	Hemangiomatosis Sarcoidosis Cat-scratch disease Bacillary angiomatosis Tuberculosis Wegener's granulomatosis
Heterogeneous on post-contrast images (with splenomegaly)	Myeloproliferative diseases Lymphoma	Sarcoidosis Sickle cell disease in cases of acute sequestration crisis Peliosis Mycobacterial infection (acute) Pneumocystis carinii Fungal infections Disseminated Kaposi sarcoma Cat-scratch disease Gaucher's disease Niemann-Pick disease Langerhans' cell histiocytosis Amyloidosis Other storage diseases Angiosarcoma (large) Hemangiomatosis Lymphangiomatosis

IV, intravenous.

Table 14.6. Abnormal signal intensity (SI) on magnetic resonance imaging (table by F. Deckers and A.M. De Schepper)

Common	Uncommon	
High-SI T1, high-SI T2	Subacute hematoma Hemorrhagic infarction Hemorrhagic metastasis	Hemorrhagic cyst Splenic sequestration Hemorrhagic lymphangioma Hemorrhagic angiosarcoma Melanoma metastasis Hemorrhagic lymphoma Niemann-Pick disease
High-SI T1, low-SI T2		Inflammatory pseudotumor
Low-SI T1, high-SI T	Lymphoma Infarction Abscess Metastasis	Cyst, primary Cyst, secondary Hemangioma Lymphangioma Wegener's disease
Low-SI T1, isointense-SI T2	Lymphoma Metastasis	
Isointense-SI T1, high-SI T2	Lymphoma Abscess Fungal abscess, acute Fungal abscess, treated Metastasis	Hamartoma Lymphangioma Niemann-Pick nodule
Isointense-SI T1, isointense-SI T2	Lymphoma Metastasis	
Low-SI T1, low-SI T2	Hemosiderosis Lymphoma Gamna-Gandy body Fungal abscess, healed Normal neonate spleen Chemotherapy	Sickle-cell disease Angiosarcoma Epithelioid vascular tumor Littoral cell angioma Sarcoidosis
Isointense-SI T1, low-SI T2	Lymphoma Chemotherapy	Inflammatory pseudotumor Gaucher's-disease nodule

Table 14.7. Abnormal patterns on Gd-enhanced magnetic resonance imaging (table by F. Deckers and A. M. De Schepper)

	No enhancement	**No enhancement, obscured on late images**
	Laceration Infarction (rim sign) Gamna-Gandy body Cyst Subcapsular hematoma Lymphangioma	Lymphoma Metastasis
	Early enhancement	**Late enhancement**
	Inflammatory pseudotumor Hemangioma (persistent) Hamartoma (persistent)	Hemangioma (centripetal) Abscess (rim) Lymphangioma (septae) Angiosarcoma (persistent)

Table 14.8. Spontaneous (non-traumatic) splenic rupture (table by F. Vanhoenacker and A.M. De Schepper)

	Common	Uncommon
Infectious disease	Infectious mononucleosis Malaria	Typhoid fever Typhus Influenza Viral hepatitis Tuberculosis Actinomycosis Brucellosis Tularemia Aspergillosis Syphilis Kala-azar Meningococcal septicemia Virus-associated hematophagocytic syndrome Yaws
Neoplastic disease	Acute leukemia Lymphoma	Metastases Hemangioma Angiosarcoma Myeloproliferative disease Plasmocytoma Plasma cell leukemia
Non-neoplastic hematologic disease		Congenital afibrinogenemia Hemophilia Hemolytic disease of the newborn Autoimmune hemolytic anemia Congenital hemolytic anemia
(Cardio)vascular disease	Splenic vein thrombosis Congestive splenomegaly Splenic infarcts	Infectious endocarditis Mycotic aneurysms Peliosis
Systemic disease		Crohn's disease Rheumatoid arthritis Felty's syndrome Systemic lupus erythematosus Polyarteritis nodosa Wegener's granulomatosis Amyloidosis Sarcoidosis Gaucher's disease Glycogen storage disease Langerhans' cell histiocytosis
Miscellaneous		Spontaneous rupture in normal spleen Ectopic pregnancy Pregnancy or during labor

Reference

Dachman AH, Coldwell DM (1993) Trauma and nontraumatic rupture. In: Dachman AH, Friedman AC (eds) Radiology of the spleen. Mosby Year Book, St. Louis, pp 88–90

J.L. Bloem, A. Split; Department of Radiology, Leiden University Medical Center, Rijnsburgerweg 10, 2300 RC Leiden, The Netherlands
P. Vanhoenacker; Department of Radiology, O. L. V. Ziekenhuis, Moorselbaan 164, B-9300 Aalst, Belgium
B. Op De Beeck; Department of Radiology, Academisch Ziekenhuis-Vrije Universiteit Brussel, Laarbeeklaan 101, 1090 Brussels, Belgium
J. Delanote, H. Rigauts; Department of Radiology, Algemeen Ziekenhuis St. Jan Brugge, Ruddershove 10, B-8000 Brugge, Belgium
L. Steyaert; Department of Radiology, Algemeen Ziekenhuis St. Jan Brugge, Ruddershovelaan 10, B-8000 Brugge, Belgium
F. Vanhoenacker, A.M. De Schepper; Department of Radiology, University Hospital Antwerp, Wilrijkstraat 10, B-2650 Edegem, Belgium
F. Deckers; Department of Radiology, St. Augustinusziekenhuis, Oosterveldlaan 24, B-2610 Wilrijk, Belgium

Appendix: Scintigraphy of the Spleen

M. De Roo

CONTENTS

A.1 Introduction

The number of indications for the scintigraphic exploration of the spleen has strongly diminished since the advent of computed tomography (CT) and magnetic resonance imaging (MRI). The position, shape and volume of the spleen and intrasplenic lesions are, in general, more accurately visualised using CT and MRI, notwithstanding the continuous improvement of scintigraphic imaging techniques by the introduction of high-resolution digital γ-cameras and of novel scintigraphic techniques, such as SPECT (single-photon-emission computed tomography). From the foregoing, it can be concluded that splenic scintigraphy can bring useful additional information only if the scintigraphic imaging demonstrates functional phenomena related to diseases of the spleen (Spencer and Pearson 1975; Peters et al. 1983).

A.2 Technical Introduction

Two items must be considered: the tracer substances and the scintigraphic technique.

A.2.1 Tracer Substances (Radiopharmaceuticals)

A.2.1.1 Tracer Substances for Spleen Scintigraphy

Sulphur or tin colloid particles (dimensions 0.2–0.5μm) labelled by ^{99m}Tc sodium pertechnetate are, after intravenous injection, homogeneously taken up by the reticulo-endothelial system (RES) of the liver, spleen and bone marrow. The scintigraphic images can be considered as a map of the functional RES, with about 85% of the radioactive particles being trapped in the liver, 5–10% in the spleen and a few in the bone marrow (in general not visible). Under normal circumstances, the images reveal, in addition to the global uptake, the mass and functional integrity of the RES system within the liver and spleen, and the shape, position and volume of these organs (Fig. A.1). Tumoral lesions or areas of parenchymal destruction are visible as zones of diminished or absent tracer uptake.

For specific imaging of the spleen, denatured autologous red blood cells are used. Red blood cells (20ml) are separated and labelled with technetium sodium pertechnetate, denatured by means of 20min incubation at 49.5°C and, subsequently, injected into the patient.

Heating produces spherocytes characterised by damage of red cell membrane and changes in levels of intracellular electrolytes. These red cells are subject to lysis and selective removal from the bloodstream earlier. These denatured red blood cells are rapidly taken up by the macrophages of the spleen.

Scintigraphic imaging shows only the spleen or delocalised spleen tissue. Unlike the case in spleen scintigraphy with colloid particles, spleen and spleen tissues are imaged without any interference of other organs (Fisher and Wolf 1967).

M. De Roo; Herendreef 26, B-3001 Heverlee, Belgium

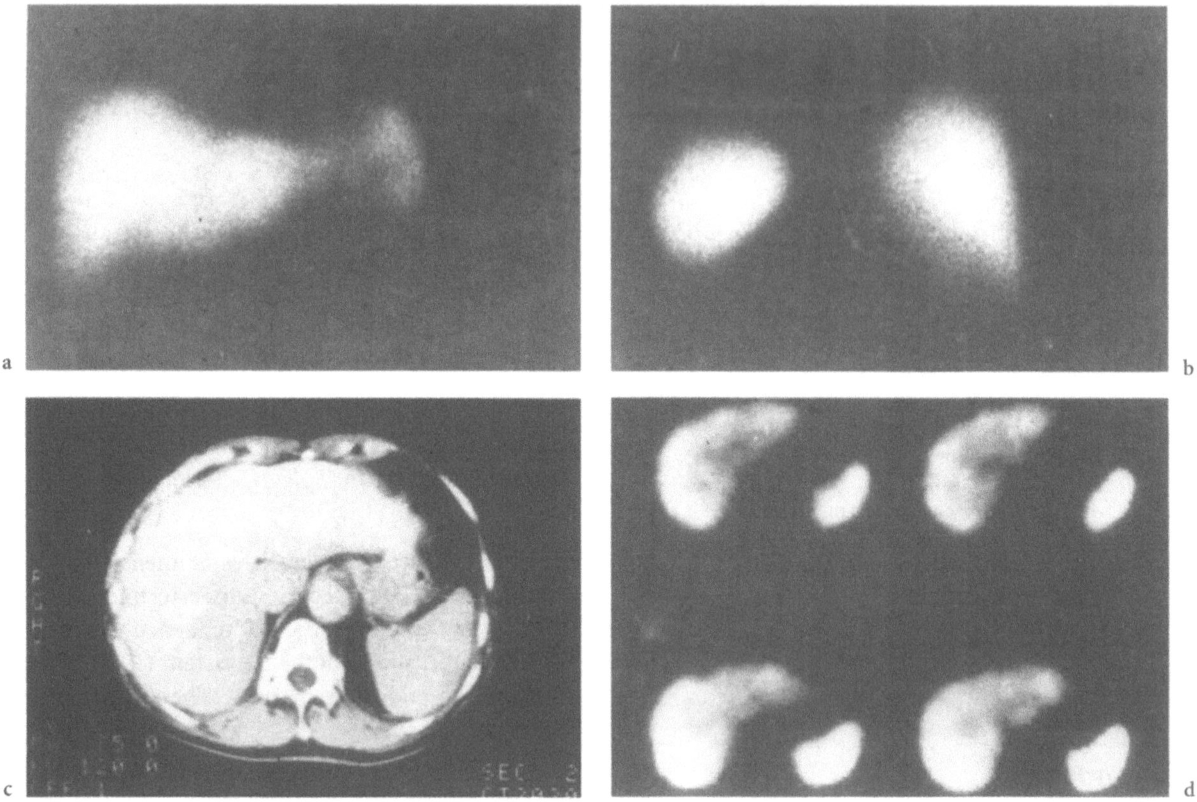

Fig. A.1. Normal colloid scintigraphy of the spleen (and liver). **a** Anteroposterior incidence, showing the liver and, less clearly, the spleen. **b** Posteroanterior incidence, showing more clearly the spleen and the right hepatic lobe. **c** Computed tomography (CT) of the liver and spleen. **d** Single-photon-emission CT at the same level as the CT image, showing the hepatic tracer distribution in a transverse slice (note the heterogeneous tracer distribution at the hilus) and, at right, the homogeneous tracer uptake in the spleen

A.2.1.2
Tracer Substances for the Bone Marrow (Secondary Spleen Visualisation)

Indium-111 chloride (indium behaves in a manner similar to iron) can be used for the exploration of the red bone marrow, but the use of labelled leukocytes is more convenient. The baseline mechanism of ^{99m}Tc HMPAO (hexamethylpropylene amine oxime) labelling of leukocytes is the lipophilicity of HMPAO, which allows the ^{99m}Tc to enter the cells, in this case the leukocytes, which must be isolated before labelling.

There are also in vivo labelling techniques for the leukocytes (and the myelocytes and metamyelocytes); in these techniques, a ^{99m}Tc-labelled anti-granulocyte antibody against the antigen substance non-specific cross-reactive antigen of the leukocyte can be injected (Becker 1995). Both labelling techniques are routinely used in scintigraphic procedures for detection and localisation of infectious foci.

A.2.2
Imaging Methods

Planar imaging (anteroposterior, posteroanterior, lateral and oblique views) is, in general, completed by SPECT when small masses of splenic tissues or small intrasplenic lesions are to demonstrated. However, for the latter indication, spleen scintigraphy is rarely useful, owing to the greater efficacy of CT and MRI.

Planar imaging is adequate for the visualisation of the functional disturbances of the different cellular constituents or the demonstration of delocalised splenic tissue. Imaging can be restricted to the abdomen or, if useful, whole-body imaging can be used.

A.3 Indications

A.3.1 Functional Spleen Scintigraphy (Using Spleen-Specific Tracers)

A.3.1.1 Trauma

The evaluation of the *volume of the residual functionally intact part of the spleen*, after surgery or restoration after splenic trauma, can provide an indication for use of spleen scintigraphy in trauma patients.

A.3.1.2 Mass Lesions

The specification of *tumoral mass or masses in the left upper abdominal quadrant* can provide an indication for use of spleen scintigraphy. If these masses take up denatured, labelled blood cells, it can be concluded that these masses correspond to the spleen, a functional intact part of the spleen or one or more accessory spleens (KOYANAGI et al. 1988).

A.3.1.3 Polysplenia/Asplenia

In *polysplenia* cases, it can be important to demonstrate the presence of functional spleen tissue. However, the absence of functional splenic tissue must be confirmed in patients with *asplenia* (sickle cell disease, leukaemia, volvulus of the spleen).

A.3.1.4 Functional Result of Surgical Intervention

In children, *splenic rupture* occurs frequently in blunt abdominal trauma, because the capsule of the spleen is relatively thin. Selective spleen scintigraphy is useful for the final evaluation of the damage to the organ. After (sometimes partial) reconstruction of the ruptured spleen, selective spleen scintigraphy is important for verification of the *functional result of the surgical intervention* (EHRLICHT et al. 1982; BOSC et al. 1984).

In case of unavoidable total splenectomy, small pieces of splenic tissue are implanted in the peritoneum in order to preserve splenic function. It has been proven, according to the literature, that susceptibility to infection after splenectomy is strongly increased (TOYOTA et al. 1986). Specific splenic scintigraphy enables one to determine whether the implants have become functional (HARDING and ROBINSON 1991).

A.3.1.5 Splenosis

Accidental implantation of splenic tissue (splenosis) can only be demonstrated in a reliable way by specific spleen scintigraphy. SPECT is recommended in order to obtain optimal results. With this technique, splenosis can be detected in 58% of the cases, while sensitivity of planar scintigraphic techniques is limited to 26% (GUNES et al. 1994).

A.3.1.6 Control of Therapeutic Splenectomy

In patients with chronic immune thrombocytopenic purpura, lymphoma or other malignant hematologic conditions, it is important to ascertain whether or not splenic tissue remains after splenectomy; this could result in a relapse of the disease (Fig. A.2).

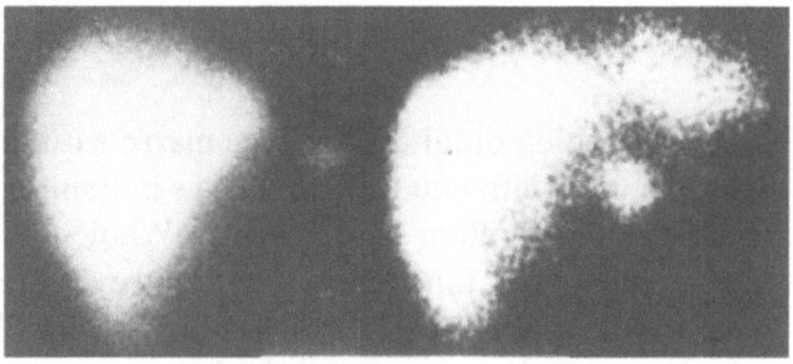

Fig. A.2. Spleen remnant (after splenectomy) caudal to the left hepatic lobe (colloid scintigraphy)

A.3.2 Non-Specific Spleen Scintigraphy

A.3.2.1 Colloid Scintigraphy

Using a colloidal tracer substance, the liver and the spleen are clearly visualised, allowing evaluation of the position and volume of both organs, the detection of focal lesions (Fig. A.3) and the visualisation of parenchymal disease of the liver, which results in a shift of the tracer accumulation

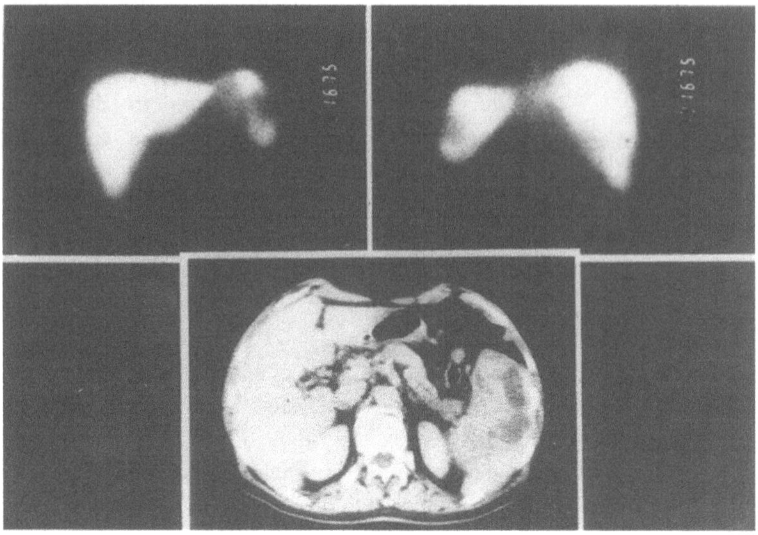

Fig. A.3. Colloid scintigraphy of liver and spleen, demonstrating expansive lesions at the lateral border of the spleen, as also demonstrated by computed tomography (lymphoma)

towards the spleen and bone marrow. For liver lesions, the overall sensitivity is about 80–85% according to the volume of the lesion; lesions less than 1.5 cm in diameter are not detected. SPECT increased the yield to approximately 90%. Until the advent of CT, liver and spleen colloid scintigraphy were the most reliable exploration methods for the visualisation of focal liver and spleen disease (Harding and Robinson 1991).

A.3.2.2 Spleen Scintigraphy in Haematology

The visualisation of functional bone marrow can be achieved using different tracers, such as indium-111 transferrin or indium-111 chloride. Whole-body images show the functional bone marrow, with only faint visualisation of the spleen. In cases with splenic myelopoiesis, the enlarged spleen shows pronounced tracer uptake.

White blood cells labelled with ^{99m}Tc HMPAO have replaced the aforementioned tracer substances (Becker 1995), enabling the exploration of the bone marrow and the role of the spleen in bone marrow diseases on a routine basis. In these whole-body images, the functional bone marrow is visible, with eventual shrinking or expansion phenomena. In normal cases, the spleen is visible owing to pooling of the labelled white blood cells. In cases of bone marrow disease (with consequently diminished bone marrow function), the volume and the tracer uptake intensity of the spleen increase, signalling extramedullary haematopoiesis (Fig. A.4).

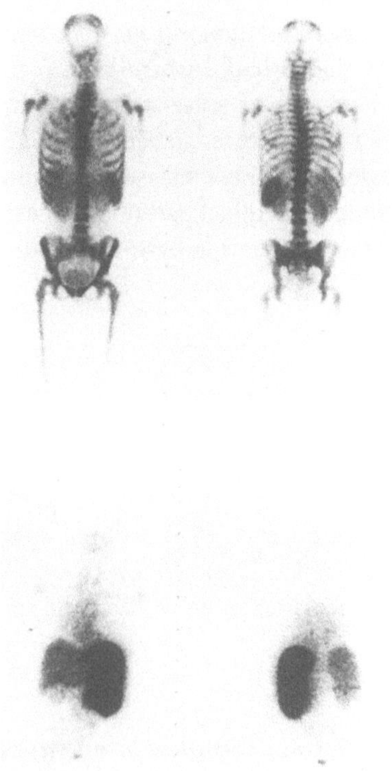

Fig. A.4. Whole-body imaging of liver, spleen and bone marrow after administration of white blood cells labelled by ^{99m}Tc anti-granulocyte antibody (Büll et al. 1996). *Upper image:* normal tracer distribution in anteroposterior and posteroanterior views, showing functional bone marrow, liver and spleen (free pertechnetate ^{99m}Tc excreted by the kidneys). *Lower image*: the same distribution in a case of osteomyelofibrosis, with extramedullary hematopoiesis in liver and spleen

References

Becker W (1995) The contribution of nuclear medicine to the patient with infection. Eur J Nucl Med 22:1195–1211

Bosc O, Bensoussan AL, Morin JF, et al. (1984) Splenic injuries: therapeutic orientation. Apropos of 46 cases. Chir Pediatr 25:1–25

Büll U, Schicha H, Biersack HJ, Knapp WH, Reiners C, Schober O (1996) Nuklear Medizin. Thieme Verlag, Stuttgart

Ehrlich CP, Papanicolaou N, Treves S, et al. (1982) Splenic scintigraphy using Tc-99m-labeled heat-denaturated red blood cells in pediatric patients. J Nucl Med 23:209–213

Fischer J, Wolf R (1967) Nuklearmedizinische Diagnostik in der Hämatologie. Hoechst, Frankfurt

Gunes I, Yilmazar T, Sarikaya I, et al. (1994) Scintigraphic detection of splenosis: superiority of tomographic selective spleen scintigraphy. Clin Radiol 49:115–117

Harding IK, Robinson PJA (1991) Clinicians guide to nuclear medicine gastroenterology. Churchill Livingstone, Edinburgh

Koyanagi N, Kanematsu T, Sugimachi K (1988) Preoperative computed tomography to facilitate the detection of accessory spleen in patients with hematologic disorders. Surg Today 18:101–104

Peters PE, Lorenz R, Fischer M (1983) Splenic imaging. Lymphology 16:90–100

Spencer P, Pearson HA (1980) Radionuclide studies of the spleen. CRC, Cleveland

Toyota S, Nakagawa T, Yamaghucci N, et al. (1986) Scintigraphic imaging of autotransplanted splenic grafts by ^{99m}Tc-labeled heat-damaged erythrocytes. Radioisotopes 35:423–428

Subject Index

List of Contributors

H. Aibe
Department of Radiology
Faculty of Medicine
Kyushu University
3-1-1 Maidashi
Higashi-ku Fukuoka, 812-8582
Japan

E.C. Benya
157 Scottswood Road
Riverside, IL 60546-2221
USA

J.L. Bloem
Department of Radiology
Leiden University Medical Center
Rijnsburgerweg 10
2300 RC Leiden
The Netherlands

H. Bortier
University of Antwerp (campus RUCA)
Groenenborgerlaan 171
B-2020 Antwerpen
Belgium

B. Corthouts
Department of Radiology,
University Hospital Antwerp,
Wilrijkstraat 10,
B-2650 Edegem,
Belgium

A.I. De Backer
Department of Radiology
University Hospital Antwerp
Wilrijkstraat 10
B-2650 Edegem
Belgium

M. De Roo
Herendreef 26
B-3001 Heverlee
Belgium

A.M. De Schepper
Department of Radiology
University Hospital Antwerp
Wilrijkstraat 10
B-2650 Edegem
Belgium

F. Deckers
Department of Radiology
St. Augustinusziekenhuis
Oosterveldlaan 24
B-2610 Wilrijk
Belgium

H. Degryse
Department of Radiology
University Hospital Antwerp
Wilrijkstraat 10
B-2650 Edegem
Belgium

J. Delanote
Department of Radiology
Algemeen Ziekenhuis St. Jan Brugge
Ruddershove 10
B-8000 Brugge
Belgium

A. Drevelengas
Department of Radiology
Papanicolaou Hospital
Thessaloniki
Greece

S.E. Falbo
Department of Diagnostic Radiology
William Beaumont Hospital
3601 W. Thirteen Mile Rd.
Royal Oak, Michigan 48073
USA

L. Hendrickx
Department of Radiology
Academic Surgical Center
Stuivenberg
Lange Beeldekensstraat 267
B-2060 Antwerp
Belgium

C.C. Hoeffel
Department of Radiology A
Hôpital COCHIN
27 Rue du Faubourg Saint Jacques
F-75014 Paris
France

H. Honda
Department of Radiology
Faculty of Medicine
Kyushu University
3-1-1 Maidashi
Higashi-ku Fukuoka, 812-8582
Japan

H. Irie
Department of Radiology
Faculty of Medicine
Kyushu University
3-1-1 Maidashi
Higashi-ku Fukuoka, 812-8582
Japan

K. Ito
Department of Radiology
Thomas Jefferson University Hospital
132 South 10th Street
1096 Main Building
Philadelphia, PA 19107
USA

Z.H. Jafri
Department of Diagnostic Radiology
William Beaumont Hospital
3601 W. Thirteen Mile Rd.
Royal Oak, Michigan 48073
USA

M. Kunnen
Department of Radiology
University Hospital Ghent
De Pintelaan 185
B-9000 Ghent
Belgium

T. Kuroiwa
Department of Radiology, Faculty of Medicine, Kyushu University, 3-1-1 Maidashi, Higashi-ku Fukuoka, 812-8582, Japan

K. Masuda
Department of Radiology
Faculty of Medicine
Kyushu University
3-1-1 Maidashi
Higashi-ku Fukuoka, 812-8582
Japan

P.J. Mergo
Department of Radiology
University of Florida College of Medicine
Health Science Center
P.O. Box 100374
Gainesville, FL 32610-0374
USA

D.G. Mitchell
Department of Radiology
Thomas Jefferson University Hospital
132 South 10th Street
1096 Main Building
Philadelphia, PA 19107
USA

K. Mortelé
Department of Radiology
University Hospital Ghent
De Pintelaan 185
B-9000 Ghent
Belgium

B. Op De Beeck
Department of Radiology
Academisch Ziekenhuis-Vrije Universiteit Brussel
Laarbeeklaan 101
1090 Brussels
Belgium

H. Rigauts
Department of Radiology
Algemeen Ziekenhuis St. Jan Brugge
Ruddershove 10
B-8000 Brugge
Belgium

P.R. Ros
Department of Radiology
Harvard Medical School
Brigham and Women's Hospital
75 Francis Street
Boston, MA 02115
USA

A. Spilt
Department of Radiology
Leiden University Medical Center
Rijnsburgerweg 10
2300 RC Leiden
The Netherlands

W. J. Stevens
University of Antwerp (campus UIA)
Universiteitsplein 1
B-2610 Antwerpen
Belgium

L. Steyaert
Department of Radiology
Algemeen Ziekenhuis St. Jan Brugge
Ruddershovelaan 10
B-8000 Brugge
Belgium

T. Tajima
Department of Radiology
Faculty of Medicine
Kyushu University
3-1-1 Maidashi
Higashi-ku Fukuoka, 812-8582
Japan

E. Totté
Department of Radiology
Academic Surgical Center
Stuivenberg
Lange Beeldekensstraat 267
B-2060 Antwerp
Belgium

R. Van Hee
Department of Radiology
Academic Surgical Center
Stuivenberg
Lange Beeldekensstraat 267
B-2060 Antwerp
Belgium

L. Van Hoe
Department of Radiology
University Hospitals K. U. Leuven
Herestraat 49
B-3000 Leuven
Belgium

F. Van Meir
University of Antwerp (campus RUCA)
Groenenborgerlaan 171
B-2020 Antwerpen

D. Vanbeckevoort
Department of Radiology
University Hospitals K. U. Leuven
Herestraat 49
B-3000 Leuven
Belgium

F. Vanhoenacker
Department of Radiology
University Hospital Antwerp
Wilrijkstraat 10
B-2650 Edegem
Belgium

P. Vanhoenacker
Department of Radiology
O. L. V. Ziekenhuis
Moorselbaan 164
B-9300 Aalst
Belgium

H. Vereycken
Department of Radiology
Academic Surgical Center
Stuivenberg
Lange Beeldekensstraat 267
B-2060 Antwerp
Belgium

G. Verswijvel
Department of Radiology
University Hospitals K. U. Leuven
Herestraat 49
B-3000 Leuven
Belgium

K. Yoshimitsu
Department of Radiology
Faculty of Medicine
Kyushu University
3-1-1 Maidashi
Higashi-ku Fukuoka, 812-8582
Japan

Medical Radiology
Diagnostic Imaging and Radiation Oncology

Titles in the series already published

Diagnostic Imaging

Innovations in Diagnostic Imaging
Edited by J.H. Anderson

Radiology of the Upper Urinary Tract
Edited by E.K. Lang

The Thymus - Diagnostic Imaging, Functions, and Pathologic Anatomy
Edited by E. Walter, E. Willich, and W.R. Webb

Interventional Neuroradiology
Edited by A. Valavanis

Radiology of the Pancreas
Edited by A.L. Baert, co-edited by G. Delorme

Radiology of the Lower Urinary Tract
Edited by E.K. Lang

Magnetic Resonance Angiography
Edited by I.P. Arlart, G.M. Bongartz, and G. Marchal

Contrast-Enhanced MRI of the Breast
S. Heywang-Köbrunner and R. Beck

Spiral CT of the Chest
Edited by M. Rémy-Jardin and J. Rémy

Radiological Diagnosis of Breast Diseases
Edited by M. Friedrich and E.A. Sickles

Radiology of the Trauma
Edited by M. Heller and A. Fink

Biliary Tract Radiology
Edited by P. Rossi

Radiological Imaging of Sports Injuries
Edited by C. Masciocchi

Modern Imaging of the Alimentary Tube
Edited by A. R. Margulis

Diagnosis and Therapy of Spinal Tumors
Edited by P. R. Algra, J. Valk, and J. J. Heimans

Interventional Magnetic Resonance Imaging
Edited by J. F. Debatin and G. Adam

Abdominal and Pelvic MRI
Edited by A. Heuck and M. Reiser

Orthopedic Imaging
Techniques and Applications
Edited by A.M. Davies and H. Pettersson

Radiology of the Female Pelvic Organs
Edited by E.K.Lang

Magnetic Resonance of the Heart and Great Vessels
Clinical Applications
Edited by J. Bogaert, A. J. Duerinckx, and F. E. Rademakers

Modern Head and Neck Imaging
Edited by S. K. Mukherji and J. A. Castelijns

Radiological Imaging of Endocrine Diseases
Edited by J. N. Bruneton in collaboration with B. Padovani and M.-Y. Mourou

Trends in Contrast Media
Edited by H. S. Thomsen, R. N. Muller, and R. F. Mattrey

Functional MRI
Edited by C. T. W. Moonen and P. A. Bandettini

Radiology of the Pancreas
2nd Revised Edition
Edited by A. L. Baert
Co-edited by G. Delorme and L. Van Hoe

Radiology of Peripheral Vascular Diseases
Edited by E. Zeitler

Emergency Pediatric Radiology
Edited by H. Carty

Spiral CT of the Abdomen
Edited by F. Terrier, M. Grossholz, and C. D. Becker

Liver Malignancies
Diagnostic and Interventional Radiology
Edited by C. Bartolozzi and R. Lencioni

Medical Imaging of the Spleen
Edited by A. M. De Schepper and F. Vanhoenacker

Diagnostic Nuclear Medicine
Edited by C. Schiepers

Springer

Medical Radiology
Diagnostic Imaging and Radiation Oncology

Titles in the series already published

Radiation Oncology

Lung Cancer
Edited by C.W. Scarantino

Innovations in Radiation Oncology
Edited by H.R. Withers
and L.J. Peters

Radiation Therapy of Head and Neck Cancer
Edited by G.E. Laramore

Gastrointestinal Cancer – Radiation Therapy
Edited by R.R. Dobelbower, Jr.

Radiation Exposure and Occupational Risks
Edited by E. Scherer, C. Streffer,
and K.-R. Trott

Radiation Therapy of Benign Diseases - A Clinical Guide
S.E. Order and S.S. Donaldson

Interventional Radiation Therapy Techniques - Brachytherapy
Edited by R. Sauer

Radiopathology of Organs and Tissues
Edited by E. Scherer,
C. Streffer, and K.-R. Trott

Concomitant Continuous Infusion Chemotherapy and Radiation
Edited by M. Rotman
and C.J. Rosenthal

Intraoperative Radiotherapy – Clinical Experiences and Results
Edited by F.A. Calvo,
M. Santos, and L.W. Brady

Radiotherapy of Intraocular and Orbital Tumors
Edited by W.E. Alberti
and R.H. Sagerman

Interstitial and Intracavitary Thermoradiotherapy
Edited by M.H. Seegenschmiedt
and R. Sauer

Non-Disseminated Breast Cancer
Controversial Issues
in Management
Edited by G.H. Fletcher
and S.H. Levitt

Current Topics in Clinical Radiobiology of Tumors
Edited by H.-P. Beck-Bornholdt

Practical Approaches to Cancer Invasion and Metastases
A Compendium of Radiation
Oncologists' Responses to 40 Histories
Edited by A.R. Kagan with the
Assistance of R.J. Steckel

Radiation Therapy in Pediatric Oncology
Edited by J.R. Cassady

Radiation Therapy Physics
Edited by A.R. Smith

Late Sequelae in Oncology
Edited by J. Dunst and R. Sauer

Mediastinal Tumors. Update 1995
Edited by D.E. Wood
and C.R. Thomas, Jr.

Thermoradiotherapy and Thermochemotherapy

Volume 1:
Biology, Physiology, and Physics

Volume 2:
Clinical Applications
Edited by M.H. Seegenschmiedt,
P. Fessenden, and C.C. Vernon

Carcinoma of the Prostate
Innovations in Management
Edited by Z. Petrovich,
L. Baert, and L.W. Brady

Radiation Oncology of Gynecological Cancers
Edited by H.W. Vahrson

Carcinoma of the Bladder
Innovations in Management
Edited by Z. Petrovich,
L. Baert, and L.W. Brady

Blood Perfusion and Microenvironment of Human Tumors
Implications for Clinical
Radiooncology
Edited by M. Molls and P. Vaupel

Radiation Therapy of Benign Diseases. A Clinical Guide
2nd Revised Edition
S.E. Order and S.S. Donaldson

Carcinoma of the Kidney and Testis, and Rare Urologic Malignancies
Innovations in Management
Edited by Z. Petrovich,
L. Baert, and L.W. Brady

Progress and Perspectives in the Treatment of Lung Cancer
Edited by P. Van Houtte, J. Klastersky,
and P. Rocmans

Springer

Printing and Binding: Stürtz AG, Würzburg